"This book saved my life. . . . I awoke at about
3:30 A.M. with a pain in my chest and I tried to
fool myself into thinking it was indigestion. . . .
but I had just read Dr. Isadore Rosenfeld's book,
SYMPTOMS. I realized that I was having the
symptoms of a heart attack and I knew I had to
get to a hospital right away."

—Jack Paar

INFORMATION THAT CAN
SAVE YOUR LIFE . . .

Will the symptom clear up on its own, or should
you see a doctor? Right now? Tomorrow? Is it safe to
wait? It may be "nothing," but then again it could be
something serious. Are you in danger? The main
reason for this uncertainty is that most people don't
always understand what a particular symptom may
mean. What's more, they often have trouble
describing it accurately. That's not only exasperating
for them, it's equally frustrating for the doctor.

The symptoms I have included are those that
patients have most frequently brought to me for
interpretation in my almost forty years as a doctor.
Having these facts available when you need them
should be reassuring. It may also improve the quality
of your life, perhaps extend it and possibly even save
it.

—Isadore Rosenfeld, M.D.

Also by Isadore Rosenfeld, M.D.:

MODERN PREVENTION

SECOND OPINION

THE COMPLETE MEDICAL EXAM

SYMPTOMS

Isadore Rosenfeld, M.D.

BANTAM BOOKS

New York   Toronto   London   Sydney   Auckland

No book can replace the services of a trained physician. This book is not intended to encourage treatment of illness, disease or other medical problems by the layman. Any application of the recommendations set forth in the following pages is at the reader's discretion and sole risk. If you are under a physician's care for any condition, he or she can advise you about information described in this book.

This edition contains the complete text
of the original hardcover edition.
NOT ONE WORD HAS BEEN OMITTED.

SYMPTOMS

A Bantam Book / published by arrangement with
Simon & Schuster

PUBLISHING HISTORY
Simon & Schuster edition published March 1989
Bantam trade paperback edition / July 1990
Bantam mass market edition / July 1994

ISBN 0-553-56813-2

Published simultaneously in the United States and Canada

Bantam Books are published by Bantam Books, a division of Bantam Doubleday Dell Publishing Group, Inc. Its trademark, consisting of the words "Bantam Books" and the portrayal of a rooster, is Registered in U.S. Patent and Trademark Office and in other countries. Marca Registrada. Bantam Books, 1540 Broadway, New York, New York, 10036.

PRINTED IN THE UNITED STATES OF AMERICA

RAD   0 9 8 7 6 5 4 3 2 1

To the most important women in my life:
my wife Camilla, my mother Vicki, my daughter
Hildi and my dear friend Mary Lasker.

CONTENTS

Before You Read Any Further . . .   1

CHAPTER 1   **Pain: A Useful Signal**   7
How and Why You Feel Pain
Headache
Pain in the Eye
Earache
Sore Tongue
Sore Throat
A Pain in the Neck
"I Have a Bad Back!"
Shoulder Pain
Leg Pain
Foot Pain
Oh, My Aching (Swollen) Joints
Pain in the Elbow
Chest Pain from the Heart
Chest Pain from the Lungs
When the Rib Cage Hurts
Pain in the Chest from Here, There and Everywhere
Heartburn
Bellyaches (Right, Left, High and Low)
Belly Pain Squarely in the Middle
Pain in the Flank
Pain in the Rectum and the Anus
Pain in the Groin
Pain in the Testicles
Pain in the Penis

Breast Pain
Painful Periods
Painful Intercourse: When the Agony Exceeds the
  Ecstasy
Pain When You Urinate

CHAPTER 2   The Lumps That Are—and Aren't   106
When a "Lump" Is Not a Growth
Swollen Tongue
Swollen Gums
Bulging Eyes
A Lump in the Neck
A Lump in the Armpit
A Lump in the Breast
A Swollen Belly—When You're Neither Fat Nor
  Pregnant
A Lump in the Groin
A Lump in the Testicle
A Lump in the Rectum
When Your Legs Swell

CHAPTER 3   Blood Should Be Neither Seen Nor
             Heard   140
Bleeding into the Skin
Why Does Your Nose Bleed?
Bloodshot Eyes
Bleeding Gums
Bleeding from the Ear
When You Vomit Blood
When You're Spitting Blood
Bleeding from the Nipple
Blood in the Urine
When You Ejaculate Blood
Blood in the Stool

Abnormal Vaginal Bleeding
Absence of Vaginal Bleeding

CHAPTER 4 Fever: How High Is High?   178
Taking Your Temperature
When You Really Do Have a Fever
Finding the Cause

CHAPTER 5 It's All in Your Mind—or Is It?   191
Seizures
Faintness and Fainting: Don't Do Something, Just
    Stand There!
Facial Paralysis: Stroke or Just a Virus?
Tremor: The Kind of Hand "Shake" You Can Do
    Without
When You're Numb and Tingling—Here, There and
    Everywhere
Lost Your Sense of Smell or Taste?
Incontinence: Wetting Yourself at Any Age
When People Act "Funny": No Laughing Matter

CHAPTER 6 Vision: When the Eyes Have It   231
The Aging Eye: Your Arms Aren't Too Short!
Spots, Blurring, Halos and Double Vision
When Your Eye Droops—and You're Not
    Winking

CHAPTER 7 Hearing Problems: Deafness,
           Buzzing and Noises in Your Ears   241

CHAPTER 8   **The Digestive System: Problems with Intake and Output**   **247**

Loss of Appetite
When You're Sick to Your Stomach
Gaining Weight for No Reason
Trouble in Swallowing
Jaundice: Yellow Is Not Necessarily Chicken
Constipation: When the Going Gets Hard
Diarrhea: When Running Is Not Good for Your
  Health

CHAPTER 9   **The Respiratory System: Is Breathing a Problem?**   **281**

Chronic Cough: Cigarettes, a Cold or Cancer?
Shortness of Breath: Out of Oxygen or Just Plain
  Nervous?
Snoring: Social Nuisance or Disease?
When You Lose Your Voice
Hiccups

CHAPTER 10   **Sexual Problems**   **307**

Male Impotence—Female "Frigidity"
Infertility: Can You and Your Partner Deliver
  Twenty Million Sperm and One Egg?

CHAPTER 11   **When Symptoms Are Only Skin-Deep**   **326**

Is There Anything Worse Than an Itch?
Becoming Bald—and You're Not Telly Savalas
Too Much Hair
When You Flush and Blush and Are Red All Over
When Your Skin Changes Color—and It's Not a
  Pigment of Your Imagination

Are You Really Pale—or Do You Just Look That
  Way?
Excessive Perspiration: Hormones, Heat or Anxiety?
What Your Fingernails and Toenails Can Tell You

CHAPTER 12 Palpitations, Pulses and an Irregular
            Heartbeat   360
How to Take Your Pulse
What Your Pulse Tells You
Is It Normal?

CHAPTER 13 High Blood Pressure: What the
            News Should Mean to You   370
Who's Vulnerable to Hypertension and Why?
Causes of Hypertension

CHAPTER 14 Sleep: Not Enough—or Too Much   379
When It's All You Can Do to Keep Your Eyes
  Open
Insomnia: Real or Imagined?
Why Are You So Tired?

CHAPTER 15 Your Urine: You Don't Have to
            Taste It to Test It   397
Testing Your Urine

CHAPTER 16 When You're Thirsty All the Time   402
Intake and Output
Finding the Cause

CHAPTER 17   Your Genetics and Lifestyle: Their
                    Impact on Your Symptoms   408
        The Effects of Age
        The "Stronger" Sex
        Equal but Not the Same
        The Health Profile of Blacks
        What Greeks, Italians, Arabs—and Some Jews—
            Have in Common
        Marital Status and Its Impact
        If It Runs in Your Family
        Is Your Job Killing You?
        Especially If You Are Gay (and Promiscuous)
        Alcohol: "How Much Is Too Much?"
        Cigarettes: The Nails in the Coffin
        Drugs (Legal and Illegal): Passport to a Permanent
            "Vacation"

A Final Word   462

Acknowledgments   464

Index   467

SYMPTOMS

BEFORE YOU READ ANY FURTHER . . .

When was the last time it happened to you? You go to bed one night feeling fit as a fiddle, and awaken the next morning deathly ill—nauseated, with diarrhea, fever and a bellyache. You're sure it's either something you ate last night or a twenty-four-hour stomach flu. But the next morning, although the diarrhea has stopped, your temperature is still hovering around 100 degrees. Just thinking about food makes you sick. The stomach cramps are no better. A simple flu should have cleared up by now, and so should food poisoning. Suddenly you remember the young woman who works at the next desk in your office. She had the same symptoms a few months ago. She also blamed them on a virus. And she waited—too long. She reached the operating room just as her appendix was about to rupture! Another few hours, and who knows whether she would have made it. Appendicitis! Maybe that's what you've got, too! Should you call your doctor right away? Should you rush to the nearest hospital emergency room?

If you're hemorrhaging, or have fallen and broken a bone, or have a raging fever or an excruciating pain, there's no question about what to do. You've got to get help—fast. It's the other kind of distress signal that presents the dilemma—something subtle and persistent: a missed period (even though you live alone, in the strictest sense of the word, and couldn't possibly be pregnant); a dry cough (particularly ominous since you're a smoker); a persistent pain in your chest (your father died of a heart attack in his early fifties).

Are you in any danger? Will the symptom clear up on its own, or should you see a doctor? Right now? Tomorrow? Is it safe to wait? It may be "nothing," but then again it could be something serious. The main reason for this uncertainty is that most people don't always understand what a particular symptom may mean. What's more, they often have trouble describing it accurately. That's not only exasperating for them, it's equally frustrating for the doctor who's trying to figure out what's going on.

I recently conducted an informal quiz in my office. After the initial pro forma "How do you feel?" I asked several of my patients the following question: "Do you have any *gribbling?*" Here are some of the verbatim responses I received:

1. "You're fantastic. I've been going to doctors for years, and no one has ever understood what's wrong with me. Gribbling—that's exactly it." (She was intolerant to milk and milk products.)

2. "I used to gribble all the time, but I don't anymore since I had my prostate fixed." (He confused "gribbling" with "dribbling.")

3. "My husband gribbles, I don't." (She turned out to be perfectly healthy.)

4. "Of course! I have lots of gribbling, but I feel better when I pass gas." (She was found to have gallbladder disease.)

5. "Only when I walk quickly in the cold weather, especially uphill. Then I get the gribbling in my chest. It goes away when I rest." (He had angina pectoris.)

Only one of my patients had the courage to say, after being pressed repeatedly about her gribbling, "I don't know what the hell you're talking about."

There's no such word as "gribbling." I made it up.

But most of my patients assumed that there was such a symptom and that they had it, even if they didn't know what it meant. Their responses confirmed a suspicion I've had for a long time: Most people are baffled by their symptoms. They don't know what they mean, and they don't know how to describe them.

That's a big problem.

Your doctor uses three techniques to determine what's wrong with you. Number one: Conversation —you report your symptoms and your doctor asks appropriate questions. Number two: Examination— your doctor feels and presses and looks and thumps. Number three: Tests—from taking your temperature to the most sophisticated diagnostic procedures. In my opinion, the first step is the most important. Nine times out of ten, an accurate description of your symptoms will lead your doctor to the right diagnosis—even before it's confirmed by a physical exam and lab tests.

If your doctor had all the time in the world to take a detailed history from you, there would be no problem. But he doesn't. And the way medical care is evolving in this country, he'll have even less time in the future. So more and more you can expect to be whisked from one technician to another, from one machine to another and from one specialist to another before the correct diagnosis is obtained. That process is not only time-consuming, expensive and often uncomfortable, but, more important, it can also delay the start of treatment. So you, the patient, are much better off if *you* can supply the clues that will instantly point your doctor in the right direction, clues based on what *you* feel, what *you* see and what *you* sense in your own body. And, in the final analysis, who is equipped to do that better than you?

You'll find in these pages all you need to know in

order to present a coherent, meaningful description of your symptoms to your doctor. You'll also have a pretty good idea of their significance, what to do about them, and how soon. In my experience, the first opinion *of an informed patient* usually turns out to be right. But remember, although this book will leave you more enlightened and better able to share in the medical decisions which affect you, it will not make a doctor out of you.

From time to time you may look for a certain symptom in these pages and find no reference to it. That may be due to an oversight on my part, for which I apologize in advance, or deliberately omitted it either because it's uncommon or because it's so critical as to preclude any speculation on your part. I have also decided not to discuss mental illness as such. I am not a psychiatrist, and it would be presumptuous for me to skim through the symptoms of psychological problems that sometimes take years to unravel. I have, however, discussed at length those behavioral changes that accompany various physical disorders ranging from nutritional deficiencies to Alzheimer's disease. One word of caution, however, is especially appropriate these days. If you observe a sudden change in personality, unusual mood swings or unexpected or inappropriate rage or depression in a previously "well-adjusted" friend or relative, always consider the possibility of drug abuse or withdrawal.

The symptoms I have included are those that patients have most frequently brought to me for interpretation in my almost forty years as a doctor. I have tried to explain their meaning to you, as I have to them, in a simple, practical and straightforward manner. In the final chapter of the book, I have also discussed the personal characteristics that are always relevant to understanding symptoms. Your age, your sex, your race, your genetic inheritance, your marital status, your occupation, your sexual orientation and your lifestyle—all contribute to your vulnerability or resistance to certain diseases and must be taken into consideration both by you and your doctor in making the correct diagnosis.

If you're the kind of person who's fascinated by medicine, who loves to read about the human body in health and disease (you may even once have harbored a secret wish to be a doctor yourself), you may read this volume straight through, cover to cover. Or you may choose to use it only as a reference when you're sick and don't know why. Whichever way you harvest the facts and opinions in these pages, having them available when you need them should be reassuring. It may also improve the quality of your life, perhaps extend it and possibly even save it.

CHAPTER 1

PAIN:
A Useful Signal

What would you do if a generous genie offered to make you pain-free for the rest of your life? No matter how sick you became, or how badly you were hurt in an accident, you would feel no pain—ever again!

Sounds wonderful, doesn't it? But if you accepted that offer, you'd be making the biggest mistake of your life. For pain, although unpleasant, is nature's most effective distress signal. When your brain senses trouble anywhere in your body, it sounds the pain alarm and continues to send it until the problem is cleared up. Imagine falling and not knowing you've broken your leg, dislocated your shoulder or fractured your skull. Think how disastrous it would be for you to sustain a heart attack and be unaware of it, going about business as usual—without the rest, oxygen and medications that can save your life. Even something as "benign" as acute appendicitis, if ignored and untreated (as it surely would be without its searing lower-abdominal pain), can progress to gangrene, rupture, peritonitis and death.

When a dog breaks a leg, veterinarians rarely give it painkillers after the limb has been set. That may sound cruel, but the pain keeps the dog off the bad leg until it's healed. In fact, it would be cruel to kill the pain with drugs, allowing the animal to walk about in comfort and so further damage the leg. Because we humans are "smart" and know how important it is to favor an injured limb, we can safely take painkillers. Sometimes, of course, we're not so smart —like the pro football player who, for the sake of one more season, has his hurt knee shot up with cortisone and novocaine so that he can continue to play, risking permanent disability.

No two individuals perceive pain or react to it in the same way. Some seem to have so high a threshold as to be impervious to pain, while others can't tolerate even minor discomfort. Almost every day I see examples of such differing responses among my patients. Take coronary artery disease, in which the blood vessels within the heart are narrowed. The usual symptom is angina pectoris—pain, tightness or discomfort in the chest induced by exertion or emotion. But in some individuals the heart disease is "silent," they have no symptoms whatsoever, regardless of how severely their arteries are clogged. That's the worst kind, because there is no warning to slow down or stop when the blood supply to the heart is not keeping up with the demand. So it should come as no surprise to learn that "silent" coronary disease is associated with a high incidence of sudden death.

Never judge the importance of any pain by its severity. Other characteristics may be more important. *How* does it hurt? Is the pain sharp and shooting, or burning, or dull? *When* does it hurt? Some diseases act up at certain times of the day or only after specific activities. *What* other symptoms are associated with the pain? Nausea, fever, vomiting, a rash? *Where* it hurts can be either a clue or a red herring, since, as you will see later, pain that's triggered in one area of the body can be referred by nearby nerve pathways to another. All these features help determine the cause and significance of your pain and what your response to it should be. In this chapter you will learn how to solve the mystery of a pain by looking for such clues.

HOW AND WHY YOU FEEL PAIN

In order for you to feel pain, two components of the nervous system must be in working order. First, the nerves that sense the trouble at the *site* of the injury or disease must be intact. Their entire pathway to the brain, to which the alarm message is conveyed, must also be unimpaired. Then the brain must be able to evaluate the message and indicate to you that something hurts—and where. Many different diseases can injure the local nerves so that they lose the ability to register and send the pain signal. Beyond that, the spinal cord, by way of which the signals make the last leg of their trip to the brain, may be severed by an accident, a tumor or disease. And even when the nerves and the spinal cord are intact, the brain itself may be damaged (as, for example, by a stroke) and unable to interpret the pain signal correctly.

The importance of intact brain function in the sensing of pain is dramatically demonstrated by hypnosis. When you are hypnotized, and instructed to feel no pain, you won't, no matter how intensely you're hurt. Although the nerves still conduct the pain signals to the brain, it does not respond to them —very much like an operator asleep at the switchboard.

Acupuncture is another example of how the brain can be rendered impervious to a pain signal. In an operating room in Shanghai some years ago, I attended a heart operation during which a young woman received no anesthesia whatsoever. Her chest was opened, her heart exposed, the operation completed and the chest closed, all while she was fully awake, smiling and sipping water. The only "painkiller" was a needle twirled in her left shoulder. Only 25 percent of people respond to acupuncture, but in those who do, this technique is quite impressive.

How and why it works is still not fully understood. It is generally believed, however, that the needle inserted in precisely the right spot sends a message to a particular area of the brain which then releases natural opiates (endorphins and enkephalins) that mask the pain.

Ultimately, the best way to ease pain is to get to its root cause and fix it—treat the pneumonia with an antibiotic, remove the inflamed appendix, release the pinched nerve in the spine. Unfortunately, we sometimes know what's wrong, but can't do much about it, as, for example, in advanced cancer or AIDS. In these terminal conditions, any means of pain control, no matter how drastic, is justified—powerful narcotics, or surgery to sever the nerves transmitting the pain, or operating on the centers in the brain that perceive it. Unfortunately, most doctors allow too many patients to suffer under these circumstances.

But most pain is not experienced in such extreme circumstances; it's either temporary, as when you break a bone, or ongoing, like arthritis. Always try to avoid powerful narcotics such as codeine, morphine, Demerol or Talwin for pain due to chronic conditions which do not shorten life. Painkillers do not cure the underlying *cause* of the pain, and you may end up with a drug habit in the bargain. I have one patient who refused to endure any pain whatsoever no matter how briefly. Her obliging surgeon gave her all the Demerol she demanded for two weeks after a gallbladder operation. That was enough to hook her for the rest of her life.

In this chapter I will help you determine the origin and significance of different kinds of pain in varying locations of your body, how serious they can be, and what you should do about them. From time to time, I'll also refresh your knowledge of anatomy—what organ is where and how it works. Don't be intimidated by that prospect. Obviously, the more you know about your body, in sickness and in health, the better you will understand its distress signals and whether they indicate a condition that is relatively harmless or one that requires medical attention. So let's start at the top and work our way down.

HEADACHE

Headaches are among the most aggravating, common and debilitating kinds of pain we experience. Entire textbooks have been written about them. Their range is a wide one. Most of us experience the occasional garden-variety headache when we're worried, hungry, stressed, tense, tired or constipated, or after straining our eyes for too long. Or we may get one after going to the dentist, or on a long airplane flight, or when we have a cold or a hangover. There is, however, another kind of headache—sudden, new, unfamiliar and unexplained. It starts for no apparent reason and either won't go away or, if it does, keeps coming back. That's the kind that worries. Let's go through the most likely possibilities and see where your kind of headache fits in.

Tension and *migraine* account for 90 percent of all headaches. The more common of the two is the *tension headache*, which can be recognized by the following characteristics:

- The pain is usually felt most in the back of the head and neck and is rarely one-sided.
- It can continue for weeks or even months, with only brief periods of respite, although it may fluctuate in severity.
- Attacks may begin at any time of the day (there are other kinds of headaches, as you will see, which

come on mostly at night or when you awake in the morning).
- The pain is usually described as a "tight band," pressing but rarely throbbing. It is never accompanied by fever.

If they're honest about it, people with tension headaches will admit to having personal problems and living under stress.

The *migraine headache* displays entirely different characteristics. Here's a typical scenario:

- There is a warning period, minutes or hours before the headache itself begins, during which the individual may be fatigued or depressed or may experience some form of visual disturbance or other neurological problem: lights flash, peripheral vision may be lost, the ability to read or even to speak is transiently impaired.
- Migraines are *one-sided,* and in any given individual it's almost always the same side. The pain is throbbing in nature, usually develops in the morning and gradually worsens after thirty minutes to one hour.
- Attacks may occur every few days or weeks, or not for months. They continue for hours but rarely last longer than a day or two.
- Migraines may be precipitated by alcohol or certain foods such as chocolate. Ironically, they often occur *after* stress, when you're relaxing.
- They are frequently accompanied by nausea and vomiting and are relieved by sleep.

A *cluster headache* is a variation of the migraine. It occurs mostly in men, while typical migraines are more apt to strike women, especially those with mitral valve prolapse, and usually clear up after menopause. The pain of a cluster headache is often situated behind the eyes, comes on very suddenly, without warning, peaks within five to ten minutes and disappears in less than an hour. It is often triggered by alcohol. Sleep doesn't help. In fact, cluster headaches awaken you. They occur several times a day for weeks and then stop.

The headache caused by a *brain tumor* also has special characteristics:

- It does not fluctuate in severity, but becomes progressively more severe as time goes by.
- It is worse in the morning.
- It is aggravated by exertion, straining, coughing, sneezing and lifting heavy objects, and is relieved by lying down. It is frequently associated with nausea and vomiting.

There is another serious kind of headache, one that occurs mostly in older people who have *temporal arteritis,* an inflammation of the arteries in the temporal area (near the sideburns). In this condition, it hurts to chew, vision is impaired and there are aches and pains all over the body, as well as fever and weight loss. However, the outstanding symptom of temporal arteritis is the headache. It lasts for days or weeks on one side of the head and is so localized you can actually touch the tender spot with your finger. A diagnosis of this disorder must be confirmed by a biopsy of the affected artery. Unless temporal arteritis is treated immediately with large doses of steroids, stroke or blindness may result.

Inflamed sinuses are a frequent cause of headaches, so much so, in fact, that they're often blamed when they shouldn't be. How can you spot a real sinus headache?

- It usually begins during or after a bad cold.
- There is a postnasal drip.

- It's localized to one specific area of the face or head, and comes on very quickly.
- It's worse in the morning, before all the mucus has had a chance to drain.
- It's aggravated by coughing, sneezing or sudden movements of the head.
- It's intensified by alcohol, sudden temperature changes and, in the winter, going from a warm room out into the cold.

There are other, less common causes of headaches:

- *Trigeminal neuralgia* (also known as *tic douloureux*) is an inflammation of a major nerve in the face. It develops mostly in elderly persons, who experience severe shooting pains which last only a few seconds. Brushing the teeth, chewing, even touching a sensitive spot on the face, can trigger these attacks.
- *Fever,* due to any illness, can produce headaches.
- *Head injuries* are a common cause of headaches.
- In older people, even a trivial knock on the head can cause bleeding under the skull. The accumulated blood, called a *subdural hematoma,* presses on the brain, and that leads to headaches as well as behavioral changes. The diagnosis is confirmed by CAT scan or magnetic resonance imaging.
- Assorted eye problems ranging from the wrong prescription for your glasses to *glaucoma* (a buildup of pressure in the eyeball) can give you a headache.
- *Medications* can leave your head hurting, too. The greatest offenders in my cardiological practice are nitroglycerin and related drugs such as isosorbide dinitrate (Isordil), prescribed to control angina. These agents not only dilate the arteries in the heart, which is what they're supposed to do, but also widen the vessels in the scalp, causing a head-

ache. If you have received *any* new medication, whether it's an antibiotic, a hormone or something for the heart, and you develop headaches, suspect the drug first.

- *High blood pressure* can produce a throbbing headache that is usually located in the back of the neck and is worst when you awaken in the morning.
- A sudden, blinding diffuse headache that persists, especially one that is accompanied by stiffness of the neck, raises the possibility of *bleeding into the brain*. In young persons, this is usually due to the rupture of an artery whose walls were congenitally weak. In older individuals, particularly those with high blood pressure, a blood vessel bursts because it cannot withstand the unrelenting elevated pressure over the long term.

Points to Remember

Symptom: Headache.

What It May Mean	What to Do About It
1. Stress, fatigue, hangover.	Rest and moderation.
2. Viral or bacterial infections (common cold).	Most clear up on their own.
3. Tension.	Muscle relaxants.
4. Migraine.	Develop and follow the best treatment regimen.
5. Cluster headache.	Medication.
6. Brain tumor.	Medication (steroids), surgery or radiation.
7. Temporal arteritis.	Biopsy to confirm the

	diagnosis, and start steroid treatment immediately to prevent blindness or stroke.
8. Sinus infection.	Requires antibiotics or drainage if it hangs on.
9. Tic douloureux (trigeminal neuralgia).	Requires specific medication (Tegretol).
10. Fever.	Acetaminophen (Tylenol), aspirin.
11. Head injury.	Prompt medical attention.
12. Subdural hematoma.	Medical or surgical treatment.
13. Glaucoma.	Medical care.
14. Side effect of medication.	Document it and report it to the doctor who prescribed the medication.
15. High blood pressure.	Must be controlled by weight loss, diet and drugs, under a doctor's supervision.
16. Brain hemorrhage.	Emergency medical treatment.

Suspect meningitis and see your doctor as soon as possible when you have a severe headache that occurs for no particular reason, is of long duration and is accompanied by fever, nausea, vomiting and a stiff neck.

PAIN IN THE EYE

Most eye pain is due to a problem in the eye itself—an infection, irritation or injury. Sometimes, however, even though it's the eye that hurts, the trouble lies elsewhere, like in the sinuses or the nose. Here are some possibilities to consider if you suddenly hurt in one or both eyes:

- *Fever* from any cause will give you soreness or pain in the eyes.
- *Generalized viral infections.* If your eyeballs hurt (both, not one), you feel lousy all over, you've got some fever, and your joints ache, you've got the flu. Eye pain associated with viral infections disappears along with the other complaints in twenty-four to thirty-six hours.
- *Conjunctivitis* (pinkeye) or any inflammation of the upper and lower lids, the cornea and the optic nerve behind the eye are all common causes of eye pain. Infection of a hair follicle on an eyelid, or a *sty,* is another culprit.
- *A tiny grain of anything,* a hair, a speck of dust, can feel as big as a boulder when it gets into the eye. A small *laceration* which you got when you were walking through some brush and were flicked in the eye will also make it hurt like the devil.
- Eye pain may be associated with several types of *headaches,* particularly *migraine* and *temporal arteritis.*
- *Shingles* (*herpes zoster*) involving the eye not only causes terrible pain, it can also lead to blindness. In this infection, especially common in older people, there is initially no redness or obvious injury to the eye. The typical ulcers appear only later.
- If your eye pain comes on for a week or two, disappears for a while, then returns, be sure to have your eyes examined. You may have a simple astigmatism, or you may be far- or nearsighted. Proper glasses will correct the problem.
- Chronic *infection of the sinuses* frequently causes eye pain, as well as headache. The face is tender,

there is often a low-grade fever, and postnasal discharge may be troublesome. Antibiotics and drainage are often required to eliminate sinusitis.

- Never forget *glaucoma,* increased pressure within the eye, as a cause of eye pain. It is easily treated, but when undiagnosed it can leave you blind.

Points to Remember

Symptom: Pain in the eye.

What It May Mean	What to Do About It
1. Fever.	Acetaminophen (Tylenol), aspirin.
2. Viral infection (generalized).	Usually clears up in 24–36 hours.
3. Conjunctivitis (pinkeye).	Medical treatment.
4. Sty.	Local treatment.
5. Injury or foreign object in the eye.	Consult your doctor.
6. Migraine.	Eye pain disappears when the headache does.
7. Temporal arteritis.	Medical treatment is urgently needed to prevent blindness or stroke.
8. Shingles.	Serious when the eye is affected. See your doctor.
9. Eye strain (improper glasses prescription).	Proper prescription and proper reading habits.
10. Sinusitis.	Antibiotics and irrigation.
11. Glaucoma.	Ongoing medical treatment is needed.

Any sense of pressure in the eye, pain, redness or swelling that persists, and especially if it affects your vision, should signal a call to your doctor.

EARACHE

There is nothing more likely to cause loss of sleep for young parents than the cry of their child with an earache in the middle of the night. Although rarely life-threatening, earaches can be serious. In a celebrated but tragic case involving a hospital in New York, an eighteen-year-old girl who came to the emergency room with fever and with pain in the ear was dead within a few hours—cause unknown.

Pain in the ear is most often due to something going on in the *outer canal*—a pimple, an irritation, an infection, an inflammation, or a blockage due to a buildup of ear wax. If you've been swimming in water which is either polluted or excessively chlorinated, the ear canal may end up inflamed or infected. A ruptured *eardrum*, due to a physical injury or an infection, is also extremely painful. Or the problem may lie in the *inner ear*, again because of an infection or after flying or diving, when the nasal passages are clogged and the pressure between the inner and outer ear cannot be equalized. You may also experience *referred pain* in the ear—the cause is elsewhere, but you feel it in the ear. For example, if you've got mumps and the parotid glands in your face are inflamed, you'll feel pain in the ears. If you've got a *sore throat* or an *infected tooth*, the warning signal is often sounded in the ear. Individuals who have an abnormal alignment of the teeth, whose jaws don't close properly or who have arthritis of the hinged joint of the jaw (*temporomandibular joint syndrome* —TMJ) will perceive the pain in the ear. *Sinusitis,* especially of the mastoids, the bony tissue behind the ears, also causes earache.

Here's some good practical advice if your child has an earache. First, look into the canal with a flashlight to see whether there is a pea, part of a toy or anything else stuck in it. You'd be surprised at how often children absentmindedly jam something into their ears. Unless the object, whatever it is, can be easily dislodged, it's a job for your doctor. *Never probe into a child's ear,* or into your own, for that matter. Physical injury to the delicate mechanism of the ear can cause permanent hearing loss.

Points to Remember

Symptom: Earache.

What It May Mean	What to Do About It
1. Obstruction (foreign object or ear wax).	Have the doctor remove it. Don't try to do it yourself.
2. Infection of the outer ear.	Medical treatment and antibiotics required (topical or oral).
3. Infection of the inner ear.	Antibiotic treatment.
4. Ruptured eardrum.	Medical treatment.
5. Tooth infection.	See your dentist.
6. Sinus infection.	Appropriate medical treatment.
7. Arthritis of the jaw.	Anti-inflammatory medication and possible bite realignment.

SORE TONGUE

"Stick out your tongue and say Aah" used to be part of the routine physical examination, even if your symptoms didn't seem to involve the tongue at all. Some old-timers still ask you to do it. Over the years, the tongue has become symbolic as an indicator of health, even though the information it yields in routine examinations is fairly limited, at least by today's hi-tech standards.

What can *you* learn by looking at your own tongue?

- *An enlarged tongue* may mean underfunction of the thyroid gland or overfunction of the pituitary, the master gland in the brain.
- *A tremor of the tongue* may be due to an overactive thyroid, multiple sclerosis or a variety of other neurological disorders.
- *A smooth and pale tongue* surface suggests nutritional deficiencies.
- *A coated tongue* may indicate dehydration, debauch or the fact that you've been taking antibiotics recently.
- *A tongue falling to one side* means that you've probably had a stroke.
- *Variations in tongue color* may reflect jaundice, anemia or a lack of oxygen.

In all the above instances the tongue is an indicator of trouble elsewhere in the body. But most often a sore tongue is caused by a viral ulcer, or *"canker sore,"* a painful lesion which appears on the tongue (or anywhere in the mouth) for no apparent reason. Some doctors think these viral ulcers are the result of emotional stress, fatigue or "lowered resistance."

Other possible causes of a sore tongue:

- *Herpetic sore.*
- *Ill-fitting dentures.*
- *Injury:* Someone with epilepsy may bite the tongue during an attack, leaving it painful. Physical injury to the tongue can also occur in an accident, or during contact sports.
- *Anemia* due to a lack of either iron or B_{12} will give you a chronically painful tongue.
- *Heavy smoking* will irritate the tongue and make it painful.
- If you can't see what's causing the pain in your tongue and the discomfort persists, have your doctor or dentist look at it. Sometimes small *cancers,* not visible to you, develop on the underside of the tongue.
- If neither you nor your doctor can find anything on the tongue to explain the pain, it's probably a *neuralgia*—an irritation of the nerves supplying the mouth. The pain feels as if it's in the tongue, but may in fact be coming from the nearby teeth and gums.
- If tongue pain occurs when you walk too quickly and ends when you rest, the trouble lies in the *heart.* I have several patients with angina pectoris whose symptoms occurred not in the chest but in the teeth, the jaws and occasionally the tongue.

A persistently sore tongue should be brought to your doctor's attention. It may be due only to a minor infection or irritation. But this accessible organ can, in fact, reveal disorders in such distant parts of the body as the bowel, the brain and the heart and even reflect the kind of diet you follow and other personal habits. So the old-time doctors who always asked you to show them your tongue may have been right after all.

Points to Remember

Symptom: Tongue trouble.

What It May Mean	What to Do About It
1. Enlargement: due to underfunction of the thyroid or overfunction of the pituitary gland in the brain.	Requires medical treatment.
2. Tremor: overactive thyroid or neurological disorder.	Medical treatment with drugs, surgery or radiation for the thyroid disorder; appropriate medical treatment for the neurological condition.
3. Smooth and pale: nutritional deficiency.	Correct your diet.
4. Coated: dehydration, debauch or antibiotic side effects.	Can be corrected by you.
5. Falling to the side: stroke.	Needs medical management.
6. Color variations: jaundice, anemia, lack of oxygen.	Correct the underlying disorder.
7. Pain:	
Canker sores (viral).	Self-treatment, or medical treatment if they recur or persist.
Herpes.	Acyclovir.
Dentures.	See your dentist.
Injury.	Medical evaluation.

Anemia.	Determine reason and correct.
Smoking.	Stop.
Cancer.	Radiation, surgery, chemotherapy.
Neuralgia.	Analgesics.
Referred from teeth and gums.	See your dentist.
Referred from the heart.	Requires cardiac evaluation.

SORE THROAT

If you wake up one morning with a sore throat, but have no fever, and you feel fine otherwise, your bedroom was probably dry and overheated. But if your throat continues to hurt as the day wears on, then the pain is due to something else. What can it be, and what should you do about it? Well, you can wait for a day or two. If it's due to a run-of-the-mill virus it will clear up on its own. But if you are running a low-grade fever and have tender, swollen lymph glands in the neck, call your doctor. He may prescribe an antibiotic over the phone or, if he knows that you have some other serious disease like diabetes mellitus, chronic bronchitis, poor kidney function or a heart murmur, he will probably have you come to the office. He'll look at your throat, swab it and send the specimen to the laboratory for "culture" to see what organisms grow out and to which antibiotics they are sensitive. Then he may give you an antibiotic while waiting for the results.

Whether or not to call the doctor when you have a sore throat depends on several factors.

- If you have fever, and your throat is sore, it's probably due to an infection of some kind. Statistically, the most likely one is a virus (*viral pharyngitis*). If you look at the back of your throat you'll find it pink, but without any coating or spots.

  The most common *bacterial* infection in children is the *"strep throat."* Unless treated with penicillin, a strep throat can lead to rheumatic fever, with all the heart problems that that entails later in life. You can recognize a strep infection by the presence of *white spots*. There is a kit now available to doctors (which I'm certain will be simplified so that patients can use it, too) which distinguishes between strep throat and other infections.

- *Infectious mononucleosis,* a viral infection occurring almost exclusively in young people, makes swallowing very painful. The throat is *very red,* but without the spots seen in a strep infection. Also, the lymph glands, especially those in the back of the neck, are very swollen, easily seen and felt. Incidentally, infectious mononucleosis is the kind of viral infection for which you should normally *not* take antibiotics. One in particular, ampicillin, may produce a nasty rash.

- When a child with a sore throat suddenly develops a fever that lasts for a couple of days, *tonsillitis* is a good bet. When you look into the throat, you'll see enlarged red tonsils, one on each side, covered with a creamy yellow coating. Don't rush to have the tonsils removed. Such surgery is reserved for very special cases of recurrent tonsillitis, which is relatively uncommon in this era of antibiotics.

- There are several different "bugs" which can give you a sore throat no matter what your age. One you may not think about is the *gonococcus,* which is responsible for *gonorrhea.* Engaging in oral sex shifts its portal of entry from the sex organs to the throat.

• A couple of generations ago, I would have included *diphtheria* on this list. Thanks to vaccination, I haven't seen a case in years. However, in view of the migration to this country of so many persons with uncertain immunization histories, it ought to be borne in mind. The diphtheritic throat can be recognized by the presence of a dirty-gray membrane or covering at the back of the throat.

Although most sore throats are due to some infection, a few are not. For example, in older persons, pain, burning and discomfort may result from *acid* from the stomach leaking up into the food pipe, the kind of thing that happens with a hiatus hernia. Also, if you or your child have inadvertently and perhaps unknowingly swallowed a fish or chicken *bone,* it may have scraped the throat on the way down and left it raw.

In general, when my patients call for advice about a sore throat, I tell them to wait forty-eight hours, even if they do have a little fever. Symptoms usually clear during that time without anything being done about it. If the patient is still sick after a couple of days, I have him or her come to my office, where I look at the throat, often culture it and usually prescribe an antibiotic. In young people, I also look for infectious mononucleosis, something that can be confirmed in a few minutes by means of a simple, inexpensive blood test. I do not normally prescribe an antibiotic for them, because it can result in a widespread rash; some doctors do, in order to prevent secondary infection. But in a child a sore throat accompanied by a fever, swollen glands or angry-looking tonsils demands immediate medical attention to make sure a strep infection is not left untreated.

Points to Remember

Symptom: Sore throat.

What It May Mean	What to Do About It
1. Viral pharyngitis.	Clears up without treatment.
2. Strep throat.	Must receive penicillin or another antibiotic.
3. Infectious mononucleosis.	Rest and self-treatment. Avoid antibiotics.
4. Tonsillitis.	Antibiotic treatment. Surgery rarely necessary.
5. Gonorrhea.	Antibiotic treatment.
6. Diphtheria.	Responds to antibiotics.
7. Acid reflux.	Take antacids.
8. Fish or chicken bone.	Treat the symptoms.

A PAIN IN THE NECK

When we're annoyed by someone or something, there are two parts of the anatomy in which we say we have a "pain." One of them is the neck. The neck enjoys this prominence in our colloquial vocabulary because it is so often the site of pain and discomfort. That's because it's especially vulnerable, constantly bending, twisting and turning, all the while supporting a head made big and heavy by eons of evolution. Small wonder, then, that we "get it in the neck" so often. But what *is* it that gives the getting? Here are some of the possibilities:

- If it hurts to swallow, not in the throat but in front, on the outside of the neck, it's probably from an *inflamed thyroid* (*thyroiditis*). (The thyroid gland is situated in the midline of the neck just below the Adam's apple.) The area is also very tender to touch. There is usually a little fever too, and overall you don't feel that great either.

    Thyroiditis is an autoimmune disorder. Although the pain in the gland itself lasts only a few days, the thyroid is often permanently damaged. So even after the acute symptoms have subsided, be sure to get a follow-up examination from your doctor to check on how well your thyroid gland is working.

- Now let's change the scenario just a little. You have pain on the outside of the throat, when you swallow or touch it, not in front, as in thyroiditis, but on either side of the neck, where you can feel a pulse. You probably have *carotidynia*—an inflammation of the carotids, the large arteries in the neck that carry blood to the brain. No one knows the cause. It's either an autoimmune process or perhaps a virus. The symptoms usually respond to aspirin and clear up after a few days, but I have known them to go on for weeks and require steroid hormones for relief.

- Here's another variation in neck pain. Your throat hurts when you swallow, and you can feel some *swollen glands* in your neck that weren't there before. These lymph nodes are filters which drain the mouth, the ears, the back of the neck and the scalp, trapping infectious material that passes through them. So any of the following will enlarge your glands and leave them tender to touch: in the front of the neck, an infected throat; under the jaw, recent dental work; at the back of the neck, infection in your scalp or the ear canal, infectious mononucleosis or German measles.

If you're worried about what your swollen glands may mean, here's a useful rule to remember: *Painful glands are usually due to infection.* In leukemia, lymphoma and other forms of cancer, they are not sore; they have a rubbery feel to them and are harder than infected glands; they are usually detected accidentally—for example, while you're shaving or applying makeup, and not because they're giving you any symptoms. But painful or not, glands that are swollen for no apparent reason, and which do not clear up in a week or two, should be reported to your doctor.

• Have you ever felt as if someone has grabbed all the muscles in the back of your neck and twisted them into a tight knot? That's *muscle spasm*, usually from tension, overexertion or sleeping or sitting for a long time in an awkward position. It responds to aspirin, rest, relaxation and physiotherapy. *Arthritis* in your cervical spine leaves the neck feeling stiff and less supple, and moving it about is uncomfortable. In addition to the neck pain itself, arthritis in that portion of the spine will also cause numbness or tingling in shoulders, arms and hands. Check it out yourself. Put your chin on your chest, and hold it there for a minute or two. Then turn it all the way to the tip of the shoulder. If either of those maneuvers reproduces the pain, the numbness and the tingling, then nerves leaving the neck are being compressed, usually by arthritic bones.

• Because the bones of the neck house the nerves to

and from the brain, any *neck injury* is a matter of real concern.

Points to Remember

Symptom: Neck pain.

What It May Mean	What to Do About It
1. Thyroiditis.	Thyroid function tests, to rule out thyroid damage, followed by appropriate treatment.
2. Carotidynia.	Usually responds to aspirin or steroids.
3. Enlarged glands due to infection, cancer, mononucleosis or German measles.	Appropriate medical treatment.
4. Muscle spasm.	Rest, relaxation and physiotherapy.
5. Arthritis of the cervical spine.	Muscle relaxants and physiotherapy.
6. Injury to head or neck.	X rays and appropriate medical treatment.

"I HAVE A BAD BACK!"

Back pain accounts for more time lost from work in this country than any other disability. Who am I to say, but it may have been a mistake in evolution for *Homo sapiens* to straighten up and stand on two feet! However, although standing upright does put added pressure on the spine, that's not the only reason for the national backache. Bad posture, obesity, poorly designed chairs and mattresses, weak abdominal and back muscles, heavy lifting or other injury, genetic predisposition and arthritis contribute more to our misery than does any fundamental error in design.

The spine is a stack of circular bones (vertebrae) separated by spongy shock absorbers called discs. The spine keeps us upright, but at the same time permits enough flexibility for us to bend, twist and move. It also protects the spinal cord, the rope of nerves that runs within it from the base of the brain down to the low back. These nerves send branches out of the spine to various organs along the way.

Crippling back pain can usually be traced to some malfunction of the spine, usually in the neck (the cervical spine) or lower down (the lumbar spine) because these sites are subject to the greatest pressure and are most frequently strained. The backache itself results from the interaction of the vertebrae, the discs, the nerves and the muscles that surround them.

Arthritis in the spine is responsible for most back problems, and it gets worse as you grow older. The gnarled overgrowth of bone that is the hallmark of arthritis affects the joints that hinge the vertebrae together, narrowing the little openings through which the nerves leave the spine. If you have enough arthritis, you'll hurt in the back itself where the bony overgrowths scrape and rub against each other, as well as suffer referred pain elsewhere from the pressure on the nerves leaving the tiny apertures in the spine.

These nerves can also be impinged upon by *discs*. When that happens, you experience pain throughout the area served by the affected nerve. The most common form of such referred pain is *sciatica,* in which a disc in the lower back irritates the nerve going down to the buttock and the thighs, giving you a dull ache in the back of the leg. So if your back hurts, but the pain stays right there without radiating anywhere, you're not likely to have a disc problem. That's also true for the neck.

Osteoporosis affects many women as they get older. Bones everywhere, but particularly in the spine, become more porous and fragile; they fracture easily and collapse. Not only does this cause considerable pain, but women so affected become shorter and their bent spine leaves them with the so-called "dowager's hump."

Few women develop osteoporosis before menopause. Those who do usually have a condition called *hyperparathyroidism,* which causes bone pain, osteoporosis and kidney stones. The parathyroids, a set of tiny glands in the neck near the thyroid, produce a hormone which helps regulate the proper amount of calcium in the bones. In hyperparathyroidism, there is an excessive amount of this hormone due to a tumor in the glands. As a result, calcium is sucked out of the bones and into the bloodstream. Not only do the bones become thin, but as blood is filtered in the kidney its excess calcium forms stones in that organ. Parathyroid tumors are too small to be felt and can be diagnosed only by routinely measuring calcium levels in the blood. So, if you're a pre-menopausal woman, and your bones break easily when you fall, and you've had a kidney stone or two, get your blood tested for a calcium level.

There are nonback causes of back pain, too. A *malpositioned uterus* can give you low back pain, especially after you've been standing for hours. Also, *endometriosis* (in which tissues normally present only in the uterus pop up elsewhere in the pelvis) may cause back pain, too, especially before or during menstruation.

A very serious cause of back pain is that due to spread of *cancer* to the bones of the spine. The most common example in males is a malignant prostate gland. The typical patient is a man over age fifty, previously pain-free, who suddenly has severe and continuing pain in one area of the back. A complete examination will reveal the cancerous prostate, while a bone scan or an X ray shows exactly where it has invaded the bones of the spine. An almost identical situation occurs in women with breast cancer. Months or years after their surgery, they may develop back pain, not because of osteoporosis, but from the spread of the cancer to the bones of the spine.

Any *disorder within the abdomen* (diverticulitis, colitis or tumors) can cause lower back pain, too.

Muscle spasm is probably the most common cause of back pain. It is most likely to occur when the spine is arthritic. In that case, the muscles become rigid as the body tries to prevent the diseased spine from moving all over the place and worsening your discomfort. However, this "protective" spasm can be more painful than the distress it is meant to avoid.

If you're under lots of tension and stress, your muscles may respond by going into spasm, even when there's nothing physically wrong with any of your bones, nerves or discs. Here's what can happen under such circumstances. A young man, then in his late twenties, was married some years ago. After the ceremony, he and his bride left for a hotel in New York City where they were to spend one night before going on to the Orient. They were excited, happy and a little anxious about the new experiences awaiting them. When they arrived in the Big Apple, the groom did not carry his bride over the threshold of the hotel room, but he did move some of the suitcases around after they had checked in. As he was lifting one of the heavy bags, his back suddenly went into spasm, leaving him twisted like a pretzel. He was in agony. The pain lasted throughout this, the first night of his married life, and he spent the better part of it in a hot tub while his wife tried to help him with a vigorous massage. They managed to leave on their trip in the morning, but for the next two weeks of his honeymoon the young man was a virtual cripple. He and his new wife didn't get much sightseeing done, let alone achieve some of their more amorous objectives. I am familiar with all these details because *I* was the ill-fated bridegroom. So, back pain not only causes time lost from work, it can even compromise some basic recreational activities.

Points to Remember

Symptom: Back pain.

What It May Mean	What to Do About It
1. Injury.	See a doctor immediately.
2. Arthritis.	Exercise, anti-inflammatory drugs, physiotherapy.
3. Disc disease.	Rest, traction, surgery.
4. Osteoporosis.	Exercise, calcium supplement, estrogen replacement.
5. Malposition of the uterus.	Possible surgery.
6. Endometriosis.	See a gynecologist for medication.
7. Cancer in bone.	Radiation, hormone treatment.
8. Abdominal disease.	Requires medical intervention.
9. Muscle spasm.	Rest, exercise, physiotherapy.

SHOULDER PAIN

You go to bed one night with an ache in your left shoulder. You may remember what did it—grabbing the overhead bar when the crowded bus lurched, throwing a football around on the weekend (after not having touched a ball since college) or lugging a sample case filled with kitchen tiles. You may actually have been fine at bedtime but simply slept with your arm awkwardly twisted under you. The next morning, as you reach over to turn off the alarm, you feel a wrenching pain in that shoulder. In any event, your acute pain is the result of an *injury*. That's the usual reason shoulders hurt.

But if it's painful and you don't know why, here are some possible explanations:

- The most common cause of spontaneous shoulder pain is *inflammation*, either of the joint itself (*bursitis*) or of the tendons in the area (*tendinitis*).
- The trouble may originate in the spine. When the nerves that supply the shoulder area are pinched by *arthritic bones* or by *bulging discs* as they leave the spine, you will feel the pain not only in the neck, but where the pain fibers end—in your shoulder.
- *Angina pectoris* and/or a *heart attack* are usually felt as a pressure, heaviness or pain behind the breastbone. Sometimes, however, because the nerves in the entire chest area are so close to each other, you may actually experience the pain in the left shoulder instead.
- Pain in either shoulder may be due to *irritation of the diaphragm*, the large muscle which separates the abdomen from the chest.

So here's the bottom line: If you have an ache or a pain in the shoulder, you can tell which of the above is causing it by looking for the wheres and whens of the pain. For example:

- If the ache came on gradually, is constant but is aggravated by moving your shoulder, it's probably due to local arthritis.
- When the shoulder pain comes on suddenly, is worsened by neck rather than shoulder movement and is accompanied by numbness and tingling in your arm and hand, the problem is in your neck. *Whiplash* is a specific kind of neck injury that may leave you with such a combination of shoulder, arm and hand pain. It can happen when you're in a car and are hit hard from behind so that your neck snaps forward and then backward. You'll be nursing a very painful neck and shoulder for some time, because the discs and vertebrae wrenched by the accident push on the nerves supplying the area.
- Shoulder pain from *inflamed or torn tendons* is felt in one spot, and certain positions of the arm make it worse. For example, it may hurt most when you raise your hand above your shoulder as when hailing a taxi, or you may have trouble getting your arm into the sleeve of your coat.
- Shoulder pain is probably referred from the *diaphragm* if moving the shoulders doesn't aggravate matters and you can't remember having injured your neck. Also, your belly aches, or you may have a cough, or a stitch in the chest when you take a deep breath. If the pain is in the right shoulder and is coming from the diaphragm, the possibilities are a "hot" gallbladder, an enlarged liver, or lung disease, all of which may be irritating the diaphragm. If it's the left shoulder, the source is usually an injured spleen or a diseased lung.

Points to Remember

Symptom: Shoulder pain.

What It May Mean	What to Do About It
1. Injury.	Diagnostic X rays followed by appropriate treatment.
2. Bursitis.	Anti-inflammatory drugs, local injection.
3. Tendinitis.	Anti-inflammatory drugs, local injection.
4. Arthritis.	Physiotherapy, pain control.
5. Disc disease.	Rest, traction, surgery.
6. Angina pectoris.	Cardiac medication, angioplasty, surgery.
7. Heart attack.	Emergency call to your doctor.
8. Irritation of the diaphragm.	See a doctor immediately.

LEG PAIN

Pain in the legs is almost as common as a bad back. The reason may be obvious, as when you get a *muscle spasm,* or so-called charley horse, after a long flight in a seat with only enough leg room for a three-month-old child. But many people suffer from chronic leg pain and have no idea why. Bad circulation is only one of the many different possible explanations. Here are some of the most important among them:

- *Diseased arteries.* The vessels bringing blood *to* the muscles of the leg are narrowed by arteriosclerosis.
- *Trouble with the veins.* The vessels returning *from* the legs to the heart (the veins) are dilated (*varicose veins*) or develop clots (*phlebitis*).
- *Neuropathy*—when the circulation in the veins and the arteries is intact but the *nerves* to the legs are irritated or diseased (as happens in a variety of neurological disorders, diabetes and tobacco or alcohol abuse). The result is pain or weakness in one or both legs.
- Joints in the leg are injured, infected or inflamed, most commonly by *gout* or *arthritis.*
- *Cramps* from muscle fatigue, strain, injury or depletion of certain minerals such as *potassium* and *magnesium* (especially if you're taking diuretics).

Here is how you can determine which of the above are causing *your* pain:

- It's arthritis or gout if the affected joint is red, swollen, tender to pressure and touch and it hurts more when you move about.
- Acute phlebitis (inflammation of a vein) involving a surface vessel leaves the area tender, red and swollen. When the deep leg veins are involved, the limb is not red, but may be swollen and is sensitive to deep pressure.
- When your arteries are narrowed due to arteriosclerosis, you may develop a cramp in the calf after you have walked a certain distance. A few moments after you rest, the discomfort disappears and you're able to continue, this time farther and at a faster pace than before. As the arteries become progressively more narrowed, it takes less and less effort to induce the pain, until finally symptoms appear even at rest.

The cramp you feel when you walk is the cry of your leg muscles for more oxygen, which is not available because of the arterial blockage. If you're experiencing such symptoms, look at your toes. They may be pale and cold to the touch, have small breaks in the skin (ulcers) which do not heal, or have areas of black skin (gangrene). When the disease is severe, pain may develop in the toes or the instep during the night.

The likelihood of poor circulation increases substantially if you happen to be at special risk for vascular disease—that is, if you're a heavy smoker, have high blood pressure or diabetes, or evidence of arteriosclerosis elsewhere (a previous stroke or heart attack).

- Your leg pain may have nothing to do with blood supply. It may be due to a *disc problem* in your spine. In that case, your back may feel fine, but one or both legs may ache and be weak or numb because a nerve leaving the spine, on its way to the leg, is being compressed either by an arthritic deformity of one of the vertebrae or by a bulging or ruptured disc.

- Diabetics and heavy smokers may develop leg pain because of *neuropathy*—that is, disease or irritation of the nerves. The leg appears entirely normal, the pulses are good, so is the color, and they feel nice and warm too. But oh, those shooting pains!

Differentiating one cause of leg pain from another ultimately boils down to three main observations which you can make yourself:

- If the pain is relieved by elevating the legs, chances are you have phlebitis.

- If you feel better when you let your feet hang down, then gravity is helping the blood flow into the legs, and your problem is arterial.

• If the pain is accompanied by numbness and tingling, the problem is in your back (although reduced blood supply can also cause such numbness and tingling, especially late in the course of the disease).

Leg pain is one complaint in which your own awareness of how and when it occurs and a simple physical exam by your doctor can often provide a quick diagnosis.

Points to Remember

Symptom: Leg pain.

What It May Mean	What to Do About It
1. Blocked arteries.	Medication, angioplasty, laser treatment, surgery.
2. Varicose veins.	Support hose, sclerotherapy, surgery.
3. Phlebitis.	Bed rest, warm soaks, anticoagulants administered by a doctor.
4. Nerve disorders.	Control diabetes, eliminate alcohol and tobacco, treat neurological disorders.
5. Arthritis or gout.	Physiotherapy and painkillers (but never narcotics).
6. Muscle spasm.	Massage and rest.
7. Low potassium and magnesium if you're on diuretics.	Replace the deficiency.
8. Disc disease.	Rest, traction, surgery.

FOOT PAIN

The next time you're in public—on a bus or a train or in a crowd—take a look at the *shoes* people wear, especially women. You will see feet squeezed into tiny containers, often set at an absurd angle, with the wearer precariously perched high atop a thin spike called a heel. Men too jam their feet into narrow pointed shoes which heap the toes one on top of the other. These are the individuals who, when they go to a play, a movie or a restaurant, remove their shoes with an audible gasp of relief and pleasure. But even if you wear sensible footgear, *overweight* will also cause foot pain.

With all this self-induced torture in the name of fashion, it's no wonder so many of us suffer chronic foot pain due to bunions, calluses, warts, corns, ingrown toenails, fallen arches and sprains. But in this section let's look at the pain that has nothing to do with what you stick your feet into. There are several other common problems involving your feet that can be extremely painful.

Suppose you suddenly feel a severe throbbing discomfort in your great toe, any time of the day or night, regardless of what you're doing. You can't remember stubbing it; no one has dropped anything on it or stepped on it, and yet it's incredibly painful. You remove your shoe and sock to look at the toe. If it's swollen, red, feels warm and is very tender to the touch, you've got a hot case of *gout*. This diagnosis is all the more likely if you've had similar attacks before, or if you regularly take a diuretic ("water pill"). These medications not only eliminate excess fluid and lower the blood pressure, they also raise the level of uric acid in your blood. The uric acid gets into your joints, most frequently those of the big toe, causing the kind of classic gout attack I've described.

Untreated, it may become so painful that even the lightest pressure, like covering it with a bed sheet at night, can be agonizing. This exquisite sensitivity is the hallmark of the gouty joint. There is no other form of arthritis, no matter how painful or debilitating, in which the affected area is so incredibly sensitive to touch.

Another scenario: If you suddenly develop severe pain in the heel while walking, you have a *bony spur*. I know from personal experience how disabling that can be. A few years ago my wife decided that my otherwise mild exercise regimen needed some bolstering. I vetoed her instructions for me to jog in New York's Central Park in the dead of winter. We compromised. Instead of braving the elements, I would run in place in our apartment. Bad move. After just two days of pounding my bare heels on a hard surface, I developed a severe pain in the left one which virtually crippled me for a year.

I had physiotherapy and cortisone injections and put inserts into my shoes to take the pressure off the heels—none of which did much good. Eventually the inflammation subsided on its own. So if you're a runner or a jogger and develop pain in the heel, get an X ray. It will likely reveal the source of your trouble—a tiny bony spur. Time is often the only thing that will predictably cure this condition, and while you're waiting take up swimming and cycling.

The foot has many joints, all of which are the target for several forms of arthritis. *Rheumatoid arthritis*, which we normally think of as involving the hands, can also affect the small joints of the foot, causing severe pain both at rest and while you're walking. This pain is chronic and, like rheumatoid arthritis anywhere, there is associated swelling and deformity.

When your foot (like the leg described earlier)

does not receive enough blood because of *clogged arteries,* you will experience pain in the instep, first while walking and later at rest. In order to tell whether such pain is due to a decrease in blood flow or to arthritis, a careful physical exam is required. You can do part of that yourself. If you place your fingers atop your foot just above the great toe, you should come across a good strong pulse. You may have to search a bit, because its location may vary somewhat. If no pulse is present, if your feet feel cold and if the little tufts of hair that men normally have on their toes have disappeared, then chances are that your pain is due to poor circulation. As with vascular leg pain, you're a candidate for this condition if you have high blood pressure, evidence of arterial disease elsewhere, as for example, a stroke or a heart attack, are a heavy smoker or have diabetes. If you used to experience the pain only on walking, but it now comes on when you're at rest or during the night, then your circulatory problem is far advanced.

If a *blood clot* (embolism) abruptly blocks off one of the vessels to the foot, the foot will *suddenly* become very painful, cold and numb, and will look blanched or blue. What has happened is that a clot or a piece of arteriosclerotic plaque higher up has become dislodged and moved down the artery. Unlike the pain on walking which you've had for months and years, and for which there's no urgent need to rush to the doctor, an embolism is an emergency because the affected limb is in jeopardy.

The arteries in the feet may go into *spasm* when exposed to the cold, in which case your toes will throb with pain and first turn blue, then white. Later, as they warm up, the flush of blood returning to the area restores their normal color, but then the pain is even worse. This disorder, which is called *Raynaud's disease, or phenomenon,* is provoked by a drop in temperature that does not affect normal individuals. It is an autoimmune condition that occurs mostly in women.

The pain in your feet may be due to nerves—physical, not emotional. As in the case higher up in the legs, the nerves that supply your feet emerge from your spine. When a disc in the spine presses on a particular nerve, you may feel the pain all the way down to your feet. One way to test that diagnosis yourself is to try walking on your heels. If the nerve is being compressed, the muscles in your legs will not support heel walking.

Nerves can malfunction in a variety of disorders, including several neurological diseases, syphilis, diabetes, alcoholism and heavy cigarette smoking. Such nerve involvement, regardless of the cause, is called *neuropathy*. The discomfort it produces is *intermittent*, sharp, shooting or burning, and not the throbbing ache of circulatory disease, or the extreme and constant agony of gout, or the chronic pain of arthritis.

Some persons suffer terribly from *neuromas*, little swellings of the nerves in the toes. They cannot be felt, or seen in an X ray. No one knows why they occur, but the only way to obtain relief is to remove them surgically. The diagnosis of neuroma is one of exclusion—that is, what's left after all other possibilities have been ruled out.

There are three things to bear in mind when you have foot pain. First, wear comfortable shoes. If you must sacrifice your feet to fashion, then do what I see smart men and women everywhere do—wear your sneakers to work, and change into fancy shoes in the office. Second, avoid injuring your feet—remember, your whole body balances on them. Third, if your foot pain is seemingly unrelated to either injury or footwear, consult your doctor, who will consider arthritis, gout, circulatory problems or nerve trouble as the possible cause.

Points to Remember

Symptom: Foot pain.

What It May Mean	What to Do About It
1. Poor shoe fit.	Wear comfortable shoes.
2. Obesity.	Weight control.
3. Acute gout.	Medication.
4. Bony spurs.	Local injections into the heel, shoe inserts.
5. Arthritis.	Anti-inflammatory drugs, physiotherapy.
6. Blocked arteries.	Lots of walking; medication; balloon angioplasty; laser treatment; surgery.
7. Vascular spasm.	Calcium channel blockers, protection against cold.
8. Nerve disease.	Treat the underlying cause.
9. Neuroma.	Surgery.

OH, MY ACHING (SWOLLEN) JOINTS

The long tube from your mouth to your anus is referred to as the gastrointestinal tract; the brain and all its nerves constitute the neurological system; everything from the windpipe down to the lungs is the respiratory tract. Believe it or not, all the joints in your body are also interrelated—regardless of how distant they are one from the other. Of course, if you wrench your knee trying to dance the hora at a wedding, or find that your elbow smarts after five sets of tennis, your joint pain is traumatic and local. But if you haven't injured yourself, and you have pain in one or more joints, you may have some generalized disease process, which, in addition to giving you arthritis (a word that comes from the Greek *arthrus,* meaning joint, and *itis,* meaning inflammation), is affecting other body systems.

When all your joints hurt, and you feel feverish, you may have some viral infection like the flu. Or you may feel fine and the pain is limited to the joints. For example, your hips ache a bit every now and again or your knee tells you when it's going to rain. Or you're sick all over, your joints are deformed, you run a low-grade fever, you're anemic and you have no energy. These last two joint-pain scenarios encompass the two most common types of arthritis. Let's deal with the more serious one first.

The symptoms of constant aching, swollen deformed joints, anemia and occasional low-grade fever are those of *rheumatoid arthritis*. But its key characteristic, that which distinguishes it from other forms of arthritis, is the overall malaise that accompanies the pain. You not only hurt, you also feel terrible. That's because rheumatoid arthritis is an autoimmune disease that affects the entire body. Indeed, it often strikes the heart and lungs too.

Osteoarthritis, by comparison, while also painful, is a totally different ball game. It is not an autoimmune disorder, is less deforming and does not involve any other organs. In other words, you feel the pain only in those joints specifically involved. Most authorities think of osteoarthritis as a "wear-and-tear process" that usually hits those joints subjected to the greatest movement and stress, such as your back, knees and hips.

These two major forms of arthritis aren't the only causes of chronic joint pain. Here are some others:

- If you have an *infection* somewhere in your body, the responsible bacteria can get into the bloodstream and penetrate a joint, usually one rather than many. The joint becomes swollen, painful and full of pus. Viral infections like hepatitis B also cause pain and swelling of several joints, but without the pus. So can bacterial endocarditis, an infection of abnormal heart valves.

- Various body chemicals can get into the joints and irritate them. Uric acid, an excess of which causes *gout,* is a good example. Almost three quarters of all gout attacks affect one joint in particular—the big toe.

- About one third of all persons with *psoriasis,* the generalized scaling skin disease that's so easy to recognize, develop pain and swelling in several joints.

- Certain *cancers, bleeding problems* (in which there is hemorrhage into the joint) and even intestinal diseases can be accompanied by some form of arthritis.

- You may develop pain in what appears to be a perfectly healthy joint—a phenomenon known as *arthralgia.* It's a complicated-sounding word which very simply means joint pain. That's what happens when you get the flu and your joints ache, though in this instance they are not also swollen, tender or red.

- Medication, both the kind your doctor prescribes and that which you buy over the counter, can produce painful, swollen joints. The list of potential offenders is a long one and includes penicillin, oral contraceptives, certain blood-pressure-lowering agents, several tranquilizers, anti-tuberculosis drugs and even the mild barbiturate taken for occasional insomnia. So, if your joints suddenly begin to hurt and blow up for no apparent reason, consider a medication you're taking as a possible cause.

Here, then, are some key questions to ask yourself to help you decide the origin of *your* arthritis:

- Are you younger than twenty, is more than one joint involved and does the pain flit from joint to joint? If the answer is yes to all three questions, you have *acute rheumatic fever*. This is all the more likely if the arthritis was preceded by a recent sore throat. Rheumatic fever is uncommon over the age of twenty-one.
- If you are a woman between twenty and forty-five with pain, stiffness and swelling in more than one joint and they are symmetrically involved, you may be unlucky enough to have rheumatoid arthritis. However, if your joint symptoms began after age forty, it's more likely that you have osteoarthritis.
- Is your large toe the only joint involved? If it's swollen, red and so tender that even the lightest touch causes pain, you almost certainly have gout. If you have been taking a diuretic, that diagnosis is pretty well clinched. If it's any other single joint like the knee or the elbow, consider *gonorrhea* (especially if you recently had a urethral discharge or some other bacterial infection).
- Is most of your trouble in your wrists? That's often a characteristic of rheumatoid arthritis.
- Is your pain most severe in your knees and hips? That's a sign of osteoarthritis.
- If the pain and swelling appeared in several joints at the same time, specifically the hands and the

feet, rheumatoid arthritis is a possibility, but so is *Reiter's syndrome*. In this latter condition, several joints become painful and swollen, and there is also inflammation of the eye and a urethral discharge. Reiter's syndrome is an autoimmune disorder usually found in young men and probably represents an unusual response to a sexually transmitted disease.

- When did the joints become swollen and tender? The "when" is important. For, while both rheumatoid arthritis and osteoarthritis cause joint tenderness and swelling, in osteoarthritis the pain often precedes the swelling and the tenderness by weeks or months. That's not the case in rheumatoid arthritis.

- Is the joint involvement symmetrical? In rheumatoid arthritis, if a joint on one side hurts, so will the one on the other. In osteoarthritis the involvement is pretty random.

- Is the joint pain worsened by activity and does it tend to disappear with rest? That's a sign of osteoarthritis.

- Are your symptoms worse in the morning and less severe as the day goes on? That's more apt to be rheumatoid arthritis than osteoarthritis, in which the pain is aggravated as the day progresses.

- If you have fever with the joint pain, and you're young, rheumatic fever is a possibility. Or the joint may be infected or involved by gout or one of the other autoimmune diseases like lupus erythematosus. A few years ago, I'd have left it at that. Today, regardless of where you live, you must consider *Lyme disease*. Transmitted by the bite of a deer tick, it classically causes fever, a rash and joint pains.

- The combination of diarrhea and joint pain may

indicate *inflammatory bowel disease* (ulcerative colitis or Crohn's disease).

Even though there are many different causes of joint disease, you can sort out the various possibilities on the basis of your age, your sex, the particular joint or joints involved, the characteristics of the symptoms, how they are affected by movement, the presence or absence of fever or of other diseases, what medication you're taking and several other factors.

Points to Remember

Symptom: Painful, swollen joints.

What It May Mean	What to Do About It
1. Injury.	X rays to detect fractures, followed by appropriate treatment.
2. Rheumatoid arthritis.	Medication, physiotherapy.
3. Osteoarthritis.	Medication, physiotherapy.
4. Acute infection.	Immediate medical treatment before there is permanent damage to the joint.
5. Acute gout.	Medication.
6. Psoriasis.	Medication.
7. Cancer.	Appropriate treatment.
8. Bleeding disorder.	Medical treatment.
9. Arthralgia due to the flu.	Joint pains will disappear when flu is over.
10. Medication.	Stop the drug that's doing it.

11. Acute rheumatic fever (in children).	Requires a doctor's care to monitor cardiac involvement.
12. Reiter's syndrome (also affects the eyes and the genitourinary system).	Appropriate medication.
13. Lyme disease.	Tetracycline.
14. Inflammatory bowel disease.	Azulfidine, steroids, surgery.

PAIN IN THE ELBOW

I have deliberately chosen to discuss elbow pain separately from pain in other joints, for two reasons: (1) because 90 percent of those who have "tennis elbow" have never set foot on a tennis court, and (2) a recent experience reemphasized to me that bone pain anywhere—the spine, the hips, the legs, the elbow—may not be due to the usual causes and should always be thoroughly evaluated.

No matter what you call it—tennis, pitcher's or taxi hailer's elbow—this is a tendinitis, an inflammation of the tendons around the elbow joint that hinges the upper arm and the forearm. (The same thing can happen to the knee joint—a condition that was once called "housemaid's knee.") It results from any repetitive movement, like a tennis serve, pitching a fast ball or some motion at work. However, you can get similar symptoms from any of the following: *strain,* sprain or misuse of nearby muscles, tendons or connective tissue; *arthritis,* whether it be osteoarthritis, rheumatoid arthritis, the acute swelling of rheumatic fever in children or an *infection* such as that caused by tuberculosis or gonorrhea. You can recognize these nonbursitis causes because they leave the elbow hot, tender, painful and swollen, whereas "tennis elbow," as disabling as it is, does not.

Here is an example of why you should never take *any* chronic joint pain for granted. A fifty-two-year-old otherwise healthy man, who loved to play tennis, developed pain in his right elbow. He denied any other symptoms. He consulted an orthopedist, who gave him a local injection for his "tennis elbow" and advised resting the arm. On this regimen the discomfort became much worse. A few weeks later an X ray was taken and revealed a *cancer* which had spread from some other part of the body to the elbow bone. The source turned out to be a tiny malignant tumor of the lung, too small to produce pulmonary symptoms (such as a cough) or even make itself visible as a shadow on a chest X ray. It had traveled to and settled in the elbow. Despite the most vigorous anticancer treatment, the malignancy spread to involve the brain, the liver, the lungs and other bones, and the patient died a few weeks later. The lesson? If you have unexplained pain in any joint or bone, and the symptoms do not clear up in short order, have it X-rayed.

Points to Remember

Symptom: Elbow pain.

What It May Mean	What to Do About It
1. Strain.	Rest and analgesics.
2. Arthritis.	Physiotherapy, local injection, analgesics.
3. Infection.	Antibiotic treatment.
4. Cancer.	Appropriate treatment.

CHEST PAIN FROM THE HEART

Chances are that at some time or another you're going to have to decide what to do about pain or discomfort in your chest. That decision may need to be made in a hurry, perhaps in the middle of the night without the immediate availability of a medical opinion. So, before discussing the many various possibilities of chest pain, let me offer one cardinal rule you must never forget: *Any adult who suddenly experiences discomfort in the chest must assume that it has something to do with the heart* and act accordingly. If it turns out to be a false alarm, you've lost nothing. But if it indeed was the heart, you may have saved your life! As you read on, you will see how cardiac pain usually does manifest itself. But it can be so variable and the stakes are so high that unless you're absolutely *sure* about what's going on, play it safe. Get your doctor on the phone immediately or go to the emergency room of the nearest hospital. Remember, a heart attack is not always "painful." It is more often perceived as a heaviness, a pressure, an awareness or a shortness of breath. I learned long ago never to ask anyone, "Do you have chest pain?" Even among known cardiac patients, the answer is frequently "No." If I leave it at that, I may miss the diagnosis. Words like "uncomfortable," "pressing" or "shortness of breath" will frequently evoke a definite "Yes!"

Let me expand on the advice to act promptly after the sudden onset of an unfamiliar chest symptom. Obviously, if you're fifteen or sixteen years old, it's most unlikely that your chest pain or pressure is due to coronary disease, and there's usually no need for you to rush off to an emergency room. But by the time a man has reached forty, a quick trip to the emergency room is a reasonable response when there is *any* doubt. It's different for women, because they are *relatively* immune to heart disease before menopause—unless they smoke and are on the Pill, have diabetes or high blood pressure, have had their ovaries removed or have very abnormal blood fats (cholesterol). For both sexes, the chances of any given chest symptom being due to coronary artery disease increase if any of these risk factors are present.

Now, if your *heart* is not the source of the trouble, what else can it be? The chest is a very busy place, with several different organs and nerves, all of which can produce symptoms simulating those of a heart attack. Among the possible perpetrators are the *lungs* (pleurisy, an inflammation of the lining of the lungs which sometimes heralds pneumonia, or an embolism, a blood clot to one of the small blood vessels of the lung, can be mistaken for a heart attack); the *esophagus* (any disturbances in the way the food is propelled down the food pipe toward the stomach can cause pain which may be virtually indistinguishable from that originating in the heart); a *hiatus hernia* (when a portion of the stomach slips up into the chest so that gastric acid gives you a burning feeling in the heart area); injury to or disease of the *rib cage* (less likely to be confused with heart pain, but nevertheless something to be considered); *nerve irritation* (from their compression as they exit the spinal column); the *muscles* of the chest wall (which can go into spasm); *gallbladder disease;* and spinal *arthritis.*

Here is a brief description of each of the various common causes of chest pain and how they can be differentiated one from the other:

It always surprises me, given that heart disease is the number-one cause of death and disability in this country, how few people recognize its characteristic symptoms. Many think that cardiac pain is sharp and stabbing or that it arises in the left side of the chest. In fact the typical pain of a *heart attack* is pressurelike in quality. It is located mainly in the center of the chest, behind the breastbone, whence it can radiate to either shoulder, through to the back, the arms or the hands (it's usually but not always the left arm, the left shoulder and the left hand), the jaw or the ears. If closure of the artery is complete, the symptoms do not disappear when you stop whatever it is you're doing. A nitroglycerin tablet under the tongue may give relief for a few minutes, but then the pain recurs. The patient is pale, weak and short of breath, breaks out into a cold sweat and is usually very apprehensive. There may be a cough, palpitations (an awareness of the heartbeat), dizziness and lightheadedness. Things may improve somewhat in the sitting position.

That's the description of a classic heart attack, but the picture may vary considerably, depending on your particular threshold for pain, as well as on the severity and the location of the damage within the heart. Indeed, a heart attack may be "silent," and unrecognized by the victim, who may either live through it despite a lack of treatment—or die.

Angina pectoris is another cardiac condition that produces chest pain similar in nature to that described above for a heart attack: pressing or squeezing, often beginning in the middle of the chest and radiating to the left arm, shoulder or hand. Angina is less severe, is not usually associated with weakness, sweating or other symptoms and, most important, is of short duration. An anginal attack is frequently precipitated by some unusual stress—physical (like walking too fast up a hill, especially in cold or windy weather) or mental (like a heated argument or an exciting football game) and disappears quickly when the exertion or stress is over. Angina usually reflects a partial blockage of the coronary arteries by arterio-sclerosis rather than the complete obstruction that causes most heart attacks. Repeated or increasing frequency of angina, especially when it comes on at rest or during the night, is a warning that a heart attack is imminent. See your doctor immediately!

Angina does not necessarily mean physical block-age of an artery. It may also indicate temporary arterial spasm. This requires treatment, because prolonged spasm can result in a heart attack, too.

The heart can generate another kind of pain, due to an entirely different disorder, one that affects the wrapper that envelops it—the pericardium. When the pericardium becomes inflamed or infected by a virus, the result is *pericarditis*. Its symptoms mimic those of a heart attack, except that the pain worsens when you take a deep breath. The only sure way to tell these two very different conditions apart is by a good physical exam and an electrocardiogram. Never make that diagnosis yourself. Simple viral pericarditis usually runs a benign course, requiring only rest and aspirin for treatment. However, the condition may also stem from more serious causes—everything from a heart attack to a cancer which has spread to the pericardium. Medical treatment will depend on the underlying cause.

CHEST PAIN FROM THE LUNGS

There will be times when you think your chest pain is coming from the heart, but it's actually originating in the lungs. That can happen in two common conditions of which you should be aware. One is dangerous and requires immediate attention; the other can make you really sick but is not usually a threat to life. Let's look at the less serious situation first. It's fairly easy to recognize in its typical form.

The lungs are covered by a two-layered envelope called the pleura, which can become inflamed, irritated or infected, a condition called *pleurisy*. If you have pleurisy, the two layers of this lung wrapper rub together so that you feel a sharp pain near the end of each deep breath. The pleura are a particularly attractive target for viruses. Viral pleurisy is often accompanied by fever and a cough. *Pneumonia* also frequently begins as a pleurisy. In either case, because it hurts so much to breathe deeply, you find yourself taking only shallow breaths. Moving about doesn't usually aggravate matters, but coughing really hurts. Viral pleurisy usually lasts for a few days, then clears up on its own. The pain goes away because the pleura produce a lubricating fluid between the two layers, so that now when you breathe they glide smoothly over each other without friction.

The outlook for and treatment of the pain of pleurisy, however, depend on what's causing it. There's usually nothing to worry about in simple viral pleurisy. However, pleurisy can result from a number of serious underlying illnesses. One such disorder, a *blood clot,* or *embolism,* to the lungs, is often heralded by pleurisy. Unfortunately, this diagnosis is not considered often enough by patients and doctors alike. A clot originating somewhere in the body (usually in the legs or the pelvis) travels along a network of veins into the lung, where it becomes lodged. In so doing, it cuts off the circulation to a portion of the lung, damaging it. The pleura are irritated in the process, causing the pain. The severity of the attack depends on the size of the blood clot and how much pulmonary tissue is injured. So the spectrum of symptoms in a pulmonary embolism can range from sudden pain anywhere in the chest, which worsens when you breathe, to spitting blood, a sharp fall in blood pressure (shock) and even death.

Just as there are factors which predispose you to a heart attack, so are there circumstances which should lead you to think of a lung embolism. They include:

- Recent *phlebitis,* an inflammation of the veins in the legs. A clot forms within the vein, and a piece breaks off and travels to the lung. This is most likely to happen if you have varicose veins, have been confined to bed for some reason or have been sitting for hours in a car or on an airplane.
- *Injury to the legs* can damage the veins too, causing clot formation. If the affected vessel is situated deep in the leg, you may not be aware of this injury-induced phlebitis—until the embolism actually occurs.
- *Prolonged bed rest* results in sludging of the blood flow and so predisposes to clot formation. This is the main reason we get patients up and about as quickly as we can after any illness or operation. In the days before we fully appreciated the risks of long-term confinement to bed, we used to prescribe six weeks of total inactivity after a heart attack. In time it became clear that this precaution was not reducing cardiac complications and was, in fact, contributing to a high incidence of embolism. As a rule of thumb: *No matter what it is that has put you to bed, get up and get moving as soon as you possibly can.*
- Almost any *operation,* especially one in the pelvis, leaves you more vulnerable to traveling blood clots.
- While *the Pill* remains one of the safest and most effective forms of contraception, it leaves some women vulnerable to blood clots, especially those

in their thirties who smoke and/or have high blood pressure.

As a general rule, chest pain which has the characteristics of pleurisy (it hurts when you breathe deeply and especially when you cough), while it may not be a medical emergency, is something that should be evaluated by your doctor quickly.

There is one rather dramatic condition which can cause sudden chest pain and shortness of breath together. That's what happens when a portion of one lung collapses, just like that! Strangely enough, it usually happens in young, healthy people who have absolutely no pulmonary disease of which they are aware. Nor is there any way you can anticipate and/or forestall such a *pneumothorax*. I recently had a typical case in my own practice. The patient was a young foreign diplomat at the United Nations, in his late twenties. He was physically fit and enjoyed working out for twenty minutes each day. The previous evening, just after dinner, he had suddenly become short of breath for no apparent reason; there had been neither cough nor fever, but there had been a "strong pain," as he put it, in the right upper portion of his chest. When I examined him, he looked fine but complained of the persistent pain, especially when taking a deep breath. I thought this was an early pleurisy, but when I examined him, instead of hearing the "rub" of pleura which I described earlier, I could not detect any air moving in that portion of the lung—virtual proof that it had collapsed. An X ray confirmed the diagnosis, and I sent the patient to the hospital. After a few days of conservative treatment, he finally needed an operation (not always necessary) to fix a small hole in his lung. He recovered completely.

Spontaneous pneumothorax is usually the result

of the rupture of a small blister on the lung, which allows air to escape into the chest cavity, where the resulting pressure can lead to the collapse of part or all of the lung. Before that rupture occurs, there are no symptoms. But in older patients who have emphysema (in which the lungs are hyperinflated because they retain too much air), such blisters, or "blebs," are common, and not infrequently burst and cause a pneumothorax, too.

Under whatever circumstances pneumothorax occurs, you must see your doctor as soon as possible to prevent more and more of the lung from collapsing.

Here's another example of the same process, but with a different mechanism. My youngest son, Herb, twenty-one at the time and at college, developed a severe pain in his right upper back after some vigorous calisthenics. I thought it was a muscle spasm and referred him to a physiatrist, who confirmed the diagnosis. He thought some tight muscles in the painful area could be relaxed by injecting them with novocaine. So he sent for a nice, long needle, which my son viewed with some trepidation. As it turned out, the procedure wasn't as painful as expected, but almost immediately after it was all over Herb noted some shortness of breath. There was pain too, but he thought that was to be expected. After the injection, he was asked to move his right arm every which way to see if his original pain was any better. It was not, and, moreover, Herb was now *extremely* short of breath. Well, you know that doctors' relatives are suspect anyway, so Herb was humored and reassured. Finally, in desperation (the doctor wanted to get on with his next patient—my boy was holding things up!) someone listened to his chest with a stethoscope. Only then was the diagnosis of pneumothorax made. This one wasn't spontaneous like the case I described above. Herb's pneumothorax was caused not by a ruptured blister, but by a small needle that went too deep and put a hole in the lung. If ever you receive an injection in the chest wall, for whatever reason, and you *suddenly* become short of breath, you'll now know why!

WHEN THE RIB CAGE HURTS

If you've cracked or fractured a rib, you're apt to know it and you expect it to hurt. However, some women with osteoporosis, whose bones are calcium-depleted and fragile, suffer such breaks after some trivial injury, or a sudden movement of the chest or a vigorous cough. They are often unaware of what could have broken their rib. As with pleurisy, the pain is sharp and is made worse by breathing deeply. The difference between the two is that rib cage pain is aggravated by bending and twisting the torso, which is not the case with pleurisy, a heart attack or a blood clot in the lung.

An even more insidious cause of rib fracture is a malignancy which has spread to the ribs from elsewhere in the body. Those cancers with the greatest affinity for bones arise in the prostate in men, the breast in women and the kidneys, the lungs, the stomach and the liver in both sexes. So, if you have been treated for a cancer anywhere, seem to be doing well and then suddenly experience a sharp pain that's aggravated by deep breathing *and movement* (but is not accompanied by fever), the cancer may now involve the ribs. A bone scan will determine whether that's what has happened.

PAIN IN THE CHEST FROM HERE, THERE AND EVERYWHERE

All the nerves that serve the chest area exit from the spinal cord very close to one another. Trouble in one organ within the chest can therefore be associated with symptoms at a nearby site. For example, pericarditis may resemble pleurisy, pleurisy may simulate a blood clot, and all three may feel like a heart attack. Irritation of the diaphragm (the muscle that separates the chest from the abdomen) and hiatus hernia can both cause discomfort behind your breastbone, mimicking coronary disease. A nerve going to the chest from the spine can be compressed by arthritic overgrowth or a bulging *disc,* causing symptoms that are indistinguishable from any of the other causes described above.

And then there's the pain of *muscle spasm,* or "pulled" muscles—after a particularly vigorous workout or lifting some heavy object. As a general rule, if it hurts when you press something on the *outside,* the problem isn't coming from the heart or the lung.

Finally, always think of *shingles* whenever you have sharp pain anywhere. I've been fooled time and again by sudden severe, localized pain which I was sure reflected a broken rib, the onset of pneumonia, a blood clot or even a heart attack. A complete physical examination and all the appropriate tests reveal nothing. Then, after a few days during which the patient, the family and I are quite apprehensive, the characteristic shingles rash finally appears on *one side of the chest.* It never crosses the mid-line of the body.

HEARTBURN

After drinking too much, or eating too many of the foods that you know from experience don't agree with you, you may hurt in the pit of the stomach. That results from an irritation of the stomach lining. But suppose you've been moderate in your eating and drinking, yet when you lie down, swallow, eat a large meal or bend over you feel a burning sensation in your lower chest and upper abdomen. Instinctively, you stand up or drink some liquids and you feel better. An antacid, preferably in liquid form, affords relief in about five to ten minutes. Diagnosis: *heartburn*. One day you may develop heartburn when you're with someone who is very "heart-minded." He or she may convince you to slip a nitroglycerin tablet under your tongue just to be sure: "Try it, you'll like it," the person will tell you. Not a bad idea, actually, but sit down before you do it. If the symptoms are due to heartburn, the nitroglycerin won't help a bit. If, however, it's angina pectoris, you'll feel better within a minute or two.

Heartburn results from the acid in your stomach backing up into your food pipe (*esophagus*). The muscle designed to prevent this from happening sometimes goes lax, causing reflux of the acid and the characteristic burning sensation. This is most likely to happen when a portion of the stomach slips up through the diaphragm and into the chest (you then have a *hiatus hernia*).

If you have "heartburn" and are in a high-risk group for heart disease by virtue of your sex (male), your age (over forty) and other risk factors (high blood pressure, high cholesterol, bad family history, diabetes, cigarette smoking), you should have an electrocardiogram and a stress test to make sure that what you're suffering from is indeed a reflux of acid into the food pipe and not cardiac pain.

Points to Remember

Symptom: Chest pain.

What It May Mean	What to Do About It
1. Heart attack.	Get to the nearest medical facility as fast as you can.
2. Angina pectoris.	Nitroglycerin under the tongue relieves in one to three minutes.
3. Pericarditis.	Medical diagnosis to determine the cause, followed by the appropriate treatment.
4. Pleurisy.	See your doctor to determine the cause and the appropriate treatment.
5. Pneumonia.	Requires antibiotic treatment as soon as possible.
6. Embolism to the lung.	An emergency!
7. Pneumothorax (collapsed lung).	Emergency!
8. Fractured rib.	No treatment, but find out why it happened.
9. Disc trouble in the neck.	Physiotherapy.
10. Muscle spasm.	Tranquilizers, antispasmodics, heat, physiotherapy.
11. Shingles.	Appropriate medication.

12. Heartburn.	Antacids, but first make sure it's not from the heart.
13. Spasm of the esophagus.	Antispasmodics, calcium channel blockers.
14. Hiatus hernia.	No emergency, but make sure it's not a heart attack!

BELLYACHES (RIGHT, LEFT, HIGH AND LOW)

The abdomen is not a single structure like a bone or the heart. It's a large container full of many different tissues and structures. They're all wonderful—until they give you pain.

Now, before going any further, remember this: The *sudden* onset of *severe,* unfamiliar abdominal pain is a red alert for you to get help immediately. I'm not suggesting that you panic with every cramp that's relieved by passing gas, or each time you have a bellyache and diarrhea. But something that's severe enough to double you up and make you short of breath, and that lasts for thirty minutes or more, may be a "surgical emergency." You can speculate about the cause to your heart's content, but only on the way to the hospital. The reason for this urgency is that many of the abdominal organs are hollow (the stomach, the bowel, the gallbladder). If one of them bursts, leaks or becomes obstructed, your life may be in danger. The perforation must be sewn up or the obstruction removed *quickly.*

In order to distinguish one cause of abdominal pain from another, you must first know what's where in the belly. You'll never recognize ovarian symptoms if you don't know that you have two ovaries and that they are nowhere near the liver. I'm not going to assume that you have this knowledge, especially after one of my male patients told me he thought all men had a uterus, a "vestigial" one, not as fully developed as a woman's, but a uterus nevertheless!

In order for you better to understand the information in the next few pages, simply draw two imaginary lines through your belly button: one vertical from the bottom of the chest to your pubic area, the other horizontal from one side through to the other. Your abdomen is now divided into four quarters, or quadrants—right upper, left upper, right lower and left lower. The location of any symptom can now be pinpointed to one of these four quadrants.

Pain in the Right Upper Quadrant

The right upper quadrant of your abdomen contains organs with which almost everyone is familiar, at least by name—the liver, the gallbladder, a portion of the gut (every part of the abdomen has some bowel in it), the pancreas and the right side of the diaphragm (the muscle which separates the lungs from the belly and which moves up and down when you breathe). Disease of or injury to any of these organs will give you pain in the upper-right-hand side of your belly. How intense and what kind it is will depend on what's going on and in which particular tissue.

Is it the liver? Anything that causes the liver to swell can make it hurt. An infection, a chemical injury or a weak heart is what usually does it. Here are the most common disorders:

• Several "bugs" or parasites can infect the liver. Whatever the cause of the inflammation or infection, the result is referred to as *hepatitis* (*hepar* means liver and *itis* means inflammation). The infectious agents which most commonly attack the liver in this part of the world are viruses (viral hepatitis). There are three main types to watch out for: hepatitis A, hepatitis B, and hepatitis C. People usually come down with hepatitis A after consuming sewage-contaminated food or water (shellfish are the prime offenders). Hepatitis B is especially common among homosexuals, IV drug users and those in close contact with them. Hepatitis C is almost always transmitted via contaminated blood transfusions, blood products or needles.

- A variety of chemicals and prescription drugs can damage the liver, too, either because they're toxic to the liver (*toxic hepatitis*) or because of a hypersensitivity reaction. The list of medicines which can do so includes everything from antibiotics to pills that lower blood pressure. So can carbon tetrachloride, a widely used cleaning fluid, and acetaminophen (Tylenol). However, the most important chemical liver poison is alcohol (causing *alcoholic hepatitis*).

- When the *heart muscle* is weak, it cannot pump out all the "used" blood returned to it. Some backs up into the lungs (making you short of breath) and later into the liver, distending it and leaving it sore.

Liver pain is constant and achy, not sharp or knifelike. You feel it over the whole right upper part of your abdomen—deep inside, not on the surface. The discomfort develops gradually and steadily, not in spasms or waves. Should you experience such a sensation, ask yourself whether you

- ate any shellfish in the past few weeks (hepatitis A);

- shared an infected needle with anyone (hepatitis B);
- drank really heavily (alcoholic hepatitis);
- received a blood transfusion recently (hepatitis C);
- are short of breath and have swollen ankles (signs of heart failure);
- are jaundiced and have dark, tea-colored urine (evidence of any kind of hepatitis).

Is it the gallbladder? Bile, made by the liver, aids in the digestive process. If you have been fasting or following a low-fat diet, the gut doesn't need all the bile the liver is constantly making. The excess is stored in the gallbladder. When you eat a fatty meal and need more bile to digest it, the gallbladder squirts out its reserve on demand.

Infection, malfunction and stones in the gallbladder are very often responsible for right upper abdominal pain (and sometimes in the midline as well). Although such disease affects both men and women, young and old, white and black, at special risk are Navajo Indians (perhaps 70 percent of whom have gallstones) and Four-F females—fat, fortyish, fertile and flatulent—as well as women taking the Pill.

Symptoms of gallbladder disease may sneak up on you gradually. A severe attack is often preceded by weeks, months or even years of feeling gassy and bloated one to two hours after eating fried or fatty foods and certain vegetables such as cabbage. However, your first awareness of any trouble may be an acute attack. When that happens, the pain is severe, unlike the mild ache of liver disease. At its peak, you may sweat and experience nausea which even vomiting won't relieve. You're not likely to have a high fever, unless the gallbladder becomes infected; in that case, your temperature may exceed 102 degrees and you'll have chills. The pain itself is most intense in the right upper quadrant, but may also spread around to the back near the right shoulder blade.

Most diseased gallbladders contain stones. If the stones are small enough, one or more may pass from the gallbladder into the ducts that carry the bile to the intestines. You will then experience *biliary colic,* whose pain starts quickly and comes in waves as the ducts try to squeeze out the obstructing stone. When they succeed and the stone is finally eliminated, you feel better. But if the stone remains lodged in the duct, it will need to be removed one way or another —by surgery, by dissolution techniques or by extraction without an operation. Obstructed bile ducts cause jaundice, which clears when the stone is passed.

Then there is the *pancreas,* a glandular organ which is located deep in the abdomen and which manufactures digestive juices and insulin. It extends from right to left; its "head" lies in the right upper quadrant, the "body" runs across the midline and the "tail" is situated in the left upper quadrant. Although the pancreas is not nearly as likely as the liver or the gallbladder to cause you pain, it certainly can do so. Most feared, and with good reason, is *cancer* of the pancreas. The most common cause of pancreatic pain, however, is inflammation, *pancreatitis,* to which heavy drinkers and people with gallbladder disease are especially vulnerable.

An attack of *acute pancreatitis* may be very, very painful and is accompanied by sweating, nausea and vomiting. The symptoms differ from those of gallbladder disease in that the pain penetrates straight into the back and you feel worse lying down and better sitting up, leaning forward. The diagnosis usually requires confirmation by blood tests to measure the level of certain enzymes released by the damaged organ.

What else could it be? Your bowel twists and turns throughout the abdominal cavity. If the portion that lies in the right upper quadrant becomes inflamed by *diverticulitis* or some form of *colitis*, you'll feel pain in that area. It's not common, but it can occur. It's usually not severe or sudden in onset, but more like a cramp. It lasts for a few minutes and then disappears for a half hour or so, and then the cycle repeats itself. You're also likely to have some diarrhea or constipation or both.

Pneumonia—in the belly? I have seen many patients who, after several days of cough and fever due to a "cold," suddenly develop right upper quadrant pain. The "cold" was actually pneumonia. The inflamed and infected lung is in contact with the diaphragm, which also becomes irritated enough to involve the nearby bowel, thus accounting for the right upper quadrant symptoms. So remember, any abdominal pain preceded by a respiratory illness may actually be due to *infection in the lungs*.

Always think of *shingles* whenever you have unexplained pain *anywhere*. Shingles is caused by an inflammation of the nerves by the chicken pox virus. After the original infection in childhood, this virus lies dormant in the nervous system for decades. Then it becomes reactivated, either by stress or because the immune system which holds it in check becomes weakened as one gets older. The released virus then inflames nerves *anywhere* in the body, causing exquisite pain in the involved area. The first symptoms are a superficial sensitivity, a burning feeling or even an itch which later evolves as a severe pain. For four or five days you simply hurt in one well-defined location. The skin appears perfectly normal, without a rash or any other telltale signs. Aside from the pain, you don't really feel sick at all. Now, if it's the right upper quadrant of the abdomen that's involved, your doctor can be led on a wild-goose chase looking for gallbladder disease, pancreatitis or even kidney stones. He or she tests and tests and finds nothing. After a few days, the reddish pimples characteristic of shingles finally pop out on the skin exactly where the pain was felt. The rash follows the course of the inflamed nerve, never crossing the midline to the other side of the body. *Such a "unilateral" rash is virtually diagnostic of shingles.*

Is it the kidney? Kidney trouble can occasionally cause pain in the right upper quadrant, too. Your kidneys are positioned more in your flank, one on each side of the body, so a kidney problem is usually reflected by pain in the flank and the back. However, should the right kidney become infected, or develop an abscess, or form stones, or be hit by a traveling blood clot originating somewhere in the circulation, the resulting pain may be experienced in the right upper quadrant as well as in the back. If the problem is due to a small stone traveling down from the kidney on its way out of the body, the pain comes in waves, is excruciating and may shoot down toward the groin and into the right testicle. (More about this later in the discussion of flank and testicular pain.)

Pain in the Left Upper Quadrant

The left upper quadrant of the abdomen contains its own organs, and in order to figure out why you're having symptoms in that area you should know what they are: the spleen, the stomach, the pancreas (remember, it lies across the upper abdomen), a loop of the bowel (it's everywhere in the belly) and, of course, the left side of the diaphragm. We don't have a liver and a gallbladder with which to contend in this location, so left upper quadrant pain is generally less frequent than distress in the right upper quadrant. But things can and do go wrong in this area.

Is it the spleen? The spleen lies quite close to the surface of the body, while the pancreas is situated deep in the belly, virtually on the backbone. When the doctor examines your spleen, he doesn't push very hard or deep, because it's right there. The main job of the spleen is to remove red blood cells from the bloodstream after their normal life span of 120 days. It traps them, breaks them up and returns their components to the bone marrow, where new red blood cells are made. When the spleen increases in size—this happens in a number of different diseases —the capsule, or wrapper, which covers it stretches. This causes pain. Also, when the spleen is all soft and enlarged, as occurs in infectious mononucleosis, it becomes vulnerable to rupture because it is situated so close to the surface. That's why people with infectious mononucleosis should avoid contact sports; in fact, it's better for them not to exercise at all (even in the unlikely event that they should feel like doing so). Any untoward motion, blow or jarring can burst an enlarged spleen—another reason why your doctor doesn't prod you too hard when he examines it. Sometimes an enlarged spleen will rupture spontaneously. *The telltale sign of a ruptured spleen, aside from the pain and tenderness in the area, is a blue discoloration around the belly button.* This Technicolor touch is due to the accumulation of blood (which, by the way, is blue until exposed to air) in that area.

Is it the bowel? It may very well be. The large bowel crosses the top of the abdomen, curves downward in the left upper quadrant, then descends along the left side of the abdominal cavity. Unlike in some other parts of the belly, left upper quadrant pain frequently doesn't indicate any disease at all and may be due to gas bubbles trapped in the bowel where it makes its very sharp downward turn. However, if you have *diverticulitis* or any other inflammatory disease of this portion of the bowel (exactly as it can happen on the right side), this is where you'll feel the pain. Your symptoms will then also include diarrhea and/or constipation, blood and/or mucus in the stool and some fever.

Here's a cardinal rule to remember: Whenever you have discomfort *anywhere* in the abdomen, always look at your stools. The presence of bright red blood indicates bleeding low down in the bowel such as you might expect from hemorrhoids; a black stool reflects bleeding higher up in the stomach or the small intestine. Another thing to remember: If your stool is black, don't panic. It may be the result of iron and charcoal in your diet; Pepto-Bismol can have the same effect. But always have your stools checked for blood, anyway.

Is it the stomach? Very possibly. Unlike the heart, the stomach is not set smack in the middle of your body. It's actually located in the left upper quadrant. Anything that irritates the stomach lining, a condition known as *gastritis* or functional dyspepsia—whether the irritant is too much alcohol, the wrong food, or daily aspirin—will cause pain in the region. The symptom itself is not usually excruciating, but is more of an ache, and is apt to be accompanied by nausea and vomiting. Antacids help a lot. If the pain persists for more than a day, see your doctor; you may have an *ulcer* or even possibly a *cancer*. Chances are overwhelming, however, that it's a simple gastritis.

Is it a hernia? The diaphragm, which separates the chest from the abdomen, contains an aperture through which the food pipe passes into the abdomen. When the muscles that control the size of that opening weaken, usually with age, the hole through which the food pipe passes enlarges, allowing the upper portion of the stomach to move freely from the abdomen (where it belongs) up into the chest cavity (where it doesn't). This condition is called *hiatus hernia*. When the stomach acid enters this hernia, you feel pain in the left upper belly, but also sometimes in the chest. This invariably raises fears of heart trouble, but there is a difference between the two symptoms: the discomfort from a hiatus hernia is almost always aggravated by bending over or lying down flat, while heart pain is generally not. But since the difference between the two is not always clear-cut, be sure to get the chest pain evaluated no matter what your instincts tell you.

Could it be the pancreas? Definitely. Remember that the pancreas stretches across most of the upper abdomen. When it is inflamed, you will feel the pain on the right, in the midline or on the left.

A variety of ailments and toxins can strike the pancreas, including *cancer* (to which heavy smokers are more vulnerable), alcohol, long-term use of diuretics or steroids (the latter commonly prescribed for arthritis, asthma, cancer, organ-transplant rejection and certain chronic diseases), inflammation caused by bile leaking from the gallbladder ducts and by the passage of stones through those ducts. You should suspect the pancreas as the source of the trouble if the pain is very severe and deep-seated and is accompanied by fever, nausea and vomiting and if you are at special risk for pancreatic disease—that is, you have gallbladder trouble, are a heavy smoker, drink excessively, suffer from diabetes or take diuretics or steroids.

What else could it be? Viral *pleurisy, pneumonia* or any process that irritates the lung results in a sharp stitchlike pain when you take a deep breath. If the irritation spreads to the diaphragm, the pain may *seem* to originate in the abdomen. Suspect this possibility if, after some respiratory infection, you develop unexplained abdominal pain. If you injure a rib on either side of the chest—whether by making too hard a tackle in your weekend football game, or because you're a postmenopausal woman and your bones were rendered brittle by osteoporosis and they fracture easily (sometimes a cough or a simple movement is all it takes)—you will have pain that may seem to stem from your belly. It's not hard to tag those symptoms. Rib cage pain worsens when you cough, sneeze, move or push on the exact spot where it hurts most. Ulcers of the duodenum often cause pain in the left upper quadrant, too.

Pain in the Right Lower Quadrant

Again, let's start with what's situated in this part of the abdomen. First, there's the *appendix,* which is a little fingerlike piece of tissue projecting from the large bowel. Then there's the bowel itself, which is potentially the seat of various disorders, including *cancer.* But we also have a whole new set of organs to consider here: the ovaries and the fallopian tubes in women and the ureters carrying urine from the kidneys to the bladder in both sexes.

Is it the appendix? Here's a good rule to remember, one I learned when I was a medical student and am reminded of very frequently as a practicing doctor: *Any pain in the right lower portion of the abdomen, statistically speaking, is appendicitis until proven otherwise.* If you can pinpoint the pain with one finger, and it has persisted for twelve hours without relief, appendicitis is almost a sure bet. This is especially true if the pain also hovers around your belly button. If you suspect that your appendix is inflamed, call your doctor immediately. If he confirms your diagnosis, he will almost certainly recommend surgery before this organ of dubious function becomes gangrenous and bursts.

The appendix isn't the only potential trouble spot in the right lower quadrant. Other possible problems include *irritability,* inflammation or infection of the bowel (by ulcerative *colitis, Crohn's disease* or *diarrhea* from organisms and parasites such as amoebae and worms picked up in underdeveloped countries and in dirty restaurants right here at home), *shingles,* and pressure on nerves which leave the *spine* and end up in this location. A *kidney stone* in the course of its trek down to the bladder will also cause excruciating pain in this area.

If you've missed your last period and are suddenly felled by severe pain in either the left *or* the right lower abdomen, think first—and fast—of a *ruptured ectopic pregnancy.* An ectopic pregnancy occurs when the fertilized egg remains in the fallopian tube instead of moving into the uterus. This misplaced egg never becomes a baby, because it eventually bursts, spilling the products of conception into the abdominal cavity and irritating it with considerable blood and other debris. The result is severe, diffuse belly pain. On the other hand, when pain develops gradually and continues for days, weeks or months at a time, it is more likely to reflect an infection within the pelvis—*pelvis inflammatory disease*—by a sexually transmitted disease such as gonorrhea or chlamydia. *Ovarian cysts,* especially when they rupture, and *ovarian tumors* can produce similar chronic pain patterns. Pain which is worst with your periods suggests *endometriosis.*

Pain in the Left Lower Quadrant

Pain in this area can result from all the conditions that affect the right lower quadrant, *except* appendicitis.

There are millions among us with a disorder that goes under a variety of names—"nervous stomach," "spastic colon," "irritable bowel syndrome." Whatever you call it, the symptoms are the same—cramping, diarrhea and/or constipation, gas and bloating in the lower abdomen. As I've indicated earlier, such persons run from doctor to doctor, desperately looking for help. There is no explanation for irritable bowel at the moment, although it often appears to be stress-related. These individuals—and their physicians—must, of course, make absolutely sure that they do not have a bowel tumor, diverticulitis, inflammatory bowel disease or lactose intolerance. Beyond that, the symptoms can sometimes be controlled by medication or by resolving any emotional factors that may be contributing to the condition.

BELLY PAIN SQUARELY IN THE MIDDLE

Upper Midline Abdominal Pain

This is classically due to an *ulcer* in the stomach or the duodenum (the initial portion of the small intestine which begins where the stomach ends). *Stomach cancer* can also cause pain in the stomach, but malignancies rarely involve the duodenum.

Do you have an ulcer? A *gastric ulcer* is an erosion in the lining of the stomach. Most ulcers respond to treatment, but then act up unpredictably. They are more apt to do so if you booze, smoke, take caffeine, regularly use aspirin or related painkillers for any

length of time or require chronic cortisone therapy.
An ulcer attack, untreated, usually lasts a few weeks
and clears up as mysteriously as it began. The pain
feels like a bad hunger pang and indeed occurs most
often on an empty stomach, when the acid normally
present in the stomach can eat away at the vulnerable gastric lining. So ulcer pain awakens you in the
middle of the night because that's when the stomach
is empty.

If you think you have an ulcer, be sure to look at
your stools (as you should anyway). Black stools indicate that the ulcer is bleeding (but not all ulcers
bleed). Though tense, nervous and stressed individuals are usually tagged as ulcer prone, seemingly relaxed and well-adjusted persons are also candidates
for this disease. *Irritation* of the lining of the upper
intestinal tract by aspirin or alcohol, without frank
ulceration, can also cause distress in the upper midline area.

Lower Midline Abdominal Pain

This usually signals something going on in the urinary tract, the bladder, the female reproductive organs, the bowel or the rectum.

With respect to the reproductive organs, *endometriosis*—in which tissues that normally belong in the
uterus are present in various parts of the pelvis or the
bowel—may be the culprit. Endometriosis is not life-
threatening; but it hurts. The misplaced tissue responds to hormonal changes, just as it does in the
lining of the uterus. So with every period you'll experience pain wherever the endometriosis happens to
be located in your particular case.

Lower midline belly pain accompanied by a fever
and vaginal discharge indicates *pelvic inflammatory
disease*. However, *the most common cause of gyne-*

*cologic pain in postmenopausal women is large fib-
roids (benign tumors) in the uterus.* Less frequent
and never to be forgotten are uterine and ovarian
cancers, as well as the perennial *irritable bowel.*

Arteriosclerosis—in the belly? We normally think
of arteries, and the diseases that can befall them, in
terms of the heart, the brain, the legs or the kidneys.
But every organ in the body is dependent on a
healthy blood supply. The bowel is no exception.

The bowel's job is to propel food along its entire
course, to carry out the process of digestion and to
absorb nutrients. In order to do that, it needs nour-
ishment—and that means blood. When one or more
of the larger vessels supplying the bowel with blood
is blocked or narrowed, that portion develops *mesenteric angina* (the arteries to the bowel are called
the mesenteric arteries). Suspect this diagnosis if
you're sixty or older, have evidence of arteriosclerosis elsewhere in your body and experience severe
cramping pain in your lower abdomen, together with
bloody stools shortly after eating. The only way to
confirm this diagnosis is by angiography—the X ray
taken after dye is injected into the abdominal circulation by means of a puncture in the groin area.

The major artery in the body is the *aorta.* It leaves
the left ventricle, the main chamber of the heart, and
bends to course down into the abdomen. On its way
it gives off major branches to the kidneys, the gut
and other organs. The aorta is particularly vulnerable to arteriosclerosis, especially in someone with
long-standing, untreated high blood pressure. Over
the years, its walls weaken (from the sustained
pounding of the elevated pressure) and form large
plaques containing cholesterol, calcium and other
substances. If the process persists unchecked, the vessel balloons out, at which point it's called an *aneurysm.* An aneurysm is "pulsatile"—that is, if you put

your hand on your belly you can feel the vessel beating in time with your heart. If it continues to expand, it will eventually leak or burst—and that's a life-threatening emergency. When that happens, the pain is so severe that the patient either goes into shock or dies within a few minutes. However, if it's a slow leak rather than a rupture, there may be some warning symptoms which consist of an ache for a few days in the midline of the abdomen. But before you panic because you can feel a pulsating in your own belly, remember that that's normal in thin people.

On a less terrifying but still serious note, progressive narrowing and obstruction of the abdominal aorta, without its forming an aneurysm or rupturing, causes poor circulation in the legs, and chronic impotence (because the penis is deprived of the blood required for an erection).

Points to Remember

Symptom: Abdominal pain.

What It May Mean	What to Do About It

In the Right Upper Quadrant of the Belly:

1. Hepatitis.	Treatment depends on the specific cause.
2. Swollen liver due to heart failure.	Medical management.
3. Gallbladder disease.	Diet, antibiotics, surgery, newer nonsurgical therapy.
4. Pancreatic cancer.	Supportive care, no cure.
5. Pancreatitis.	Emergency treatment.
6. Diverticulitis.	Diet, antibiotics, occasionally surgery.

7. Colitis.	Medication, occasionally surgery.
8. Pneumonia.	Antibiotics.
9. Shingles.	Medication.
10. Kidney trouble.	Medication.

In the Left Upper Quadrant:

1. Enlarged spleen.	Determine cause and treat.
2. Diverticulitis.	Diet, antibiotics, occasionally surgery.
3. "Gastritis."	Diet, medication.
4. Stomach ulcer.	Medication.
5. Stomach cancer.	Surgery.
6. Hiatus hernia.	Diet, antacids.
7. Pancreatitis.	Emergency treatment required.
8. Pancreatic cancer.	Supportive care, no cure.
9. Pleurisy.	Medication.
10. Pneumonia.	Antibiotics.

In the Right Lower Quadrant:

1. Appendicitis.	Emergency surgery.
2. Bowel cancer.	Surgery.
3. Irritable bowel.	Medication (antispasmodics).
4. Colitis.	Medication, occasionally surgery.
5. Crohn's disease.	Azulfidine, steroids, surgery.
6. Infectious diarrhea.	Antibiotic treatment.
7. Shingles.	Medication.

8. Disc disease in the spine.	Physiotherapy, surgery.
9. Kidney stones.	Lithotripsy, surgery, medication.
10. Ectopic pregnancy.	Emergency surgery.
11. Pelvic inflammatory disease.	Antibiotic treatment.
12. Ovarian cysts and tumors.	Surgery.
13. Endometriosis.	Medication.

In the Left Lower Quadrant:

1. All of the above *except* appendicitis.	As above.
2. Irritable bowel.	Medication (antispasmodics).

In the Upper Midline:

1. Stomach ulcer.	Medication.
2. Duodenal ulcer.	Medication.
3. Stomach cancer.	Surgery.
4. "Gastritis."	Diet, medication.

In the Lower Midline:

1. Bladder infection.	Antibiotic treatment.
2. Kidney stone.	Lithotripsy, surgery, medication.
3. Endometriosis.	Medication.
4. Pelvic inflammatory disease.	Antibiotic treatment.
5. Uterine fibroids.	Hysterectomy.
6. Uterine cancer.	Surgery.
7. Ovarian cancer.	Surgery, chemotherapy.

8. Irritable bowel.	Medication.
9. Arteriosclerosis.	Medical and dietary management.
10. Abdominal aneurysm.	Surgery, depending on the size.

PAIN IN THE FLANK

Most people assume that flank pain means kidney trouble. That's often but not always the case. (The flank lies between the right or left upper abdomen and the back.) An *arthritic spine* and/or a *muscle spasm,* neither of which has anything to do with the kidney, can cause discomfort in that area. So can a *bulging disc* pressing on nerves that wend their way from the spine to the flank area. And, of course, there's *shingles,* in which you suffer unexplained, localized pain for a few days, followed by the appearance of the characteristic one-sided rash. However, if, along with the pain, you have fever, chills and urinary problems, the kidney is the likely source.

There are several disorders to which the *kidney* is vulnerable, any of which can result in flank pain. A *stone* which obstructs the outflow of urine can cause it to back up into the kidney, ballooning it and leaving you with an aching flank. The kidney may become *infected,* develop an *abscess,* be struck by a traveling blood clot, or *embolism,* or suffer a *hemorrhage.* Persons receiving blood thinners (anticoagulants) should bear this possibility in mind. How can you distinguish one cause from another?

• If you have flank pain and suspect that the kidney is the source, be sure to look at your urine to see whether it's frankly bloody (a brownish color may also indicate the presence of blood) or cloudy, possibly reflecting infection.

• When the trouble is due to a kidney stone (one American in seven has such stones) the pain is agonizing, comes in sharp stabbing waves or spasms and is usually not limited to the flank. It spreads down the entire course of the ureter—the duct that carries the urine from the kidney to the bladder—into the groin and, in males, the testicles as well. During such an attack, you'll pace and fidget, trying (in vain) to assume a comfortable position. If the stone is in the very end of the ureter as it "tunnels" into the bladder, frequent, urgent urination often results.

• Kidney pain due to infection is accompanied by high fever, chills, nausea and vomiting.

• Pain, fever and a frankly bloody urine indicate bleeding and/or infection within the kidney.

Points to Remember

Symptom: Flank pain.

What It May Mean	What to Do About It
1. Spinal arthritis.	Anti-inflammatory drugs, physiotherapy.
2. Muscle spasm.	Rest, physiotherapy, exercise.
3. Disc disease.	Rest, physiotherapy, possible surgery.
4. Shingles.	Medication.
5. Kidney disorders:	Medication or surgery.
Stone.	Observation, lithotripsy, surgery. If small, the stone may pass on its own.

Infection.	Antibiotic treatment.
Abscess.	Antibiotic treatment, surgery.
Embolism.	Determine the source, anticoagulants, medication.
Hemorrhage.	The cause determines the appropriate treatment.

PAIN IN THE RECTUM AND THE ANUS

During or after an especially hard and large bowel movement, one at which you had to strain a great deal, you may experience pain in the rectal area. You may also notice some bright red blood on the surface of the stool, on the toilet tissue or in the bowl. The pain may last for a few days, clear up and then return intermittently. This picture is quite typical of *hemorrhoids* (enlarged or varicosed veins in the rectal area), which account for most cases of rectal and anal pain. Hemorrhoids are usually the result of chronic straining at stool by persons with long-standing constipation or women who have had several babies. But anything that stretches, tears or otherwise *injures* the tissue in and around the rectum and the anus will cause pain: an abscess, a cut (fissure) from the distention of a particularly large and hard stool, lacerations in persons who engage in anal intercourse or insert foreign objects into the rectum, frequent enemas in which the anal or rectal tissue is damaged by the nozzle. The liquid in the enema can also be irritating and the source of chronic pain.

No matter how obvious the cause of your rectal symptoms, never make the diagnosis yourself, especially if you have noted *any* change in the quality or the frequency of your bowel movements. Remember that cancer of the colon often masquerades as a benign condition.

Here are some characteristics of rectal and anal pain that can help you identify its cause:

- When the pain is accompanied by diarrhea, there may be a problem higher up in the abdomen: *colitis, diverticulitis,* a *polyp* or a *tumor.*
- *Inflammation of the prostate gland* frequently results in a specific type of rectal discomfort. It feels as though you're sitting on a golf ball. Add to that the other features of prostatitis—frequent and painful urination with interludes of fever—and the "golf ball" sensation is clarified. If you're a woman and are experiencing rectal pain, in addition to the disorders mentioned above (excluding prostatitis) think of an *ovarian cyst* and *pelvic inflammatory disease.*

Sometimes an *inflamed appendix* will give pain in the rectum rather than in the belly; that's why doctors always do a rectal exam when they suspect appendicitis.

Points to Remember

Symptom: Rectal and anal pain.

What It May Mean	What to Do About It
1. Hemorrhoids.	Local treatment, lubricated wipes or suppositories to alleviate symptoms, stool softeners, rubber banding, injections; laser therapy or surgery in more serious cases.

2. Rectal damage or infection (ulcers).	Medical therapy, hot sitz baths, surgery. Make sure it's not sexually transmitted (antibiotics if it is).
3. Colitis.	Sigmoidoscopy for a definite diagnosis, and appropriate medical treatment.
4. Diverticulitis.	Dietary and medical management. Surgery in more serious cases.
5. Polyp.	Removal by endoscopy or surgery.
6. Tumor.	Surgery.
7. Prostatitis (in men).	Antibiotic treatment and/or surgery if the gland is enlarged.
8. Ovarian cyst.	Surgery.
9. Pelvic inflammatory disease.	Antibiotic treatment.
10. Appendicitis.	Early surgery.

PAIN IN THE GROIN

Most people use the terms "groin" and "testicle" interchangeably, but what causes pain in one won't necessarily do so in the other. So let's be specific. The groin is the area where your abdomen ends and your legs begin. When you hurt in the groin on either side, always think *hernia* first. Hernias occur when the local support tissues weaken, permitting loops of bowel to slip from the belly into the groin. (Normally, the space between the two areas allows only for the passage of blood vessels and nerves into the scrotum, and not loops of bowel.) A hernia becomes apparent as a swelling in the groin, most marked when you stand. At some point, it may begin to ache. But you can have the ache without a visible bulge. Your doctor can find the hidden hernia by inserting one finger into the scrotal sac in men. He'll always ask you to cough, because that raises the pressure in the belly and forces the loop of bowel into the hernia opening. A weakness of the muscles which causes a hernia is equally simple to find in women.

If you have a hernia, it's important to know it. Sometimes the piece of bowel is very small in relation to the opening through which it slips in and out. In that case, there's no immediate threat. But if the aperture is relatively small and the loop of bowel big, the latter can be pinched or trapped in the opening. When that happens, the condition is called an "incarcerated" hernia. (One of my patients who developed this complication called in panic to tell me, "My hernia is burning me. I think it's incinerated!") Such entrapment constitutes a surgical emergency because the blood supply to the loop of bowel is cut off in the tight squeeze, resulting in destruction of the affected bowel.

Almost any infection in the pelvic area, the feet or the legs may cause enlargement and pain of the *lymph glands* in the groin. You can actually feel the tender glands yourself. If they are swollen but not painful, they're more likely to indicate a malignancy or a tumor than an infection.

If your groin pain is due neither to a hernia nor to swollen lymph glands, it may result from a *disc in your spine* pressing on nerves that extend to that area. A low-lying *kidney stone* may also cause pain in that location. Frequent urination and blood in the urine (visible or under the microscope) are often the tipoff to this problem.

Points to Remember

Symptom: Groin pain.

What It May Mean	What to Do About It
1. Hernia.	Medical examination and surgery if there is risk of "incarceration."
2. Enlarged lymph glands.	Medical examination to determine the cause, and appropriate treatment.
3. Disc disease in the spine.	Physiotherapy, surgery.
4. Kidney stone.	Medical management if it does not pass without intervention.

PAIN IN THE TESTICLES

If you wake up one morning to the throbbing ache of a swollen, tender testicle, the reason may not be a mystery to you. You may have injured yourself recently in a contact sport or caught an errant baseball there. Under those circumstances, you expect it to be swollen and painful. A dilated vein within the sac (a *varicocele*) may become painful as the day wears on, especially if you're on your feet for long hours. But if you ache in this area, haven't been injured there, and don't see or feel anything unusual, then the problem may have other causes. The ducts through which the sperm leave the body can become inflamed (*epididymitis*) and painful. These inflammations usually respond quickly to rest and antibiotics. A *hernia* into the scrotum, which happens when the tissues separating the abdomen and the scrotum weaken, causes a fullness or a swelling in the area, most noticeable when you stand up. Such a hernia may become inflamed and tender, indicating the need for surgical repair, sometimes urgently.

Testicular aches and pains are, surprisingly, not usually cause for alarm. But there are two specific circumstances which warrant your close attention. The first is *mumps*. This viral infection almost always runs a harmless course. The swelling in the parotid glands of the face (in either cheek) usually disappears without complication. Occasionally the testes are also involved, especially when the disease occurs later than in childhood. In that event, they are painful. The best way to deal with mumps is to prevent it from happening in the first place—that is, by getting vaccinated early in life.

Another potential cause of testicular pain and swelling is *testicular torsion*. The cord that suspends the testicle becomes twisted, suddenly cutting off the blood supply to the testicle. If this situation is allowed to continue for more than a few hours, the gland may become gangrenous and have to be removed. Testicular torsion can be very insidious, occurring from time to time in otherwise healthy young men, then resolving spontaneously so that there never seems to be any reason to do anything about it. I have one such patient who went through college with three or four attacks of severe testicular pain. Each time the gland became progressively swollen and tender to the touch, the doctors at the university infirmary told him he had a "virus." Then one day the pain didn't clear up but became worse, and he developed nausea and vomiting. His parents drove to the university and brought him home to his own doctor, an eight-hour trip. When he was finally seen by a urologist, he was in severe pain. An incision in the scrotum by the surgeon exposed the testis, which was now black with gangrene and had to be removed! Had the diagnosis been made earlier, the knotted, twisted structures could have been "unwound" by a simple surgical procedure, and the testis might have been saved.

Interestingly enough, testicular torsion is not a random accident! Certain individuals are prone to it, so much so that when the surgeon fixes the involved testicle he will always do a minor procedure on the "healthy" one to prevent torsion there too.

Another cause of testicular pain is unrequited love and unfulfilled passion. The resulting congestion of the scrotal tissues causes pain. The condition, known among its sufferers as "blue balls," is easily remediable—but not by a doctor!

A *kidney stone* sliding slowly and painfully down the main ducts from the kidney to the outside world can cause your testicles to hurt, too. This referred pain comes on quickly, and ends after the stone has been passed.

Cancer of the testis, the major malignancy in men between the ages of twenty and thirty-five, is usually painless, at least initially. So if you feel a lump which doesn't hurt, don't ignore it. The fact that it doesn't hurt is not good news.

Points to Remember

Symptom: Testicular pain.

What It May Mean	What to Do About It
1. Injury.	Supportive care, possible surgery.
2. Varicocele.	May require surgery.
3. Epididymitis.	Antibiotics, rest, support.

4. Hernia.	Support or surgery.
5. Mumps.	Supportive care.
6. Testicular torsion.	Diagnose early and treat surgically. Delay may result in loss of the testis.
7. Kidney stone.	Pain will clear when the stone is passed.
8. Cancer of the testicle.	Usually painless. Must be removed. High rate of cure.

PAIN IN THE PENIS

There's nothing funny about having pain in or on your penis—"Just ask the man who owns one." One of the major causes of penile pain is *trauma* of one kind or another, usually from excessive manipulation. Bites (human as well as insect), pimples or any *surface lesion* are all frequent causes of pain.

Another common source of pain in the penis is *genital herpes.* The actual eruption is sometimes preceded by five or six days of burning, itching or pain at the site of infection, followed by the visible lesions. After these blisterlike sores close over and heal, the pain disappears. After the first attack, some herpes sufferers remain symptom-free for months, years and occasionally forever. Others have frequent recurrences. Acyclovir, an antiviral drug, very effective when taken orally, not only lessens the intensity of the attacks but reduces the number of recurrences. In the days before AIDS, genital herpes caused quite a hysterical reaction in both sexes. Today it is viewed more calmly, especially when compared to the lethal AIDS epidemic.

Inflammation of the prostate gland frequently causes penile pain. This may be due to infection or to irritation. In the former case antibiotics are needed; in the latter, simply resting will make things better.

Syphilis can produce a penile sore, but this one is painless. Other sexually transmitted infections which *can* cause penile pain are *nonspecific urethritis* (an infection or inflammation of the urethra usually caused by chlamydia) and *gonorrhea,* which, despite penicillin and other antibiotics, still plagues mankind. Infection under the foreskin of uncircumcised men (*balanitis*) can also produce penile pain and swelling. Treating the underlying disorder will, in most cases, do away with this symptom.

The following are less common causes of penile pain:

- *Cancer* of the penis. Its recognition is not a problem, because you can see the growth right there on the surface of the organ. Penile cancer does not usually cause pain unless it becomes infected. It is treated surgically.
- *Prostheses* for the treatment of impotence are now being widely used. Tubes are surgically implanted in the penile tissue to make it erect, and when the prostheses function well the patient can enjoy satisfactory and pleasurable sexual activity. However, from time to time, such implants become infected and result in pain.
- There is one disorder in which penile discomfort is associated with—believe it or not—red eyes and joint pain. This unlikely combination is called *Reiter's syndrome,* an autoimmune disorder. (I referred to it earlier in the section on painful joints.) So, if your penis hurts and has a discharge and you have a low-grade fever and aching joints, look at your eyes in the mirror. If they're red, you've got yourself a diagnosis. The condition usually subsides without treatment after several weeks.

- Penile pain can also stem, paradoxically enough, from a source of pleasure—an erection. If a clot forms in the arteries of an erect penis, blood is prevented from leaving the organ. The result is an erection maintained long after it is needed, or wanted—and extreme pain. This state of affairs, called *priapism,* may require surgical measures for relief. It is most commonly seen in such blood-sludging diseases as leukemia and sickle cell anemia (but healthy people get it, too).
- A more common cause of painful erection is *Peyronie's disease,* in which scar tissue forms within the penis (no one knows why), causing it to curve when erect and making sexual intercourse difficult and sometimes impossible. Surgical intervention may help.

Points to Remember

Symptom: Pain in the penis.

What It May Mean	What to Do About It
1. Trauma.	Local treatment.
2. Skin infections.	Antibiotics.
3. Genital herpes.	Acyclovir.
4. Inflammation of the prostate gland.	Antibiotics.
5. Sexually transmitted diseases.	Appropriate antibiotics.
6. Infection under the foreskin (balanitis).	Antibiotics. If chronic, it may require circumcision.
7. Cancer of the penis.	Surgery.

8. Infected prostheses used in the treatment of impotence.   Removal of the prosthesis.

9. Reiter's syndrome.   Medical management.

10. Priapism (persistent erection).   Treat the underlying disorder.

11. Peyronie's disease.   Surgery occasionally helps.

BREAST PAIN

There is so much concern with breast cancer (one of every seven women in this country will develop it) that any breast symptom raises the specter of this malignancy. If you hurt in one or both breasts, you must, of course, determine the cause. But while you're doing so, remember that breast cancer is usually painless. The reason for your breast pain will probably turn out to be one of the following:

Chronic cystic mastitis—one of the most frequent causes of breast pain. If your breasts are lumpy to begin with, they may become tender either at midcycle or just before your period, when estrogen levels are at their peak. When the period begins, these levels fall, and the pain is diminished. In chronic cystic mastitis, *both* breasts are usually involved. Some of my patients tell me that abstaining from caffeine and taking vitamin-E supplements help reduce this discomfort. So does a low-fat diet rich in complex carbohydrates. But the breasts don't necessarily have to be lumpy in order to hurt. Nor is age a factor. A teenager may have breast tenderness when she starts *menstruating*, as may older women approaching *menopause*. Breasts often become engorged and tender very early on in *pregnancy*. In fact, if you suddenly develop breast pain for no apparent reason and have not been keeping track of your periods, don't be surprised to learn that you're pregnant. After *childbirth,* when the breasts are filled with milk, they may ache, too.

Female hormones (*estrogens*), whether used for contraception in the Pill, for prevention of osteoporosis or for control of menopausal symptoms, often leave the breasts full and painful. Indeed, a whole slew of drugs will enlarge the breasts and make them sore, both in men and in women. These include digitalis preparations (digitoxin, digoxin); Aldomet (alphamethyldopa), used to control high blood pressure; Aldactone (spironolactone), a mild diuretic; Inderal and the beta blockers; and several mood-altering medications such as chlorpromazine.

Male *alcoholics* often have a high level of female hormone in their blood (because their *damaged liver* is unable to break down this hormone, which all normal men produce in tiny amounts). As the unwanted estrogens accumulate, these men become "feminized"—they lose their sex drive and potency, they shave less often, their hair distribution is altered and their breasts enlarge and become painful. The same complications occur in men with advanced cancer of the prostate whose testes have been removed or who are receiving estrogen therapy.

Of course, your breasts may hurt because they have been *injured* in some way. A bite from anyone for whatever reason can also lead to infection and pain. For example, a hungry baby may have bitten a nipple, infecting the surrounding tissue (mastitis).

Shingles can result in severe pain in only *one* breast because the virus never crosses the midline of the body.

Finally, whenever you have pain in the breast, always examine your nipples for evidence of discharge.

If you see any, report it to your doctor. It may reflect cancer.

Points to Remember

Symptom: Breast pain.

<u>What It May Mean</u>	<u>What to Do About It</u>
(Remember that cancer of the breast is not usually painful.)	
1. Chronic cystic mastitis.	Avoid caffeine. Try vitamin-E supplements, low-fat, high-carbohydrate diet.
2. Normal hormonal fluctuations.	If the pain is troublesome, it may respond to bromocriptine or small doses of danazole.
3. Sign of early pregnancy.	Medical confirmation and consultation.
4. Milk engorgement after birth.	Normal.
5. Estrogen therapy.	Medical management to adjust dosage.
6. Medication.	Discuss with your doctor the drugs you're taking. Switch or discontinue the offending agent.
7. Liver damage caused by alcoholism.	Colchicine, supportive care.
8. Injury, such as a bite.	Treat with antibiotics at the first evidence of infection.

PAINFUL PERIODS

Every month the walls of the uterus become engorged with nutrient-rich blood in anticipation of the arrival of a fertilized egg. When conception does not occur (or there has been a miscarriage), the now blood-filled lining is no longer necessary and is shed. Even though monthly menstruation is a normal function, it often leaves otherwise healthy women feeling miserable and uncomfortable and in pain (dysmenorrhea). Just as they do in so many other unsolved mysteries in medicine, doctors may tell such women that their dysmenorrhea is psychosomatic or due to stress. Personally, I don't believe that at all. In my opinion, if there is no evidence of any other local cause, painful periods are the result of prostaglandins acting on the pelvic tissue. Prostaglandins are secreted by the lining of the uterus, and their release can now be blocked by antiprostaglandin medicines.

Regardless of why they happen, menstrual cramps are such a common phenomenon that most women consider them inevitable. They needn't be, because a treatable cause of the *excessive* pain is frequently found after a careful diagnostic search. For example:

• Any condition which interferes with the elimination of menstrual blood will cause pain. Remember that this flow must pass from the uterus out through its narrow neck, the *cervix*. Occasionally, the cervical opening is abnormally small, so the blood has a hard time getting out. Some of it backs up and is retained for a while within the uterus, where it clots. When the uterus then tries to expel these clots (very much like what it does with a baby ready to be born), the contractions cause pain. Dilating the cervix eliminates the narrowing as well as the cramps. Sometimes one or more *polyps* in the cervix may also obstruct the flow of blood out of the uterus each month and make for painful menstruation.

- *Endometriosis* is another common cause of painful menses. In this disorder, tissue which should be found only in the uterus appears elsewhere in the pelvis, for reasons that are not understood. Every period is accompanied by excruciating pain as this aberrant tissue reacts to hormonal influences.
- What with all the sexually transmitted diseases now rampant in our society (everything from chlamydia to gonorrhea), *pelvic inflammatory disease* is quite prevalent. The presence of such chronic disease almost invariably causes or aggravates menstrual pain.
- *Polyps* or *fibroids* within the uterus itself can leave you uncomfortable, too, if they interfere with its ability to contract. Also, periods may be painful when the uterus is malpositioned—tilted either too far back or too far forward. Finally, several ovarian disorders, including benign *cysts,* can result in menstrual pain in response to cyclical changes in the hormone level.
- *Intrauterine devices* (IUDs) are often associated with severe menstrual cramping, probably because of low-grade pelvic inflammatory disease which they induce.
- In women who use *the Pill* and then stop it when they want to have a baby, the first few periods are apt to be more painful than normal. Again, a hormonal effect.

If your periods *always* hurt, get a thorough gynecological examination early on to rule out a correctable cause. Don't resign yourself to the false folklore that menstruation has to be a "curse" every month.

Points to Remember

Symptom: Painful periods.

What It May Mean	What to Do About It
1. Some pain is normal, excessive pain is not.	Gynecological examination to determine the cause and the appropriate treatment.
2. Cervical obstruction.	Dilatation of the cervix.
3. Endometriosis.	Medication.
4. Pelvic inflammatory disease.	Antibiotics.
5. Polyps (cervical or uterine).	Surgery.
6. Uterine fibroids.	Surgery if the symptoms are severe.
7. Ovarian cysts.	Surgery.
8. Intrauterine device.	Removal.
9. After you stop the Pill.	Symptoms are temporary.

PAINFUL INTERCOURSE: WHEN THE AGONY EXCEEDS THE ECSTASY

Most well-adjusted women who love their mates have no pain during intercourse, but sex can hurt for physical reasons, even when the relationship is a perfect one. If your lovemaking is marred by discomfort (dyspareunia), here are some possible explanations:

- There are several *vaginal malformations* of which a woman may not be aware that make intercourse painful. These range from a vestigial (poorly developed) vagina to one which is double (but each half is too small!). Since most pediatricians do not perform routine vaginal examinations on their prepubertal patients, it is most important for every adolescent female to have a gynecological checkup *before* she becomes sexually active.

- In a pre-menopausal woman, the most common reasons for painful intercourse are *infections:* local vaginal infection—like a boil on the vulvae (vaginal lips); inflammation of the urethra from sexual friction; cystitis (the so-called "honeymoon" disease); and chronic infection in the pelvis. Large *hemorrhoids* can also lead to painful vaginal intercourse in certain positions. So will *tumors* of the genital tract, although they are rare. *Endometriosis* (displaced uterine tissue) also accounts for many cases of dyspareunia.

- *After a pregnancy* during which a couple has abstained from sex for what seems like an eternity, premature resumption of lovemaking may cause pain. This is especially true if any surgery, however minor, was needed during the delivery, if labor was difficult and the vaginal tissues were injured, or if the mother is lactating. In the latter circumstance, the estrogen level is low, and so the lining of the vagina becomes dry, very much like what happens after menopause. In any event, sex should always be very gently performed for a few weeks after delivery.

- *Menopausal women,* or those about to be, secrete less female hormones, so their vaginal lining loses its normal moisture and becomes dry. Under these circumstances, despite continued and even heightened sexual desire and arousal, intercourse becomes painful. Local application of estrogen creams alleviates the problem and is really a must.

- Very often, in trying to discover why a patient finds intercourse painful, I have found that it stems from lack of experience and education—on both her part and that of her partner. When there are no vaginal malformations or infections, when hormone levels are adequate and natural lubricants plentiful and when there are no emotional problems, the cause of painful intercourse may be traced to an excessively exuberant or impatient partner. The cure, in that case, is simple: care, patience and an understanding of mutual needs.

- Just as discussions of sexual "performance" are traditionally limited to the male and his potency (or lack of it), so is painful intercourse usually considered only in terms of women. But the sex act can also be painful for *men*. Usually it's because of an infection on the surface of the penis, as, for example, a herpes sore. Most males will want to abstain anyway at such times, for fear of infecting their partner. Also, when the prostate gland is infected or inflamed, intercourse may be uncomfortable. A disorder to which I have referred earlier, Peyronie's disease, is often associated with painful intercourse. Scar tissue forms in the shaft of the penis so that when it becomes erect it looks like a boomerang. The cause is unknown, but it is presumed to be an autoimmune condition. Treatment is generally unsatisfactory, although surgical correction occasionally results in some relief of symptoms.

Points to Remember

Symptom: Painful intercourse.

<u>What It May Mean</u>	<u>What to Do About It</u>
1. Vaginal malformation.	Surgical correction.
2. Genitourinary tract infections.	Antibiotics.
3. Hemorrhoids.	Removal.
4. Genital tumors.	Surgery.
5. Endometriosis.	Medication. If the pain is intolerable, surgery.
6. In postpregnant women.	Patience and gentleness.
7. In menopausal women.	Estrogens, lubricants.
8. In men:	
Infection of penile skin.	Antibiotics.
Herpes.	Acyclovir.
Prostatitis.	Antibiotics; sitz baths. Avoid alcohol and caffeine.
Peyronie's disease.	Possible surgery.

PAIN WHEN YOU URINATE

Making urine and passing it comfortably requires the normal function of several different organs and structures. The kidneys are the body's filters which extract waste products from the blood and make urine in which to eliminate them. The urine passes from the kidney down a long tube, the ureter, which empties into the urinary bladder. After a certain amount has been accumulated there, the stretched bladder wall sends a message to your brain, which tells you it's time to "go." The news is insistent enough to awaken you from sleep. The longer you ignore it, the more uncomfortable you become. When circumstances permit, you empty your bladder. In order to be able to do so normally, certain muscles must relax and others contract. The urine passes out of the body through the urethra, the duct that leaves the bladder to the exterior. Quite a complicated procedure for such a simple act.

When it hurts to get rid of the urine, you've probably got a *genitourinary tract infection.* If you're a woman, it's most likely a bladder infection (cystitis). In males, it's more apt to be an infection of the prostate. Whatever its origin, an active urinary tract infection not only is painful but is accompanied by fever and chills.

You can pinpoint the location of the infection by paying attention to where it hurts and when. For example, if you feel a burning, as if you were passing hot water, *while you're actually voiding,* the trouble is likely to be in the urethra itself. If, however, it hurts *after* you've finished, the focus is probably in the bladder. In any event, your doctor will want a urine culture to make the diagnosis and select the right antibiotic.

In women, painful, frequent urination may be due to mechanical irritation of the urethra and is often associated with vaginal infection. Then there is *interstitial cystitis,* the cause of which is unknown. This is an inflammation of the bladder which we used to think was the result of infection. We're not so sure anymore.

In men, if, in addition to the pain, the stream of urine is thin, weak or split, there may be some obstruction to its outflow, almost certainly by an *enlarged prostate.* But it may also be due to a neurological problem causing paralysis of the muscles which control bladder function.

Look at your urine, too. If it's obviously bloody, you're almost always dealing with a *kidney stone,* a tumor or a severe infection somewhere in the urinary tract. Urine that looks clear to the naked eye may nevertheless be infected; conversely, if it's cloudy, that may be due to phosphates in your food—a perfectly normal finding.

Points to Remember

Symptom: Painful urination.

What It May Mean	What to Do About It
1. Infection anywhere in the genitourinary tract.	Antibiotics.
2. Interstitial cystitis.	Palliative medication.
3. Enlarged prostate.	Surgery, eventually.
4. Kidney stones.	They'll probably pass, because the pain is low down.

CHAPTER 2

THE LUMPS THAT ARE—AND AREN'T

Run your hand over your scalp. Do you feel one or more bumps on your skull of which you were previously unaware? Don't worry. These are *exostoses*—harmless overgrowths of bones. Women often have them removed for cosmetic reasons. My favorite aunt had such a bony lump right smack in the middle of her forehead, almost like a horn; it didn't hurt and it wasn't dangerous, but she chose to be rid of it anyway because she didn't like the way it looked. Now feel under your armpit. You can make out something hard and painless there. Is that serious? Very possibly, especially if you're a woman and haven't had a mammogram recently.

Finding a lump anywhere in your body can be a frightening experience. It needn't always be. In this chapter you'll read about some of the more common lumps, when you really need to worry—and when you don't. In most cases, however, you will want to have the lump checked out anyway, just to be sure.

Here are several categories of lumps and swellings of which you should be aware:

Lipomas are aggregations of fat that form under the skin of especially well-padded persons. The lumps feel soft and roll easily under your fingers. Leave them alone unless, of course, they begin to hurt (which they sometimes do if they become too large) or are cosmetically unacceptable.

Fibromas, another type of benign lump, generally feel firmer than fat. Now and then, a *cancer* originating elsewhere spreads to and accumulates beneath the skin as a lump. In such cases, the overlying skin is pigmented or discolored, and the lump itself also feels harder and is not as freely movable as the benign variety.

Superficial *bleeding* just under the skin can leave a discolored lump due to the congealed blood. It's the kind of thing that usually happens after an accident, no matter how trivial it seemed at the time. But here's another common cause, more frequent than my venipuncture technicians admit: When, in order to draw blood for testing, a standard-sized needle is introduced through your skin, it makes a tiny hole in the wall of the vein. After the needle is withdrawn, and before nature closes the hole, blood continues to ooze out of the vein into the surrounding tissues. Depending on the size of the leak, a firm collection of blood is left behind and a few days later feels like a lump. This is most likely to happen if you bleed easily (which you will if you're taking aspirin regularly or are being treated with anticoagulants), if the needle which was used had a defect in it, a microscopic burr which made the hole in the vein a little too large, and, of course, if the technician doing the job had trouble finding the vein and ended up poking more than one hole into it. In any event, these lumps all eventually disappear.

A similar complication can result from an angiogram—when dye is introduced into the circulation in order to see your blood vessels on an X ray. Any leak that occurs after such a procedure is much more substantial than that following a simple blood test, because here the punctured vessel—usually in the area of the groin—is an artery, not a vein. Arteries bleed more vigorously than veins. After the catheter through which the dye is injected has been removed, blood seeps out of the artery into the tissues of the upper leg and the lower abdomen. The entire area becomes red, black, blue and yellow (the colors change with time) and swollen. Most of the blood is reabsorbed, but for weeks and sometimes months a hard lump remains. If that has happened to you, don't panic. It too will disappear. But if you can feel it *pulsing,* that means the artery is actually pumping blood out. Call your doctor immediately.

Bleeding can also occur within an *injured or diseased organ* and so enlarge it that it feels like a lump. A good example is hemorrhage into the spleen because of some disease process. When you feel your belly, you think you've got a lump.

When fluid is trapped in a closed space from which it cannot escape, and becomes infected, it forms an *abscess.* Most of us have had such abscesses at one time or another, whether external and visible (in the gums or in a hair follicle in the skin), or internal and invisible (in the liver, the lungs or the gallbladder). Depending on its location, such an abscess may be felt as a lump that "gives" when you push it —because of the pus it contains.

You cannot usually feel the *lymph nodes* in the neck, the groin, under the armpit and behind the elbow, unless they become enlarged. These glands function as filters, and anything they trap in the course of doing their job—viruses, bacteria or cancer cells—makes them swell. If you do detect such a gland, here's a useful rule of thumb. If it's hard and painless, it is likely to reflect a malignancy somewhere; if it's soft, freely movable and tender, it is probably an infection. But remember, the only way you and your doctor can be absolutely certain about that distinction is by means of a biopsy.

Sometimes a "lump" is simply a matter of altered body "geography"—an organ situated where you don't expect it. The best example is a "dropped kidney"—one that is positioned lower than normal in the flank and so can be felt in the belly. I have had many patients—and known several doctors—who were very concerned on discovering a "lump" in the abdomen, which turned out to be a perfectly healthy kidney that had "gone south." Sometimes a cancer migrates (metastasizes) into previously healthy tissue from elsewhere in the body and is detected as a new lump. The liver particularly attracts such malignancies. When they spread to this organ, a hard, irregular (as opposed to smooth), painless lump appears in the right upper quadrant of the abdomen. That's bad news.

Several body organs are sacs whose contents reach the "outside world" via *ducts*. When a duct draining one of these organs becomes obstructed, the material being secreted backs up into the organ, dilating it. The result is a "lump" or swelling. A familiar example is the salivary glands (one on either side of the jaw below the ears). The saliva they produce reaches the mouth via the salivary ducts. When a stone forms in one of these ducts, or they become obstructed by infection—as they do when you have mumps—your face swells because the gland continues to make saliva that has no place to go but back!

The same kind of thing, although less dramatically apparent, happens in the tiny glands under the skin that secrete oil. If their little ducts leading to the surface become infected, the secretions back up, resulting in a small painful lump we call a *boil*. If it attains a more respectable size, then it's an *abscess*.

The gallbladder stores the bile produced within the liver and squeezes it out to the intestine on demand through its ducts. When these bile ducts are chronically obstructed—usually by a tumor growing nearby in the belly, most commonly in the pancreas —bile backs up and distends the gallbladder. You're not likely to feel it, but your doctor will if he examines you carefully. The swelling is usually painless and is typical of cancer of the pancreas. Stones blocking the gallbladder don't usually enlarge it enough to be felt, because they are generally repositioned in a matter of days.

WHEN A "LUMP" IS NOT A GROWTH

Another example of a "mass" in the abdomen that resembles a cancer is a bladder full of urine. Remember that the bladder stores urine. When a certain amount is present, you receive a signal that lets you know it needs to be emptied. The emptying is done through the urethra, which, in men, travels close to the prostate. When this gland becomes enlarged, as it often does in older men, it obstructs the urethra, so that urine backs up and is retained in the bladder. Over a period of time, the bladder dilates and its walls thicken to accommodate this abnormally large urine reservoir. I'll never forget one patient in whom I felt a large, hard, painless "mass" in the lower central abdomen. I suspected cancer and quickly admitted him to the hospital for a work-up. We found nothing more than a thick, large bladder, the result of a chronically enlarged prostate. The patient had his prostate removed, the obstruction to his urinary outflow was relieved and the possible "cancer" disappeared!

A similar sequence of obstruction, backup and swelling occurs in *veins and arteries*. When a large clot forms in a varicose vein, wherever it happens to be, the flow of blood out of the vessel is compromised and backs up, causing a swelling. If the vein happens to be in a testicle, it will become a "varicocele"; in the rectum, you end up with hemorrhoids; in the legs, varicose veins cause your feet to swell.

Most lumps and swellings are benign, some are cancers, others are due to infection, inflammation or obstruction to the flow of blood or some other fluid. As we look in greater detail at some specific lumps and swellings, remember this one rule: *When a swelling appears suddenly and hurts, it's likely to reflect an injury or an infection. One that comes on gradually and painlessly may be a tumor.* Let me also share with you something I learned a long time ago: the rule of sevens, according to which any lump that has been present up to seven days is probably an inflammation; for seven months, a cancer; for seven years, something with which you were born. What's congenital that might fit the bill? A *cyst* anywhere in the body. How do you recognize a cyst? It gets larger and smaller as its contents are cyclically expelled and refilled.

Points to Remember

Symptom: A lump or a swelling.

What It May Mean	What to Do About It
(Whatever *you* may think of any lump, always check it out.)	
1. Exostoses (hard bony overgrowths on the skull).	Harmless.
2. Lipomas (fatty lumps under the skin).	Can be removed for cosmetic reasons.
3. Fibromas (smooth growths under the skin).	Benign.
4. Cancer under the skin.	Appropriate cancer therapy.

5. Discolored nodules under the skin after a blood test or an injury.	Harmless, will disappear.
6. Internal organ enlarged by hemorrhage.	Diagnosis and treatment.
7. Abscess.	Antibiotics and drainage.
8. Enlarged lymph glands (may be infectious or malignant).	If infectious, antibiotics. If malignant, appropriate treatment.
9. Migrating organs.	Leave them alone.
10. Obstruction of a duct leading from an organ such as the gallbladder or the salivary glands.	May need surgical "unplugging."
11. Obstructed urethra, causing backup of urine.	Treat the enlarged prostate that's causing the obstruction.
12. Obstructed veins or arteries, causing backup of blood.	Medical or surgical treatment.

SWOLLEN TONGUE

I know people who first thing in the morning go through the ritual of examining their tongue in the mirror. Most of them haven't the faintest idea what they're looking for. They usually end up confirming what they already knew, that the coating on the tongue, the pounding in the head and the churning in the stomach reflect a hangover. They rarely pay attention to the *size* of the tongue, because any subtle increase is not easy to appreciate. But the next time you evaluate the status of your tongue, note whether it does appear bigger than the last time you looked. If it does, the most likely cause is an *allergic reaction* to something you've eaten or to a medication you've taken. Aspirin, for example, will often cause the tongue to swell. The presence of hives elsewhere on the body clinches the allergic origin of the enlargement.

Other causes of a swollen tongue include:

- *Very low thyroid function.*
- A tumor of the *pituitary gland* which causes the gland to produce too much growth hormone and leads to massive enlargement of the tongue, as well as the fingers, the toes and the jaw (the condition known as acromegaly).
- A bad *strep infection* in the mouth. This occurs only rarely these days, but when it does the tongue becomes very enlarged—and painful. Yeast infections, after prolonged use of antibiotics, can also increase the size of the tongue.
- A condition called *amyloidosis,* in which an abnormal protein in the body settles in the tongue, making it bigger than normal. This material also affects the heart, the liver, the kidneys and indeed virtually every organ in the body. It's a serious disease.
- *Leukemia* and other malignancies can infiltrate the tongue, dramatically increasing its size.

Points to Remember

Symptom: Enlargement of the tongue.

What It May Mean	What to Do About It
1. Allergic reaction.	Antihistamines. Avoid the offending food or drug.
2. Low thyroid function.	Thyroid supplements.

3. Overfunction of the pituitary gland (acromegaly).	Surgery, radiation.
4. Infection.	Antibiotics (except if the enlargement is caused by yeast).
5. Amyloidosis.	No satisfactory treatment at present.
6. Tumor.	Surgery, radiation.

SWOLLEN GUMS

As long as you're looking into your mouth, check your gums too. If they're swollen, almost overhanging the teeth, they're probably infected by some *virus* or *fungus*. After taking antibiotics for any length of time, you may develop monilia, a yeast infection, which is responsible for this characteristic appearance. *Leukemia* too gives the gums an easily recognizable swollen look. *Ill-fitting dentures* or other dental appliances can irritate your gums so that they swell and hurt. *Gingivitis*, an infection of the gums, leaves them bleeding and sore. Your *mouthwash* or *toothpaste* can irritate your gums and give you gingivitis very much the same way as something that you apply to your skin can result in a contact dermatitis. Occasionally an *abscess* in the gums will result in a localized swelling, too. *Dilantin* (widely used in the treatment of epilepsy) and certain barbiturates frequently cause thickened gums. And if you've been on a crash or fad diet for any length of time, nutritional deficiencies will also make your gums swell. I've seen several patients oh so pleased with their weight loss until they see what they look like when they smile.

Points to Remember

Symptom: Swollen gums.

What It May Mean	What to Do About It
1. Infection.	Antibiotics, except if it's a fungus *due* to antibiotics.
2. Poorly fitting dentures.	Dental correction.
3. Sensitivity to toothpaste or mouthwash.	Change the brand.
4. Reaction to a drug (Dilantin, phenobarbital).	Use substitutes.
5. Malnutrition.	Proper diet.
6. Leukemia.	Chemotherapy.

BULGING EYES

Prominent eyes are usually just a personal or familial characteristic. But sometimes you will notice that a friend looks "different" because the eyes appear to have become more protuberant. The most common cause of bulging eyes (both, not just one) is an *overactive thyroid*. People with these "pop" eyes don't blink them very often and have a staring quality to their gaze; you can see the whites above and below the cornea, and to the sides. The eyes can, in fact, become so prominent that it's hard for the eyelids to cover them.

If only one eye bulges, either it's not hyperthyroidism or it's just the initial stage. You then have to think of something in the socket, behind the eyeball, pushing it out. The usual cause is a growth of some kind or a hemorrhage in the socket due to a vascular problem.

Points to Remember

Symptom: Bulging eyes.

What It May Mean	What to Do About It
1. Hyperthyroidism (both eyes).	Medication, radioactive iodine, surgery.
2. Disease in the eyeball socket (hemorrhage, tumor).	Evaluation and treatment of the cause.

A LUMP IN THE NECK

Lumps in the neck are most commonly due to lymph-node enlargement, just as they are in the armpit. Local problems likely to swell the neck glands (and make them hurt) are sore throats of various kinds, and a visit to the dentist at which he drilled, filled, extracted or merely cleaned your teeth or poked around your gums. If you have *infectious mononucleosis,* glands will puff up throughout the neck—front and back; *German measles* will do the same thing. Lymph nodes in the neck can also swell in a generalized *allergic reaction* to certain drugs. Years ago, I used to see patients with enlarged, tender, draining glands due to tuberculosis; thanks to modern therapy, I haven't come across such a case in twenty-five years. As in other glandular areas, the worrisome lumps in the neck are painless, hard and don't go away.

In addition to diseased lymph nodes, an *abnormal thyroid gland* can also produce swelling of the neck.

The thyroid gland is about two inches high. It lies over the windpipe (trachea), below the Adam's apple, and is shaped like a shield, with two elongated lobes on either side of the midline connected by a broad band of tissue. (The name "thyroid" comes from the Greek word for "shield-shaped," *thyreoeides*.) Normally, the thyroid gland cannot be felt except in very thin people. Also, it's the only gland in the neck that moves when you swallow. So if you see or feel a lump in the front of the neck, swallow some water. If the tissue in question moves under your fingers, it's in the thyroid. An enlarged thyroid is called a *goiter*. When it feels soft, it is often associated with overactivity of the gland. But it may be hard, smooth or lumpy. That creates diagnostic problems. The size of the goiter has nothing to do with the function of the thyroid gland, which may be normal, low or overactive. Regardless of its hormonal action, a goiter may become so big that it presses on neighboring structures, causing hoarseness or cough. It may even push on the food pipe, making it difficult to swallow. When that happens, it's usually removed surgically.

Sometimes the overall size of the gland may be normal, but in passing your hand over it, perhaps while shaving, you may feel a small lump. This may simply be an extra piece of thyroid tissue, working just like the rest of the gland. But such a *nodule* may produce too much hormone independently of the rest of the gland, in which event we call it "hot." A thyroid nodule may also be "cold"—that is, not making any hormone at all. Hot thyroid nodules are almost never malignant; a cold one may be, especially in a man. A radioactive scan can distinguish between these two types. Cold nodules are often removed just to be sure—again, more so in men than in women. Most cancers of the thyroid gland, which can also be seen or felt, are extremely slow-growing and often curable by surgery even after they've been present for several years.

Points to Remember

Symptom: Swelling in the neck.

What It May Mean	What to Do About It
1. Enlarged lymph gland due to:	
Local infection.	Antibiotics.
Viral illness (mononucleosis, German measles).	Medical supervision.
Generalized allergic reaction to drugs.	Avoid what did it.
2. Thyroid goiter.	Medical management or, if the enlarged gland compresses nearby structures, surgical removal.
3. Thyroid nodule.	Radioactive scan to determine whether it consists of functioning tissue (hot) or not (cold). Sonogram, CAT scans and needle biopsy may help in assessing the diagnosis and treatment.

A LUMP IN THE ARMPIT

You're most likely to find a lump in your armpit if you're a woman who's in the laudable habit of examining her breasts. A proper breast self-examination should always include the armpit because cancer can enlarge the lymph nodes there even when the breast itself seems perfectly normal. Remember that lymph nodes are filters, trapping malignant tumor cells or infectious organisms. When they do, they increase in size and are easily felt. That's why, whenever a cancer is removed from any part of the body, the surgeon always checks for "involvement" of the glands in the area. They are usually the first port of call for traveling cancer cells.

The above notwithstanding, if you do find a lump in the armpit, don't panic. It's probably the result of *infection* somewhere in your arm draining into the glands of your armpit. In that event, the lump appears suddenly and is painful or tender, in contrast to the big, hard, painless *cancerous* glands.

If you find an enlarged gland in one armpit, always check the other, as well as the lymph nodes in your groin and neck. *Viral infections* such as German measles, chicken pox, infectious mononucleosis and many others frequently cause widespread glandular enlargement. Unfortunately, so do certain malignancies like Hodgkin's disease and other serious lymphomas.

A generalized *allergic reaction,* such as to sulfa drugs, iodine, penicillin and a host of others, can also produce glandular swelling.

Occasionally, what seems like a lump in the armpit is not a lymph node at all. It may simply be some perfectly normal *breast tissue* that has "lost its way" and ended up in the armpit. Such a "mass" may also be a benign *cyst,* or a harmless fatty tumor (*lipoma*).

It's not a good idea for you to try to diagnose an armpit lump or lumps yourself, unless the cause is right there staring you in the face, as when you've cut yourself removing underarm hair and have an obvious infection. Interpreting the significance of any swollen gland can present dangerous pitfalls. Even your doctor may have trouble deciding the cause of the particular glandular enlargement after a thorough physical exam and appropriate blood tests. Very often the only way to solve the problem is to have a biopsy done. That will confirm the diagnosis.

Points to Remember

Symptom: Lump(s) in the armpit.

What It May Mean	What to Do About It
1. Infected gland (painful).	Treat the underlying infection.
2. Malignancy (especially of the breast)—hard, painless.	Appropriate anticancer management.
3. Generalized viral infection.	Will ultimately disappear without therapy.
4. Allergic reaction.	Will subside after the provoking agent is removed.
5. Aberrant normal breast tissue.	No treatment needed.
6. Cyst.	No treatment needed unless it troubles you or becomes infected.
7. Lipoma.	Harmless, unless it grows so large that it causes discomfort.
8. Not sure?	Biopsy.

A LUMP IN THE BREAST

Ninety percent of all breast *cancers* are discovered, not by doctors or by mammograms, but by women

themselves. But casually feeling your breasts when
the spirit moves you is not the way to do it. For
breast examination to be effective, for you to find a
lump when it's still small enough to cure, you've got
to learn how to do it correctly. You can do that by
asking the American Cancer Society to send you its
booklets demonstrating the technique. Practice it,
then ask your doctor to see whether you're doing it
the right way. Keep practicing. You can never become
too good at it. After you've learned how, check your
breasts every month, especially if there is a family
history of breast cancer. You should also be examined
at regular intervals by your doctor. Have your first
mammogram at age thirty-five, then repeat it every
two years between forty and fifty, and annually thereafter. In my view, all three—a good self-examination
technique, regular professional evaluations and mammography—offer the best chance of finding a breast
malignancy *early enough to cure*.

Of course, only a minority of breast lumps are
malignant. Most are either simple *cysts* or the benign
"lumpy" breast condition *chronic cystic mastitis*. But
you can't be absolutely sure about which is which—
and neither can your doctor! Both of you can suspect
that what you feel is not a cancer—you can be *"almost* sure," but that's not enough. *Every lump demands a complete investigation—at least once*. When
the doctor examines your breasts, he or she will define the characteristics of the lump—its size, degree
of hardness, whether or not it's tender or it dimples
the overlying skin, so that it resembles that of an
orange. He will search for lumps in the other breast
and both armpits, and ask you whether your siblings
or maternal relatives had breast cancer. He will want
to know about your drinking habits, because of the
suspicion that alcohol may be associated with a high
instance of breast malignancy. At this point, the doc-

tor will have a pretty good idea what that lump is all about, *but he may still not be certain*. So you will probably be advised to have a mammogram. That's not foolproof, either, but cancer does show certain typical features on this X-ray picture. If there is the *slightest* doubt about the lump after the physical exam and the mammogram, your doctor will (or should) order a biopsy—either a needle aspiration (the contents of the lump are drawn out through a needle and analyzed for malignant cells) or an open biopsy (the lump is actually removed surgically or a piece cut out of it, and examined under the microscope).

There are several characteristics of a breast lump which make the diagnosis of cancer more likely. First of all, cancerous lumps are usually painless. If your breast hurts, chances are that either you've *injured* it or you have an *infection* there. If the enlargement feels like a cyst, that is, like a little sac with fluid in it, your doctor may shine a beam of light through it in a darkened room. Fluid will illuminate; if the enlargement is solid it won't. The solid kinds are the ones to worry about. Unfortunately, this test is far from foolproof, because the breasts often contain various sebaceous (waxy) cysts, fatty tumors and other conditions which mimic a solid tumor. When the skin above the mass is dimpled or irregular and orange-peel-like in appearance, you can be almost sure it's cancer. Lumps in *both* breasts suggest some process other than cancer. When the nipple bleeds, suspect a malignancy.

An important reminder: Although uncommon, breast cancers do occur in men. I discovered two cases in my own practice just this past year.

Certain *drugs* can cause the breasts to swell and even leave them lumpy and painful. These agents include Aldomet (alphamethyldopa—used in the treatment of high blood pressure), chlorpromazine (a psychotropic drug), Aldactone (a mild potassium-sparing diuretic), digitalis (commonly prescribed for a variety of heart disorders) and the beta blockers (for angina, hypertension, cardiac-rhythm disturbances). This side effect occurs in both men and women, but is more noticeable in men because men's breasts are smaller than women's to begin with. When you discontinue the offending drug, the breasts slowly return to normal—but it may take weeks for them to do so.

The three cardinal rules for breast cancer are: (1) have them checked three ways—by self-examination, by your doctor and by routine mammography; (2) any new breast lump, especially if painless and located in one breast, should be presumed to be cancer until proven otherwise; (3) most breast lumps should be biopsied just to be sure.

Points to Remember

Symptom: A lump in the breast.

What It May Mean	What to Do About It
1. Cancer, especially if painless and present in only one breast.	Biopsy and then appropriate treatment: modified radical mastectomy, lumpectomy, radiation, hormones or chemotherapy—or a combination of treatments.
2. Benign cyst.	Biopsy to be sure.
3. Chronic cystic mastitis.	Biopsy to be sure; vitamin E; no caffeine; low-fat, high-carbohydrate diet.

| 4. Injury. | Will clear up eventually. |
| 5. Drug reaction. | Stop the offending agent. |

A SWOLLEN BELLY—WHEN YOU'RE NEITHER FAT NOR PREGNANT

You know the feeling: You've just finished a heavy meal, maybe washed it down with a carbonated drink, and your trousers, skirt or belt are just a bit too tight. In a few hours (with or without the release of gas via the northern or southern route), most of the bloating is gone. Such aftermeal distention is not usually a medical problem. When, then, should you worry about a bloated belly and why?

When abdominal fullness is recurrent, *on again, off again,* it's almost always due to *swallowed air* or gas formation in the gut. Most air swallowers deny doing it, because it's neither deliberate nor conscious on their part, but simply a nervous habit. The air, gulped down in large amounts almost as if it were water, distends the stomach and leaves a feeling of fullness which begs to be relieved by what doctors politely refer to as "eructation" (read "belching"). Such individuals invariably blame their excess belching on something they ate, or on the fact that they're "gas formers." Actually, in only a small minority of cases is bloating due to gas-forming carbohydrates (cabbage is a good example). When it is, change of diet and avoiding sweets will do away with the gas.

In certain "functional" disorders of the gut such as *"nervous stomach," "spastic bowel"* and *"irritable colon"* (in which there is often no physical disease of the intestinal tract), large amounts of gas are generated within the bowel, resulting in the rise and fall of the abdominal wall. Again, a change in diet or antispasmodic medication may help.

There is one disorder in which distention after eating does reflect physical disease—and that's *gallbladder trouble*. One or two hours after a meal, you feel bloated and are relieved by belching. This is how it is believed to happen, although we're not really sure: a healthy gallbladder can squirt out enough bile to digest the fatty foods you eat; a diseased one (with or without stones) cannot, so the undigested fat just sits there in the intestine, leaving you feeling full and gassy.

Remember that when it is air distending your belly, the fullness and tightness come and go. By contrast, when your girth *increases and does not recede*, it's due either to simple weight gain or to *fluid* that has accumulated in the abdominal cavity. Fluid in the belly *looks* different from air. When your belly is full of fluid, your flanks bulge as the liquid is pulled down by gravity. Air, however, is uniformly distributed; so the flanks are not distended. If fluid accumulates in your abdomen, contrary to what you might expect, you won't necessarily gain weight, because the conditions that cause such fluid accumulation are generally associated with severe illness and malnutrition.

The most common cause of fluid in the abdomen (ascites) is advanced liver disease (*cirrhosis*), a late manifestation of either long-standing alcoholism or chronic viral hepatitis. Of course, if you're an alcoholic, a swollen belly won't be the first sign of the problem—unless you've missed the red bulbous nose and the spiderlike red spots on the abdomen, chest and upper arms. Regardless of the cause, in men the sick liver's inability to deactivate the tiny amounts of female hormone present in all males results in shriveled testes, a decreased sex drive and the appearance of feminine characteristics, such as increased breast size and the loss of facial hair.

Heart trouble as well as cirrhosis of the liver can result in accumulation of fluid in the abdomen. A weak cardiac muscle cannot expel all the blood returned to it from the rest of the body. Some of it backs up, first into the lungs, and later to the rest of the body, including the belly and the legs. You can tell that the problem is due to the heart if you are very short of breath, especially when lying flat. Also, in cirrhosis the belly swells *before* the legs do; in heart failure, the reverse is true.

There's another cardiac condition, in addition to weakness of the heart muscle, that can cause the abdomen to fill with fluid: disease of the *pericardium*, the tissue that envelops the heart. If the pericardium has been inflamed by a virus, by tuberculosis or by some other infectious agent, and sometimes after open-heart surgery, it may become scarred and hardened. This tough tissue compresses the heart, acting like a steel band around it. Even though the underlying heart muscle itself may be strong and healthy, it cannot contract strongly enough in this viselike grip. So it is unable to expel all the blood it contains, much the same as what happens when it's weak. This condition, called *constrictive pericarditis*, causes blood that can't be pumped out of the heart to back up into the abdomen, making it swell. When fluid rather than scar tissue accumulates around the heart in the sac enveloping it, the same sequence of events occurs.

When a *cancer* is growing in the belly, no matter where it originated, there is an accumulation of fluid in the abdomen. *Cancer of the ovary* results in particularly impressive fluid formation. I have actually seen the increased girth of a belly which was the result of an ovarian cancer mistaken for pregnancy—at least for a while—in women of childbearing age.

Pregnancy is such an obvious cause of belly swelling you'd think no woman would ever miss that diagnosis. After all, she has nine months in which to make it! Believe it or not, some women have been known to go right down to the wire and into labor without ever having even suspected they were pregnant. I met one such woman just a few months ago on a TV talk show. She told me she thought she was simply getting fat and never gave her periods any "mind." One day she felt some cramping in her abdomen. She sat down on the toilet—and gave birth to a healthy baby! Such women usually do not understand the physiology of menstruation or of conception. So, if you have had intercourse and are of childbearing age, always consider the possibility of pregnancy if your girth is increasing for no apparent reason.

The other side of the coin is a condition called *pseudopsiesis*. This is a psychiatric problem, admittedly rare, in which a woman is mistakenly convinced she's pregnant. Her waistline increases as you might expect it would, but then after nine months there's nothing to show for it. I've never seen such a patient myself, and I don't know by what mechanism the belly gets big, but the disorder does exist.

Abdominal swelling needn't involve the entire belly. It can be localized. The asymmetry may be due to a cyst within the abdomen or, if it's in the lower portion, it may be the result of retained stool when you're severely constipated. If you have noticed an abdominal lump, refer back to the four quadrants that I mentioned in Chapter One. If it's in the upper-right-hand quadrant, it's most likely due to the liver or to something within it. In the upper left, it's probably an enlarged spleen caused by a variety of ailments including infectious mononucleosis, leukemia, lymphoma and other blood disorders. A swelling in the lower midline may be due to a distended urinary bladder, to a uterus enlarged by pregnancy or *fibroid tumors,* to ovarian cysts or to other growths. If you had an abdominal operation years ago, you may find a lump along the line of the incision where the scar tissue has stretched so that the abdominal contents beneath it bulge out. Such *incisional hernias* sometimes need to be surgically repaired.

So abdominal swelling that's not the result of simple weight gain or pregnancy usually reflects either air or fluid retention. Air comes and goes, while fluid accumulates insidiously. The bottom line: You needn't run to your doctor if you have to loosen your belt after a heavy meal, but you should see him or her if your increase in girth is progressive and unrelenting.

Points to Remember

Symptom: Swollen stomach.

What It May Mean	What to Do About It
1. Transiently, after a heavy meal.	Eat in moderation.
2. Air swallowing (a nervous habit).	Awareness often leads to self-control. Eat slowly, avoid carbonated beverages, don't chew gum or suck candies, avoid drinking through a straw or sipping the surface of a hot beverage. A pencil held between the teeth will prevent you from swallowing air.

3. "Nervous stomach" or "irritable bowel" with gas formation.	Change your diet, reduce carbohydrate consumption. Antispasmodics.
4. Gallbladder disease.	Low-fat diet, small meals. Stones and/or gallbladder may require removal. Avoid long fasts followed by heavy meals.
5. Cirrhosis of the liver.	Supportive care, diuretics.
6. Heart failure.	Treat the underlying cause.
7. Constrictive pericarditis.	Surgery.
8. Generalized cancer.	Supportive care, chemotherapy.
9. Ovarian cancer.	Appropriate treatment.
10. Pregnancy.	Medical confirmation.
11. Uterine fibroids.	Hysterectomy.
12. Any large tumor in the abdomen.	Surgery.

A LUMP IN THE GROIN

Like enlarged glands anywhere, a swelling in the groin is most frequently due to lymph glands enlarged by *infection* (sometimes sexually transmitted), a generalized *drug reaction,* a *viral illness,* tumors of the lymph nodes (e.g., Hodgkin's disease) or *cancers* that have spread from other parts of the body. But in this area you must also consider the possibility of a *hernia.* This is usually a soft, large bulge in the groin on one or both sides. It's bigger when you stand up, it recedes when you lie down and you can often push it back in with your finger.

Points to Remember

Symptom: A swelling in the groin.

What It May Mean	What to Do About It
1. Enlarged lymph glands due to:	
Local infection.	Identify the cause and treat.
Generalized drug allergic reaction.	Discontinue the drug.
Viral illness.	Usually runs its course.
Malignancy.	Appropriate medical treatment.
2. Hernia.	Support or surgery.

A LUMP IN THE TESTICLE

Earlier, in the section on testicular pain, I discussed the various conditions that could leave you hurting there—local injury; dilated veins in the sac; *infection* of structures within the scrotum such as *epididymitis; mumps;* and a condition called *testicular torsion.* In most of those situations, the pain is usually accompanied by some swelling. But a testicular lump that doesn't hurt is suggestive of *cancer,* especially in young men aged twenty to thirty-five.

Cancer of the testis is the most common malignancy in this age group. That's the bad news. The good news is that it is easily detected and is often curable even after it has spread. Of course, as with tumors anywhere, the sooner you find it, the better off you are. It amazes me how few young men know how to look for lumps in their testes or take the trouble to do so. Just as most women now appreciate the importance of routinely and thoroughly examining their breasts, so should vulnerable men be educated to the need to examine their testes and taught how to do it by their doctors.

Another frequent cause of "testicular swelling" is a *loop of bowel* that has made its way into the groin or the scrotum. It's the only "lump" I know that will disappear just by being pushed in. But if you have a *hydrocele,* a large cyst in the scrotum which looks very much like a loop of bowel, you won't be able to get rid of it by any manipulation. Another way to differentiate one from the other is to shine a light through the swelling. The water-filled hydrocele will illuminate, the loop of bowel will not.

Remember, too, that the scrotum, the sac of skin that contains the testes, is vulnerable to the same problems as skin anywhere. It may be the site of a carbuncle or a boil; a rash can cause swelling of the entire area, with resultant swelling of the testes. The rich network of veins throughout the scrotum and the testes is subject to the disorders that can affect veins anywhere—phlebitis (inflammation) and *varicosity* (engorgement).

Points to Remember

Symptom: Swollen testicle.

What It May Mean	What to Do About It
1. If painful:	
Infection of the scrotal sac.	Antibiotics.
Mumps.	Medical management until the disease runs its course.

Epididymitis.	Antibiotics.
Testicular torsion.	Surgery.

2. If painless:

Cancer.	Surgery, radiation, chemotherapy.
Loop of bowel.	Surgical evaluation.
Hydrocele.	Management depends on the symptoms. Can be surgically corrected.
Varicocele.	Management depends on the symptoms. Can be surgically corrected.

A LUMP IN THE RECTUM

When a man feels *as if* he has a fullness in his rectum, it's almost always due to an inflamed prostate gland. But male or female, if you think a normal bowel movement is incomplete, yet nothing further comes out even after you bear down, you almost certainly have an internal *hemorrhoid.* You may actually be able to feel it with your finger in the anal canal. Hemorrhoids ("piles") don't always hurt. They become painful only when clots form within them.

There are other "things" you may detect around the rectum (usually when you're wiping after a bowel movement) that don't seem quite right: *skin tags* from old "burned-out" hemorrhoids (they're painless); an *abscess* (an infection that is very likely to hurt); and *venereal or genital warts,* due to a contagious viral infection, which are painless and usually disappear without treatment.

All the above notwithstanding, the sensation of a lump in the rectum can also mean a *growth* in that area, benign or malignant. But don't ever screen yourself for a rectal malignancy. That diagnosis should always be made by your doctor when he performs the appropriate examination after you've described your changing bowel habits: ribbonlike stools, alternating diarrhea and constipation or the presence of blood in your movement.

Points to Remember

Symptom: A lump in the rectum.

What It May Mean	What to Do About It
1. Hemorrhoids.	Ointments, suppositories, rubber banding, sitz baths, injections, laser therapy, surgical removal.
2. Skin tags.	Harmless.
3. Abscess.	Surgical drainage, antibiotics.
4. Venereal warts.	Topical medication or laser therapy if they do not disappear.
5. Rectal tumors.	Surgery.

WHEN YOUR LEGS SWELL

Your feet may puff up from time to time given conducive circumstances, even when you're in the best of health. Mine do on long airplane flights. (I always carry a small shoehorn to help me get my shoes back on as we're about to land.) Some women retain water during their menstrual period, and so their feet swell. If you've been in the sun too long, your feet may become swollen; a generalized allergy can do it, too; and, of course, so will varicose veins or any injury or sprain of the ankle or foot. But aside from these obvious causes, there are several disease states in which there is persistent swelling of the legs, the ankles and the feet.

Statistically, *chronic* swelling of the legs and feet is most likely to be due either to *heart failure* or to *phlebitis* of the leg veins. It's easy to tell these two conditions apart. Phlebitis generally involves just one leg, congestive failure affects both; phlebitis is painful, swelling due to heart failure is not. The various causes of swelling each have their own mechanisms and features. Consider heart failure first.

The left side of the heart (left ventricle) pumps blood to the entire body via the arteries. This blood is delivered to the tissues, where it discharges its oxygen and collects carbon dioxide and other waste products. This oxygen-depleted blood then travels back through the veins to the right side of the heart, which pumps it into the lungs for reoxygenation. It is then returned to the left side to complete the cycle.

When the heart muscle has been weakened by a heart attack, by long-standing, untreated high blood pressure, by a virus or by a diseased valve, it is not strong enough to pump out to the lungs all the blood returned to it from the veins. So after a while it begins to back up into those veins. As a result, the liver, situated downstream from the heart, becomes congested with blood, and it enlarges. Eventually, the *veins* as far away as the legs are also distended. At some point, the fluid component of the blood seeps out into the tissues, causing them to swell.

When the *left* side of the heart is weak, fresh blood from the pulmonary tree cannot be accommodated, and so it backs up into the lungs. This "pulmonary congestion" leaves you short of breath and coughing. The right and left sides of the heart usually weaken together, which is why somebody with heart failure has swollen legs *and* is short of breath.

Let's look at how some other conditions cause swelling of the lower extremities.

- *Phlebitis* occurs when one or more veins, either on the surface of the leg or deep within it, become inflamed or obstructed by a blood clot. The inflammation makes for pain, swelling and redness. The blockage in the vein forces the blood to back up and seep out of it into the surrounding tissue, its walls having become more permeable because of the inflammation. In contrast to heart failure, which affects both legs, phlebitis usually involves only one.

- Persons with serious *kidney disease* are swollen all over—in the legs, face and hands (they can't get the rings on or off their fingers). This generalized swelling is due to a wholesale loss of the protein *albumin* in the urine. Albumin is made by the liver and circulates in the bloodstream. A healthy kidney does not allow it to escape into the urine. However, when the kidneys are diseased, albumin pours out. Insurance companies ask for a urinalysis before they sell you a policy, looking for the presence of this protein as evidence of kidney trouble. Now, albumin is found not only in the blood, but in the surrounding tissues as well. Normally, there is a balance of the albumin content in these two compartments. But when lots of albumin is lost, nature tries to restore the equilibrium, and so fluid in the bloodstream diffuses out into the surrounding tissues in order to equalize the concentration of the albumin. That extra fluid is what causes the swelling everywhere.

- *Liver disease*—the advanced stage, not the mild

hepatitis you get from eating contaminated shell-fish—causes the legs to swell by two mechanisms. First, the damaged liver cells can't make enough albumin; the net result is the same as if the kidneys had allowed it to pour out: The tissues swell in the body's attempt to equalize the albumin concentration within the blood vessels and the surrounding tissues. Second, the liver is scarred, so that blood returning from the legs to the heart can't get through and so backs up. Large glands or tumors in the abdominal cavity can also press on these veins, causing the feet to swell.

- *Starvation.* Have you ever wondered why starving children have potbellies? The abdominal swelling is due to the lack of protein (albumin) in the diet. So fluid seeps out of the blood vessels and into the tissues—in this case, the abdomen—just as it does in kidney and liver disease.

- *Severe underfunction of the thyroid gland* will result in generalized swelling, including the legs. As with the protein imbalance of kidney and liver disease, the swelling is due to loss of fluid from the bloodstream into the tissues in search of a balanced level of albumin.

- In recent years, another cause of swollen legs has literally exploded on the scene. It occurs in persons who have undergone *coronary-bypass surgery.* This operation utilizes vein strips from one or both legs as new conduits to bypass the obstructions in the coronary arteries. When substantial lengths of vein are removed, the legs swell. That's neither serious nor uncomfortable and usually clears up in a few months as the veins that are left accommodate to the increased demand.

- Several *medications* can result in swelling of the legs: testosterone (most commonly prescribed for impotence); long-term steroid therapy (for arthritis, asthma, cancer); estrogen (the female hormone); the Pill; certain antidepressants (Nardil); blood-pressure-lowering drugs like Apresoline, reserpine, Aldomet, Esimil, and the most recent addition to the list, nifedipine (Adalat, Procardia—given for a variety of vascular conditions).

• When the *pericardium,* the outer lining of the heart, becomes diseased, usually by viral or other infections, or after cardiac surgery, it may become thick and rigid, like a suit of armor around the heart. This prevents normal contraction and relaxation of cardiac muscle. As a result, less blood reenters the heart's right ventricle, so it backs up, swelling the neck veins, the abdomen and eventually the legs.

You now have a general idea of how and why your legs and feet puff up. The following may help you decide which particular condition *you* have:

• If the swelling is one-sided, you're not dealing with one of the generalized disorders such as a lack of protein in the blood, heart failure or liver or kidney disease.
• In heart failure, it's usually just the legs that are swollen, and not the eyes, the face and the fingers.
• If your belly *and* your legs are swollen, chances are the problem lies within your liver rather than your heart, especially if the abdominal swelling came first.

Here are some other observations you should make:

• Push your thumb hard into the swollen leg for a few seconds, then remove it. If it makes an indentation that persists for a minute or two, it's called "pitting." Pitting is never present in swelling due to low thyroid function, but it is in most other causes.

- If you are a male and, in addition to your swollen legs, you're jaundiced, your breasts are enlarged, you don't need to shave more often than every second or third day, your palms are red and you are short of breath, you can be certain that you have severe liver disease.

- If your face is swollen as well as your legs, it's probably not from heart or liver disease. Think instead of low thyroid function, some generalized allergic reaction, the constriction of the heart by its covering (the pericardium) or trichinosis, the infection you get by eating improperly cooked pork infected with the trichina worm or kidney trouble.

- If your swollen legs have a brown pigmentation, especially around the ankles, then your problem is a long-standing one, usually from chronic varicose veins. The pigmentation is from the blood that has left the vein wall and seeped into the nearby tissues.

- If the swelling is painful, red and warm, you must have injured the leg, or it's infected, or you have acute phlebitis. Uncomplicated heart failure or diseases of the kidney or the liver do not cause pain.

- Suspect heart failure if *both* legs are swollen and you're also short of breath.

- Are your legs swollen all day, or just in the evening? If it's a twenty-four-hour affair, than a protein disturbance or a vein problem is a good possibility. If it's worse at bedtime, then it's more likely to be due to heart failure.

- If the swelling came on quite suddenly, it's more likely due to an obstruction, thrombosis, or an infection in the veins than to a generalized protein problem.

- If your belly swelled before your legs did, the cause

probably lies in the liver or in a thickened pericardium. But if the legs were first, followed by the presence of fluid in the abdomen, then there is either a kidney or a heart problem.

Whatever its cause, don't take your friend's "water pills" for a quick fix of your swollen legs. A real cure is possible only after the proper diagnosis is made and the appropriate treatment begun.

Points to Remember

Symptom: Swollen legs.

What It May Mean	What to Do About It
1. Heart failure (both legs).	Treat the heart condition.
2. Phlebitis (one leg).	Heat, rest, elevation of the legs, and (usually) anticoagulants.
3. Varicose veins.	Support hose, sclerosing injections, surgery.
4. Kidney disease (swelling is generalized).	Medical treatment, dialysis.
5. Liver disease.	Diuretics, steroids, diet.
6. Starvation (or food faddism).	Proper diet.
7. Low thyroid function.	Thyroid replacement.
8. Coronary-bypass surgery using leg veins.	Support hose.
9. Medication.	Remove the offending drug.
10. Pericarditis.	Drugs, surgery.

CHAPTER 3

BLOOD SHOULD BE NEITHER SEEN NOR HEARD

The sight of blood, especially your own, is usually frightening. Except for menstruation, the general idea is for blood to remain *inside* the body. We possess a very intricate mechanism that insures a balance between the blood's ability to clot (so that you don't bleed to death when you prick your finger or nick your face while shaving) and the need for it to remain sufficiently fluid in order to keep flowing. Anything that upsets this delicate balance will result in either a clot blocking a blood vessel (when the blood is "too thick") or a hemorrhage somewhere (when it's too thin).

Here are some situations in which this balance can be disrupted:

- You may bleed after an *injury* to an artery or a vein. (Veins ooze, arteries spurt.)
- *Several medications* can make you bleed by affecting the bone marrow (where blood is made), the liver (where chemicals that control its "clottability" are produced) and components within the blood itself. These drugs range from simple aspirin to anticoagulants like Coumadin (warfarin).
- *Allergic states,* in which the blood-vessel walls become so permeable that the blood simply leaks out.
- *Malignancies* can erode blood-vessel walls, causing them to bleed. For example, a cancer in the bowel will result in blood in the stool when it invades a

small artery or vein in the course of its wild growth. Such bleeding may be either visible to the naked eye or only chemically detectable. You can't always tell just by looking.

- If you've had *hypertension* for years, and it has been inadequately treated, or not at all, the high pressure pounding the artery walls weakens them and ultimately results in their rupture. The result is a hemorrhage, usually into the brain, the eye or the abdomen.

These are some of the basic causes of bleeding. If it's internal, you may not be aware of it. But if blood leaves the body in the stool, the sputum, the urine, or from the nose, the bowel or the vagina, you'll usually see it if you look (except for the bowel and the urine, where chemical testing may be necessary when the bleeding is very slight). Regardless of where it happens, however, there are some cardinal rules to remember about bleeding:

- If your *stool looks black* and tests positive for blood (either with your own home testing kit or the doctor's test), it's almost certainly coming from high in the intestinal tract (the stomach or the duodenum) rather than lower down (from hemorrhoids). Its black color results from the fact that blood is chemically altered during its long journey from the stomach down to the rectum.
- *Bright red blood* on the *outside* of the stool is apt to come from *hemorrhoids*. But beets can also color the stool red for twelve hours after you've eaten them.
- If you're *spitting dark brown blood,* chances are you have *pneumonia,* especially if you also have a fever and it hurts to take a deep breath. But if you're a heavy smoker with a chronic cough and

begin to spit blood without an accompanying fever, *lung cancer* is a possibility.

- If you are in your thirties, are taking the Pill or have varicose veins, and you suddenly feel a pain in your leg and spit red blood, you've probably suffered a *blood clot to your lung*.
- If you see blood in the urine, and voiding is painful, it's likely that you have *cystitis,* a common inflammation and infection of the bladder that attacks women of all ages. Men get it, too, but much less frequently.

Now let's look in greater detail at some actual bleeding situations.

BLEEDING INTO THE SKIN

Bleeding under the skin doesn't usually pose a problem in diagnosis. For example, if you've bumped into something and blood from the injured vessels seeps into the surrounding tissue, you expect to see a bruise. If you're stung by an insect and can't avoid scratching the area, you know why there is some local bleeding. If every time you have your period you notice little hemorrhages under your skin, you probably know that that happens in many women, and you're not alarmed.

But if you suddenly bleed into the skin for no such apparent reason, you've got to think of other possibilities:

- A *drug reaction.* Anticoagulants or aspirin "thin" your blood, making you bruise or bleed more easily when you injure or cut yourself. Suspect *any drug* (quinine in the tonic water you mix with your gin, or in tablet form to prevent leg cramps; quinidine for your heart, antibiotics, diuretics) when you start to bleed under the skin or bruise more easily.

- An *allergic reaction* may leave your blood vessels more permeable, permitting blood to ooze out of them and seep under the skin. Many of the *autoimmune disorders* also have this particular effect.
- *Leukemia* (cancer of the blood) invades the bone marrow, replacing the healthy cells, which help control clotting, with cancerous ones that don't.
- A *viral* illness may reduce the number of platelets (components of the blood which play an important role in clotting), causing bleeding into the skin and, more important, internal hemorrhage as well.
- If superficial bruising can be easily produced in your child by a trivial blow, he or she may have some *congenital defect* of the blood-clotting system. But if the bleeding is deep under the skin and occurs after the mildest trauma, then *hemophilia* is a possibility.
- Bleeding that keeps recurring *in the same area,* as for example the nose or the bowel, may reflect a hereditary abnormality of specific small blood vessels. By contrast, when the hemorrhages are *widespread,* but most marked in the legs, you're probably dealing with some generalized disorder of the blood or the blood vessels.
- *Family history* is important. If you suspect a hereditary disorder like hemophilia or weakened small-blood-vessel walls, knowing whether any of your "blood" relatives has a bleeding tendency is crucial. If you marry a blood relative, you greatly increase the risk of your children having such hereditary bleeding abnormalities.
- If you've begun to bleed easily under the skin and also develop jaundice, it's probably due to *liver*

disease—the liver is not making enough vitamin K to clot your blood properly.

- Older people sometimes develop large purple blotches just under the skin, predominantly on the arms and legs. This is what happens when *aging skin* loses some of its fat padding and leaves the underlying blood vessels more vulnerable to injury. These hemorrhagic areas in the skin do not mean you're bleeding internally too.

- Sometimes the purple blotches are due not to aging but to *Cushing's syndrome,* caused by an overproduction of cortisone by the adrenal glands. This may be due to disease within them or in the pituitary gland of the brain. Also, if you take too much *cortisone* for too long, you may experience the same bleeding phenomenon; the body can't distinguish between the cortisone in a pill and that which it produces in excess itself.

Points to Remember

Symptom: Bleeding into the skin.

What It May Mean	What to Do About It
1. Local injury.	Stop the bleeding.
2. Drug reaction.	Identify and discontinue the drug.
3. Allergic reaction.	Antihistamines, steroids.
4. Leukemia (affecting the bone marrow).	Chemotherapy.
5. Viral illness affecting the coagulability of the blood.	Cortisone, removal of the spleen if the condition persists.
6. Congenital defect in the blood-clotting system.	Medication.

7. Hemophilia.	Medication.
8. Liver disease.	Diet, medication.
9. Aging skin.	No treatment.
10. Cushing's syndrome.	Surgery, medication.
11. Excessive cortisone intake.	Reduce the dosage.

WHY DOES YOUR NOSE BLEED?

You're not likely to worry about a garden-variety nosebleed which stops in a few minutes and whose cause is obvious. Nose-picking is the number-one reason for such bleeds. Or if someone throws a Frisbee a little too hard and you catch it not with your hands but with the bridge of your nose, a trickle of blood won't worry or puzzle you. And if your child has the rather interesting hobby of shoving small portions of a toy into his nose just to see whether they fit, again a little blood is no surprise. If you live in a dry, overheated home or spend much time in airplanes (notorious for their desertlike lack of humidity), your nose may bleed spontaneously.

If you have *repeated* nosebleeds, see a doctor anyway, even if the cause is obvious. For there are many different local disorders, including a *tumor* (uncommon), chronic cocaine sniffing, swollen, *allergic membranes,* nasal *polyps* (very common) and warts, all of which may need to be diagnosed and treated. The first thing the specialist will do is shine a light up your nostrils to look for a bleeding point—a tiny vein or artery that has been irritated. If one is found, cauterizing it (somewhat painful but necessary) will heal it and put an end to the bleeding. If such a focus is not found, the search will be expanded to include either X rays or CAT scans.

You may be able to tell where in the nose the blood is coming from (but not why). To do so, pinch your nostrils closed and lean forward. If the bleeding stops within five minutes or so, the source is in the front of your nose. But if the blood continues to gush down the back of the throat, then there is a bleeding artery in the back of your nose. In that case, the doctor will likely pack your nose with gauze or cotton to stop the hemorrhage—a most unpleasant experience.

Should your nose bleed without an obvious local cause or injury, and you don't spend lots of time in a dry environment, have your *blood pressure* checked. In middle-aged and older persons, sudden onset of nosebleeds may indicate hypertension. If your blood pressure is normal, then have your *coagulation mechanism* studied to see whether or not you bleed and clot normally.

A word of caution: A nosebleed after you've injured your head may indicate a *skull fracture*. X rays should be taken no matter how trivial the blow seemed to be at the time.

Points to Remember

Symptom: Nosebleed.

What It May Mean	What to Do About It
1. Local injury or irritation.	Bleeding will stop without treatment.
2. Polyps, tumors, chronic allergy.	Removal or treatment.
3. High blood pressure.	Medical treatment.

4. Bleeding disorders.	Medical diagnosis and treatment.
5. Head injury.	Medical diagnosis is imperative.

BLOODSHOT EYES

You wake up one morning feeling perfectly hale and hearty. While brushing your teeth, you happen to glance in the mirror—and you spit out your toothpaste in surprise. You've got a big bloody blotch in one of your eyes! It doesn't hurt, but it's frightening. Relax. In most cases, such a subconjunctival "hemorrhage" is due to *eyestrain,* a long plane flight or *fatigue.* But it often happens for no reason at all. In any event, it does *not* indicate high blood pressure or any ocular problem and soon clears up on its own (although it often gets larger the second day).

"Red eye," on the other hand, in which one or both eyes are diffusely red and *painful,* is a different matter. The cause is usually a viral or bacterial infection, glaucoma or a foreign body. Unlike the painless blotch, "red eye" usually affects your vision. See an ophthalmologist right away.

Points to Remember

Symptom: Bloodshot eyes.

What It May Mean	What to Do About It
1. Fatigue or eyestrain.	No treatment necessary.
2. "Red eye."	Medical treatment.

BLEEDING GUMS

Your gums are most likely to bleed because the bristles of your toothbrush are too hard. Poking around with a toothpick will also do it. And if you don't brush often enough and properly, the tartar that builds up around the teeth makes the gums bleed, too.

Chronic gum inflammation (*peridontitis*) gradually erodes the gums and the bone and, if left unchecked, can eventually lead to the loss of your teeth.

In general, if your gums continue to bleed even after you've changed to a softer brush, see your dentist. He'll look for evidence of local infection, he'll check your dentures to make sure they're not irritating the gums, and he'll give your teeth a good cleaning and teach you proper dental hygiene. If that doesn't help, then see your doctor. He may remind you that you're taking some *medication*, like an anticoagulant, that's making the gums bleed, or you may have a *vitamin deficiency* (C or K) or a bleeding disorder. If you're diabetic, your gums are more prone to infection and therefore to bleeding. There are some other exotic and even ominous conditions that can involve the gums, but they are so infrequent that I don't want to worry you about them.

Points to Remember

Symptom: Bleeding gums.

What It May Mean	What to Do About It
1. Improper dental hygiene.	Good dental care, with periodic visits to your dentist for a thorough cleaning.

2. Infection.	Dental treatment.
3. Effect of medication (e.g., anticoagulant).	Adjustment of the dose or using substitute drugs.
4. Vitamin deficiency.	Proper diet and/or vitamin supplements.

BLEEDING FROM THE EAR

If you're an adult and your ear bleeds from time to time, you've probably got eczema or some other skin irritation in the ear canal. I hope that you're not in the habit of trying to clear wax out of your ear with a bobby pin or—and I cringe just thinking about it—a toothpick. *Cardinal rule: Never put anything in your ear smaller than the tip of your little finger.* Even cotton swabs should be used only to clean the visible outer part. Children particularly should be taught this rule because they like to jam all sorts of objects into the ear canal, any number of which can irritate it, cause bleeding and injure the eardrum.

If the eardrum becomes *infected,* there may be a trickle of blood from the ear. *Injury* too, such as a blow to the head, loud concussive noises (a gun going off very close by) and a sudden change in pressure on an airplane (especially when you have a head cold) can damage your eardrums and cause them to bleed. If your nose also bleeds, or there is evidence of hemorrhage elsewhere, then the problem is more than just a local one in the ear. Either that "trivial" head injury may have fractured your skull or your *clotting/bleeding mechanism* is out of whack.

Points to Remember

Symptom: Bleeding ear.

<u>What It May Mean</u>	<u>What to Do About It</u>
1. Inflammation or infection.	Local treatment with ear drops.
2. Injury from a foreign object, loud concussive noises or sudden pressure changes.	See your ear doctor.
3. Head injury.	See your doctor immediately.
4. Clotting/bleeding disorder.	Medical treatment.

WHEN YOU VOMIT BLOOD

When you vomit because you have an upset stomach or have eaten tainted food or have a "virus," you'll see the contents of your last meal. If you continue to throw up after the stomach is empty, there will be green bile. There should be no blood visible, unless, of course, you've had prolonged and vigorous retching, which may cause a tear in the small blood vessels of the throat or the esophagus, producing streaks of blood in the vomitus.

However, if you vomit blood, there's a 95 percent chance that you've got one of the following three conditions—a *peptic ulcer* (in the stomach or the duodenum); *irritation* or erosion of the lining of your food pipe or stomach; or advanced liver disease with *cirrhosis*. Stomach *cancer* is a much less likely cause, but one always to be considered. So is a bleeding disorder which renders you vulnerable to hemorrhage anywhere.

If you have a peptic ulcer, you may or may not have experienced gnawing, hungerlike pain and/or been nauseated before the vomiting and the bleeding began. This is also sometimes true in cancer of the stomach. Erosion of the upper gut is most often due to excessive alcohol, and to certain drugs. The most common among the latter are aspirin and all the related nonsteroidal anti-inflammatory drugs (ibuprofen, Naprosyn, Indocin) when taken regularly, and steroid hormones.

Chronic *alcoholism* or *hepatitis* (the latter usually following a type-B infection) can scar the liver (*cirrhosis*). This forces the blood to back up into the veins of the esophagus, which become dilated. As this increased pressure continues unabated, the veins eventually rupture, and when they do there is a sudden massive, spontaneous and explosive hemorrhage from the mouth—a horrifying experience for both the patient and the onlooker.

Here are some other factors to consider when you vomit blood:

- Before blaming your gut, make sure that the blood you see isn't what you swallowed during an earlier heavy nosebleed or after a tooth extraction, or coughed up from your lung and then swallowed. If it's frothy, chances are it is from the lungs.
- If the blood is dark red or black or looks like coffee grounds, the bleeding must have started hours or even days earlier and remained in the stomach, during which time it was chemically altered by the gastric acid, which changes the color from red to black.
- What should you do if you're at home and vomit some blood during the night? *Call your doctor right away*. Don't wait until morning. You can't depend on how much blood you see, for the

amount in the vomitus does not reflect how much was actually lost. If you're lightheaded or thirsty, are sweating or feel faint lying down, then the internal bleeding is substantial. The lightheadedness means that your blood pressure has dropped. All these symptoms constitute an emergency. Go to the hospital as quickly as possible—but do not drive yourself.

Points to Remember

Symptom: Vomiting blood.

What It May Mean	What to Do About It
1. No matter what you think caused it, this is an emergency!	Seek immediate medical care.
2. After prolonged retching: irritation of the throat or the esophagus.	Soft foods, antacids.
3. Peptic ulcer.	Antacids, H2 blocking drugs (Tagamet, Zantac, Pepcid). Avoid alcohol and caffeine.
4. Irritation of the upper intestinal lining.	Avoid alcohol, caffeine, aspirin and related drugs. Use antacids.
5. Cirrhosis of the liver.	A major life-threatening emergency.
6. Cancer of the stomach.	Surgery.
7. If associated with lightheadedness, thirst, sweating or feeling faint when lying down, an internal hemorrhage.	Immediate medical care.

WHEN YOU'RE SPITTING BLOOD

Spitting blood is usually the aftermath of a *nosebleed* or irritation of the gums from vigorous *brushing*. Or some part of the respiratory tract, which begins in the vocal cords and ends in the lungs, may be infected, irritated or congested. More serious and less likely causes of blood in the sputum are a traveling blood clot to the lungs and cancer.

If you see blood in what you've coughed up or spit out, the following observations will help you decide what it means.

What is the color of the blood and the sputum? Under what circumstances did it appear? Here are some common scenarios:

• You're forty years of age or older, either male or female. You've been smoking cigarettes for a long time and have had a hacking "smoker's cough" for years. One day you see some blood in the sputum, either as streaks or mixed with it. The cough itself wasn't any different from usual, nor was it particularly violent either. You decide to ignore this episode, as many cigarette smokers do. Then it happens again—and again. Now, here's what to look for—fever, chest pain and discomfort in the legs. Then reflect on whether you have a heart condition or had a bad cold recently.

• If you can answer no to all those questions, the odds are you've got *cancer of the lung*. The key features are your *age* (over forty), your *smoking history,* the *absence of fever* and the *chronic cough* that preceded the blood. As the tumor spreads to involve more and more of your lung, you will become short of breath and may develop chest pain, especially when you breathe deeply because the cancer has seeded the pleura (the envelope that covers the lungs). Sound awful? It is. Stop smoking now—and chances are you'll avoid the whole tragic mess. Of course, when I deduce that the blood in these circumstances means cancer, I'm talking statistical probability. You may be lucky. The tumor may not be malignant, especially if you're younger than forty and otherwise healthy, and have previously had benign growths (*polyps*) in the respiratory tract.

- You're a woman in your late twenties or early thirties and you're on the Pill. You probably smoke, but not necessarily. You suddenly develop a sharp pain in the side of your chest when you take a deep breath. You may or may not have a fever. You feel as if you've got a charley horse in the calf of one leg. The blood you spit up is bright red and is substantial—more than streaking. Over the next day or two, it becomes darker. You're also aware of being a little short of breath, and may even be experiencing some palpitations. One of your legs is slightly swollen and a little tender to the touch. All of these symptoms point to a *pulmonary embolism*—that is, a blood clot in the lungs.

- Supposing, however, you're older, you're not on the Pill, and you don't smoke—and you develop these same symptoms. Think back. Have you had an operation recently? Been confined to bed? Had a broken leg? Been on a long flight? Have your varicose veins become painful? All these circumstances make you vulnerable to a traveling blood clot.

- You notice some minor blood streaking in the sputum which has persisted for days and weeks. Some years ago, when *tuberculosis* was much more common than it is today, that's the first thing we would have suspected. (It's still a possibility, especially if you live in a nursing home where you may have been exposed to someone with TB.) A far more common cause of such streaking is *bronchiectasis,* a chronic lung condition, sort of an advanced chronic bronchitis, where the bronchial tubes become widened or weakened in one or more portions of the lung. Such patients may have sinus trouble too. Once it develops, bronchiectasis is virtually forever, and requires long-term antibiotic treatment and chest physical therapy. Persons with this condition cough up substantial amounts of foul-smelling sputum which may contain blood, particularly when infection occurs.

• Any *lung infection,* whether it's bacterial or viral, can make the sputum bloody. Chronic bronchitis —infection of the bronchial tree—is an example. Here, the sputum is streaked with blood; in lung cancer, it's more likely to be mixed with the blood. In pneumococcal pneumonia (the classic kind of pneumonia that older people get), the sputum has a rusty color because the blood in it is old—the bleeding within the lung having occurred days before it was coughed up. Pneumococcal pneumonia also causes fever, chills and pain on breathing.

• If you have any type of *cardiac condition* that has weakened your heart over the years, you may suffer from congestion of the lungs. You require several pillows or actually sit up in a chair in order to breathe comfortably. Cough is common in such circumstances, and what you spit up is likely to be frothy and blood-tinged.

These are some of the major causes of blood in the sputum. What I worry about is the patient who coughs up blood from time to time because of a chronic condition like bronchitis, and who takes it for granted. It's easy to overlook a lung cancer which has developed concurrently. So, if your chronic cough changes in any way, that is, if it's more frequent or there is substantially more blood in the sputum, ask your doctor for a pulmonary reevaluation.

A final note: If you've been *coughing heavily* because of a bad cold or flu, the violence of the cough itself can produce small tears in the throat which will result in blood in the sputum. But never take that possibility for granted, especially if the bleeding persists.

Points to Remember

Symptom: Blood in the sputum.

What It May Mean	What to Do About It
1. Recent nosebleed.	No treatment necessary.
2. Vigorous tooth-brushing.	Proper dental hygiene and care.
3. Cancer of the lung (especially if you're over forty and a smoker).	See your doctor.
4. Benign lung polyp.	Surgical removal.
5. Pulmonary embolism.	Immediate medical treatment.
6. Tuberculosis or other lung infection.	Appropriate antibiotics.
7. Heart condition.	Cardiac care.
8. Irritation of the throat from violent coughing.	Cough suppressants plus specific treatment of the underlying cause.

BLEEDING FROM THE NIPPLE

This paragraph, as you see, is short. If you're bleeding from your nipple, see your doctor as soon as you can. You've got to make sure you don't have a tumor there. If you do, it may or may not be malignant.

BLOOD IN THE URINE

Blood in the urine means trouble somewhere in the urinary system—beginning in the kidneys (where urine is made) and ending in the urethra (where it leaves the body).

When trying to determine where in that system the blood is coming from and why, start with the kidney. It will bleed if you *injure* it, as, for example, in a fall or a car accident. *Kidney tumors* are another source of blood in the urine. So are *infections* and *stones*. But kidney tumors are usually painless, while stones and infections hurt. An embolism—a traveling blood clot—can also end up in the kidneys and make them bleed. Whatever the condition responsible for it, the blood from the kidney courses down the urine ducts (ureters) into the bladder and out the urethra—when you finally see it.

The bleeding may originate in the ureters. A stone lodged within them or slowly moving down toward the bladder irritates the walls of these ducts, makes them bleed and gives you excruciating pain in the process.

Farther down the line is the bladder, which stores the urine until it's voided. *Bladder tumors, polyps, infections* (cystitis) and *inflammations* can all cause blood in the urine. Tumors and polyps don't hurt, infection and inflammation do.

The *urethra* itself may be infected by anything

from a sexually transmitted disease to a virus. Or it may have been injured by a foreign object (usually inserted during masturbation), or by a doctor poking around with an instrument (cystoscope) trying to make a diagnosis, or by a catheter introduced in order to relieve you of urine which you cannot pass unassisted.

An enlarged and infected *prostate* can also give you blood in the urine as a result of congested blood vessels in the area. And finally, if your blood isn't clotting properly for whatever reason (you may be taking anticoagulants), bleeding can occur anywhere in the body—including into the urine.

If your urine is red and *apparently* bloody, don't jump to any premature conclusions. If you're a woman, either pre- or postmenopausal, the blood may *appear* to be in the urine when in actual fact it's coming from the vagina. In men, the urethra carries both urine and semen out of the body and what may be mistaken for urinary bleeding is often a bloody ejaculation usually due to an infection or congestion of the prostate.

Keep this in mind, too. Red urine does not necessarily mean blood. If you've been constipated and took a laxative you found on the pharmacist's shelf, and started seeing "blood," look at the label. A dye called phenolphthalein, present in several popular laxatives, will turn the urine red. Pyridium, prescribed by doctors to relieve painful urination, makes the urine orange-red, while beets (which confer a red color to your stool, too) may produce a reddish-brown hue in the urine resembling old blood. Rifampin, the antibiotic that cures TB, also turns the urine orange.

A cardinal rule in medicine is that *the source of blood in the urine must be established quickly and accurately*. Report your observation to your doctor and be sure to give the following clues:

- If passing blood in the urine is totally painless, chances are there's a tumor somewhere in the urinary tract.
- If your urine is reddish or brown, the source of the bleeding is high up in the kidney. If it's bright red, it's more likely lower down, possibly from a tumor or a stone in the bladder, an infected prostate or an inflamed urethra.
- If the blood becomes visible just as you begin to urinate, the problem, as you might expect, is in the urethra. But if the urine remains yellow until you're almost through voiding and then the blood appears, it's coming from the bladder. If blood is present from beginning to end, then it's very likely from the kidneys. Men can obviously make this distinction more easily than women. The latter can get around the problem by using three containers to collect the urine while voiding, noting at which point and in which container the blood appears.
- Male or female, if you see blood leaking out of the urethra even when you're not urinating, then it's surely from the urethral wall.
- The presence of blood clots in the urine indicates that a considerable amount of bleeding has occurred and will alert your doctor to search for a tumor.
- If the blood is accompanied by waves of pain (colic) in the abdomen, the back or the flank, it's usually from a kidney stone. By contrast, if the pain is steady and stays right there in the back, you've probably got glomerulonephritis (an autoimmune disorder of the kidney) or some other kidney infection.
- If you experience a burning pain or a feeling of

heat when you empty your bladder, or have trouble getting the urine out, then the blood is probably coming from the lower urinary tract and may be due to a stone or to an infected prostate or bladder.

- If you urinate very frequently, never seem really to empty your bladder and have fever and chills as well, the blood reflects a urinary tract infection involving either the kidney or the prostate.
- If various parts of your body are swollen (feet, face and fingers) and there is blood in the urine, acute-glomerulonephritis (the kidney-damaging autoimmune disorder) is a good bet. If, in addition, your joints hurt, another autoimmune disease, systemic lupus erythematosus (SLE) may be the cause.

After you've given your doctor all this pertinent information, he or she will begin a targeted work-up to determine where the blood in your urine is coming from and why. This evaluation will include most of the following: a direct look at the urine specimen under the microscope; laboratory tests for identification of any infecting organisms that may be present and a Pap test for cancer cells; cystoscopy (in which a telescopic viewing device is introduced into the urethra and the bladder, permitting a direct look); and an intravenous pyelogram (X ray of the urinary system after it has been injected with dye to make it all visible). A sonogram or a CAT scan of the kidney and the pelvis may be recommended to fine-tune the diagnosis.

Points to Remember

Symptom: Blood in the urine.

What It May Mean	What to Do About It
1. Injury.	Medical treatment, possible surgery.
2. Kidney tumors.	Surgery.
3. Infection or autoimmune disease.	Medical treatment.
4. Kidney stone.	It may pass or it may need to be fragmented or removed.
5. Bladder trouble (tumor, polyp, infection).	If a growth, surgical removal. Antibiotics for infection.
6. Urethral injury or infection.	Antibiotics.
7. Enlarged and infected prostate.	Antibiotics. Surgery later if the infection recurs and is due to enlargement of the gland.
8. Discoloration from drugs or foods.	Make sure of the origin of the red color.

WHEN YOU EJACULATE BLOOD

Blood in your ejaculate can be a terrifying experience. It shouldn't be, because it's usually due either to congestion of the veins in the prostatic area or to a low-grade infection of that gland (rarely is an important problem like a tumor present). I've never seen a case of bloody ejaculate amount to anything more than that, and it never comes from eating beets!

BLOOD IN THE STOOL

The intestinal tract is one long tube that winds its way down from the food pipe to the anus. It's narrow in some places, wide in others. Blood in the stool can originate anywhere along its course. Its color tells you whether the bleeding occurred high up (in the food pipe or the stomach) or low down (in the large bowel or the rectum).

A black stool usually means that the blood is coming from the upper portion of the tract—food pipe (esophagus), stomach or duodenum. Blood turns black during the time it takes to pass from the beginning of the gastrointestinal tract to the end. But if you have diarrhea and your intestinal tract is very active so that its contents are moved along quickly, the blood emerges red, because it hasn't been sitting around the gut long enough to turn black. At least two teaspoonsful of blood must have been lost in order to make the stool black. That may not seem like much, but continued over a period of time such "slight" blood loss can cause severe anemia. *Gastritis* due to excessive alcohol, daily aspirin or other irritant drugs that erode the stomach lining may be associated with such bleeding. So are *peptic ulcers* and *cancer*. In fact, conditions which make the stool black are also generally those that cause vomiting of blood. The only difference is that in one case the blood takes the northern route, and in the other the southern passage.

Do not assume, however, that a black stool always means blood. The discoloration may be from something as harmless as the *iron supplement* you're taking. Stools black from blood are tarlike in their consistency. *Charcoal* (commonly taken for control of excessive gas) will turn the stool black, too, as will licorice (real licorice, not the fake red stuff they sell at movie theaters) and blueberries. Stomach-settling preparations and those for prevention of traveler's diarrhea that contain *bismuth*—the most popular is Pepto-Bismol—leave the stool looking greenish black.

Bleeding from the middle portion of the intestinal tract, that is, the small bowel, is apt to be intermediate in color—maroon.

Blood originating in the colon or the rectum is bright red. However, just as black stools may be caused by iron and not blood, red stools may result from the beets you ate last night.

Whatever the color of your stool, don't rely on your impressions. Always test it to know for sure. You can easily do this yourself with one of the home kits available at your drugstore, or, if you prefer, send a specimen to your doctor.

Here's another cardinal rule: *A bloody stool means cancer until proven otherwise.* Now, statistically it's far more likely that the blood is coming from hemorrhoids. But you're not a statistic and it's easy to be fooled. The most dangerous situation is one in which you've had hemorrhoids for years and have coincidentally developed a cancer higher up in the intestinal tract. The cancer is signaling its presence with the blood, which you naturally continue to assume is from your piles.

So, if you're a chronic bleeder from the bowel, get yourself checked from time to time. That doesn't mean that you have to see your doctor every time you find blood in your stool, but a checkup at least annually is a good idea.

The appearance of blood in the stool *demands* a work-up, and that will usually include a flexible sigmoidoscopy, a colonoscopy or a barium enema. The diagnosis may end up to be some local irritation, piles, inflammatory bowel disease (ulcerative colitis or Crohn's), a bacterial infection or a parasite you may have picked up on a recent trip out of the country. Certain antibiotics (Clindomycin, Gentamicin, erythromycin and lincomycin) can cause ulcerations of the bowel—and bleeding. So can enteric-coated potassium tablets (given to replace potassium lost from diuretics), anal intercourse or the insertion of any object into the anus. Certain vascular malformations in the gut, of which you may not be aware, can also cause bleeding.

When *arteriosclerosis* narrows the arteries that nourish the bowel, the gut is deprived of oxygen in the same way as are the heart and the brain. Among the resulting symptoms are abdominal pain—and blood in the stool. So, suspect such arteriosclerosis if you're elderly, have pain in your belly after eating and are bleeding, and if all the usual tests performed in a gastrointestinal work-up are normal. But remember that blood supply to the bowel can also be cut off by other mechanisms, as for example an embolism or a blood clot.

Diverticulosis, a condition which occurs most often among the chronically constipated, is caused by the presence of small fingerlike pouches (diverticuli) in the bowel. As long as these little projections are not inflamed, there's no problem. But from time to time they become infected, and diverticul*osis* becomes diverticul*itis*. Then you feel sick—with fever, pain and occasionally blood in the stools. Diverticulitis can sometimes end with perforation of the bowel. We used to think it was caused by eating nuts and seeds and a lot of fiber, but that theory is apparently all wrong. Today we admit that we don't know what causes attacks of diverticulitis and that fiber actually helps prevent them.

What clues, then, can lead you to the proper diagnosis when you see blood in your stool?

- If the blood is in streaks on the surface of the stool and not present throughout it, and if, in addition, it's on the toilet paper and in the toilet bowl, then the problem is probably in the rectum or the anal canal—a hemorrhoid, or a tear that occurred after passing a large, hard stool.

- If the blood is an integral part of the stool, not just on its surface, suspect a malignancy, although polyps can also cause streaking. A cancer is all the more likely if, in recent weeks or months, the stools have begun to look narrow, like ribbons, and your bowel habits have changed (you used to be regular and now you alternate between diarrhea and constipation). Also, when any growth, benign or malignant, is large and low down in the colon, you may feel as though you still have some stool left after completing your movement.

- If it hurts to move your bowels, you probably have hemorrhoids or a tear (fissure) in the rectum or the anus. But if you have abdominal pain unrelated to your bowel movements, then the blood in your stool may indicate colitis, infection, a vascular problem in the gut or a tumor.

- If you have diarrhea that comes and goes, the blood you see is more apt to be due to cancer, infection or colitis than to hemorrhoids. The latter generally bleed when they are irritated by hard stools or by straining to eliminate.

- If you feel weak or pass out after losing blood from the bowel, that's a bad sign. It usually means you've lost more than 20 percent of your total blood volume. Get taken to the hospital as fast as you can!

There are other color changes in the stool that have nothing to do with bleeding but may, nevertheless, be important. If you've recently had a barium enema or taken barium orally for an upper-GI series, you'll notice that your stool is either frankly *white*, pink or at least light in color for days. How long this persists depends on how active your bowel movements are. Rest assured, they'll eventually assume their normal color. But the stool may appear to be white because it is covered by mucus due to colitis or an irritable bowel.

If your stool is *gray* or greenish black, either you've been taking preparations containing bismuth (Pepto-Bismol) or you're lacking bile pigment in your stools. It's this pigment which colors them brown. Bile is made in the liver, stored in the gallbladder, then sent down a duct into the intestine, where it mixes with the by-products of digestion, giving them their normal brown color. Anything that interferes with the passage of bile from the liver or the gallbladder into the intestine will leave your stools looking like clay. What will do this? A gallstone in the duct is one cause. In that case, you may have pain in the right upper abdomen, fever and, because the blocked bile pigment backs up into your bloodstream, jaundice. When the stone has either passed spontaneously or been removed, the jaundice and the clay-colored stools disappear. If the gray coloration of the stool has developed gradually and is not accompanied by the symptoms of gallbladder trouble, then it's not a stone but something else obstructing the duct from the outside. That is worrisome, for the most common cause is cancer of the pancreas.

Get into the habit of looking at your stool (as well

as your urine, your sputum and, indeed, any bodily discharge). It may provide you with the earliest clue to correctable trouble. In fact, it's probably the single most important bit of self-examination you can do.

Points to Remember

Symptom: Blood in the stool.

What It May Mean	What to Do About It
1. If black: gastritis, peptic ulcer, a fissure from retching, cancer of the stomach, cirrhosis of the liver.	Medical diagnosis and appropriate treatment.
2. If maroon, inflammatory bowel disease, tumor in the small bowel.	Surgery or medical management.
3. If bright red: hemorrhoids, anal fissures, bowel tumor, ulcerative colitis, Crohn's disease.	Proper diagnosis and treatment, surgical or medical.
4. Drug side effects (aspirin or other irritant drugs, certain antibiotics, and potassium supplements).	Substitute or discontinue.
5. Arteriosclerosis of abdominal arteries.	Small, frequent meals rather than large ones; vascular evaluation; possible surgery.
6. Diverticulitis.	High-fiber diet; medication.
7. Other bowel disorders.	Diagnosis and treatment.

ABNORMAL VAGINAL BLEEDING

Bleeding may be something to worry about unless you're a healthy female between the ages of thirteen and fifty (or so). Then you expect to bleed, regularly, every month. If you don't menstruate, *that's* abnormal. But vaginal bleeding that's too heavy, or too little, or at the wrong time of the month, can pose a diagnostic problem. The various possibilities depend on your age (before or after menopause), whether or not you're taking birth-control pills, the state of your health and how active you are physically.

If you have abnormal vaginal bleeding, you can be certain it's coming from somewhere in the genital tract and is due to infection, hormonal changes and sometimes cancer. The risk of malignancy increases with age. The likelihood of infection depends to a large extent on your sex life. Hormonal levels fluctuate in response to signals from the brain, the ovaries, the thyroid and the adrenal glands. But make sure that the blood you see is in fact from the vagina and not the urine or the stool.

Let's start with a review of the various sites in the female genital tract from which vaginal bleeding can originate.

The *lips* at the entrance to the vagina (the *introitus*) can be injured, most commonly by vigorous intercourse. Sometimes, however, if you look carefully, you may see a small polyp there, or a little ulcer, a wart or even varicose veins—all of which can bleed. When the hymen is broken, expect some bleeding, too.

The *interior of the vagina* can become inflamed or infected or can host a malignancy, all of which may cause bleeding. Various foreign objects inserted into the vagina, usually during masturbation, can cause bleeding. (The astonishing variety of such objects indicates imagination if not prudence.) After menopause, when the level of estrogen hormone drops, the vaginal walls become dry and there is less lubrication during sex, which may cause pain and bleeding.

Continuing upward from the vagina, we reach the *cervix,* the opening into the uterus. It can bleed when infected (herpes sores located there are a fairly common cause), when bruised by profound penetration during intercourse, or after insertion of an IUD. Polyps or malignant tumors of the cervix also cause bleeding. (Women should have Pap tests regularly to detect such tumors in their earliest curable stage.)

Bleeding frequently occurs from the uterus, where a pregnancy may have gone wrong, or cancer, polyps or fibroids have developed or an abortion (spontaneous or induced) may have occurred. Foreign bodies may have made their way up from the vagina. Hormone fluctuations, birth-control pills and either stopping or starting estrogen-replacement therapy may all cause uterine bleeding.

In pre-menopausal women, every month the ovaries release an egg, which then enters the *fallopian tubes,* where it meets the sperm. The fertilized egg then travels to the uterus, where it is implanted. If it remains in the tube instead of entering the uterus, the result is called an *ectopic pregnancy*. It has no future there and eventually ruptures through the fallopian tube wall, causing severe pain and bleeding. That's as serious as it sounds. More commonly, bleeding occurs when the fallopian tubes become infected and inflamed due to a sexually transmitted disease.

Ovarian malignancy, infection or cysts can all produce vaginal bleeding. So can *low thyroid function,* or a malfunctioning pituitary gland in the brain, or other glandular problems.

Whenever you wonder *why* you have abnormal vaginal bleeding, always remember that nongynecological factors can be responsible, too—blood thinners, drugs and disorders of coagulation, all of which render you vulnerable to abnormal bleeding not only from the vagina but from anywhere in the body.

Vaginal bleeding in *postmenopausal women* has a variety of causes. Suppose that you've either just entered menopause or are well into it. You've almost forgotten what it was like to have a "period" when, suddenly, you see blood coming from your vagina or find it on your panties. What can it be? Statistically, there is a significant chance that it's due to cancer of the cervix or the uterus. Indeed, most uterine cancer occurs in postmenopausal women. The likelihood of such a tumor is greater when the bleeding is scanty and not profuse and if you've not had any children. The tumor may, of course, be a benign polyp, but you can't tell for sure without a biopsy.

Here's another scenario. You're in your early fifties and your periods have become so irregular you can no longer predict them with any accuracy. What's more, you've begun to have hot flashes, cold sweats and some *painless* bleeding. Chances are this is simply the tail end of your normal menses. The bleeding will stop within the next few months. But, with the strong *statistical* probability of cancer, you've still got to double-check it with your gynecologist.

If you've developed pain in your lower abdomen along with the bleeding, cancer is a possibility, but it's at least as likely to be due to *fibroids*. These large benign tumors in the wall of the uterus are a very common cause of bleeding in pre-menopausal women and one of the main reasons for a hysterectomy.

In *pre-menopausal women,* vaginal bleeding may simply reflect a variation of the normal twenty-eight-day menstrual cycle. That cycle can be as short as twenty-four or twenty-five days or as long as thirty to thirty-two days. Blood flow usually lasts anywhere from three to seven days, and most women require four or five sanitary napkins per day. If your flow can be dealt with by a tampon, it's probably normal in amount. What, then, constitutes abnormal vaginal bleeding? Excessive flow *during your period* even though it occurs regularly and on the button every twenty-eight days. The usual cause is a fibroid tumor (more common in menopausal women, but by no means limited to them), or an underactive thyroid gland (hyperthyroid women have a scanty menstrual flow).

Vaginal bleeding *between periods* is abnormal, but that's sometimes difficult to determine if your cycles are very irregular. Here are some additional clues to help you clarify what's happening:

- If you're on the Pill, expect your bleeding to be unpredictable.
- The presence of clots in the menstrual blood indicates that heavy bleeding has occurred in the uterus.
- If your periods have always been normal and you suddenly start to bleed heavily, you may have been pregnant without knowing it—and aborted spontaneously.
- "Spotting" between periods may be due to cancer of the cervix or uterus, or a polyp.
- If you're bleeding and your lower abdomen hurts, you probably have a pelvic infection (especially if the pain came on gradually and is accompanied by fever and a vaginal discharge).
- If you're an alcoholic and/or have severe liver disease, there's too much estrogen present in your body, which can cause vaginal bleeding.

Regardless of your own diagnosis, always tell your gynecologist if you're bleeding. While you're waiting for an appointment, here are some additional clues to which you may draw his or her attention.

- Is your skin dry and rough? Are you tired and sleepy? If so, the abnormal bleeding may be due to underfunction of your thyroid gland.
- Have you had a fever, one that comes and goes? As luck would have it, it won't be there when you finally get to the doctor. So tell him or her about it. Fever usually means infection.
- If you've had little hemorrhages in your skin, or bleed a little too easily in other parts of your body, the problem may lie in a generalized clotting disorder of which the vaginal bleeding is only one manifestation.

After listening to your history and doing a careful physical exam, the doctor's work-up may then consist of anything from a pregnancy test to a Pap smear, a CAT scan or a pelvic sonogram. But by making the observations outlined above, you can simplify the diagnostic process and speed it along.

Points to Remember

Symptom: Abnormal vaginal bleeding.

What It May Mean	What to Do About It
First, make sure it's coming from the vagina, and is not from the rectum or in the urine.	
1. Injury or disease of the vaginal lips (intercourse, infection, polyp, wart, ulcer, varicose veins).	Appropriate medical treatment.

2. Vaginal injury from insertion of foreign objects, from malignancy or from infection.	Appropriate medical treatment.
3. Dry vaginal walls due to lack of estrogen after menopause.	Estrogen replacement, either orally, by transdermal patch or inserted into the vagina.
4. Cervical infection, cancer or polyps.	Appropriate antibiotics. Surgery.
5. Uterine cancer, polyps or fibroids.	Appropriate treatment.
6. Abortion (spontaneous or induced).	Requires a diagnostic dilatation and curettage.
7. Fluctuation in hormone levels.	Appropriate medication.
8. Stopping and starting the Pill or estrogens.	Discuss with your gynecologist.
9. Ectopic pregnancy.	Emergency medical care.
10. Ovarian cancer, infection or cysts.	Appropriate medical or surgical treatment.
11. Low thyroid function.	Thyroid replacement.
12. Coagulation disorder.	Medical treatment.

ABSENCE OF VAGINAL BLEEDING

What about the other end of the spectrum—when there's too little vaginal bleeding or none at all? Suppose you are at the age when most girls start menstruating—twelve to fourteen or so. All your friends have begun their periods, but you haven't. Don't worry about it. Many perfectly normal females begin to menstruate later than most. But if you're pushing fifteen, here are some possible causes for the delay.

Considering how young so many women are when they become sexually active these days, a girl may become *pregnant* just before her very first period. That would stop menstruation for the next nine months. A long shot, granted, but possible. A more likely cause is an *imperforate hymen,* one without any opening, so that blood can't get out of the uterus. There are other congenital abnormalities that can block the exit of the menstrual fluid, as, for example, marked narrowing of the cervix, a double uterus or the absence of a uterus altogether. Also, some hormonal problem may be interfering with the production and interaction of the various glandular secretions which make for normal menstruation.

In women who have been menstruating normally right along, a sparse or absent menstrual flow is a different matter. If you miss your period, the most likely cause is always the obvious one, pregnancy, even if you took all the necessary precautions or thought you were too old to become pregnant. There's always a small chance of failure in every method of birth control.

Diseases and disorders not directly related to menstruation may also reduce or arrest your periods. *Drastic weight reduction* because of severe malnutrition, whether unavoidable (due to poverty), deliberate (fad dieting) or a result of psychiatric disorders (anorexia nervosa and bulimia in young women), results in a loss of body fat and an imbalance of hormonal levels which shuts down the menstrual cycle. An overactive thyroid gland will also cause decreased vaginal bleeding. There are some *glandular tumors*— especially of the adrenal or the pituitary—which cause an overproduction of testosterone, the "male" hormone, and produce "masculinization" of the female. In addition to growing hair like a man, women with this condition also lose their periods.

The world is on an *exercise binge*. Women now participate in almost every sport with the same vigor, determination and excellence as men. The price they often pay is cessation of their menstrual cycle. The reduction of body fat in a female athlete is accompanied by a corresponding drop in estrogen levels. All of this is reversible, however, and it appears that such exercise is protective against certain forms of cancer.

Here are some additional circumstances in which menstrual flow is absent or reduced:

- If you've had a recent life crisis—the death of someone very close to you, a broken love affair, the loss of your job—the *emotional response* may affect your hormone levels so that you will skip a period or two. If it's any more than three, have yourself tested to exclude other possibilities.

- If your normal periods don't start up again after you've had a baby, the *pituitary gland* in your brain may have been damaged.

- If you've had a *dilatation and curettage (D&C)* to correct excessive bleeding, and your periods never resumed, the curettage may have produced scar tissue which is now interfering with normal menstruation.

- A *brain tumor* may cause severe headaches or a change in vision—and loss of periods.

- Have your breasts been shrinking since you stopped having periods? Are you losing your pubic hair, but growing hair on your face, arms, legs and body? You can be sure you have a *generalized glandular disorder* affecting your hormone-producing glands. Determining which one it is requires a sophisticated work-up. However, your doctor will have a pretty good idea of where the trouble lies by making certain observations. For example, a decrease in your skin pigmentation, especially if accompanied by a secretion of milk from your nipples, indicates underfunction of the pituitary gland in the brain. On the other hand, an increase in skin pigmentation points to underfunction of the adrenal gland.

- If you've become nervous, jumpy, "hyper," can't tolerate the heat and perspire a lot, your problem is due to an *overactive thyroid gland.*
- If you have purple streaks on your skin and bruise easily, think of *Cushing's syndrome,* an overproduction of steroid hormones by the adrenal gland, or excessive intake of this hormone by mouth or injection.
- Lastly, an easy one: If your periods have begun to dwindle, you have hot flushes and you're pushing fifty, think *menopause.* That and pregnancy are, in the final analysis, the two most common causes of decreased or absent vaginal blood flow.

Points to Remember

Symptom: Decrease or absence of normal menstrual flow.

What It May Mean	What to Do About It
1. Normal delay of onset—to age fourteen.	Patience.
2. Pregnancy.	Medical confirmation and consultation.
3. Imperforate hymen.	Surgical correction.

4. Congenital abnormalities of the genital system.

Surgical correction.

5. Drastic weight reduction.

Proper diet.

6. Glandular tumors.

Surgery or medication.

7. Vigorous athletics.

Normal and reversible.

8. Emotional distress.

If it is prolonged, medical treatment to rule out a possible physical cause.

9. Damage to the pituitary gland in the brain after pregnancy.

Hormonal therapy.

10. Following a D&C, with formation of scar tissue.

Difficult to repair. The condition may be permanent.

11. Brain tumor.

Appropriate management of the underlying problem.

12. Glandular disorder.

Hormone replacement.

13. Overactive thyroid.

Medication, surgery or radiation.

14. Cushing's syndrome.

Surgery or medication.

15. Menopause.

Normal.

CHAPTER 4

FEVER:
How High Is High?

Patients often call to ask what to do about their "temperature." Of course they mean "fever" (everyone has a temperature—if you don't, you're in serious trouble!). Semantics aside, how hot must you be to justify calling it fever?

In a healthy person, oral temperature ranges between 97.5 degrees and 99 degrees Fahrenheit. You awaken with the lower reading. The higher ones occur later in the day, usually between 6 and 10 P.M. But if your temperature stays *above 99 degrees Fahrenheit* (37.2 Celsius) for more than a day or two without ever dropping down to 97.5, then you do in fact have fever. Keep in mind, though, that the upper limit of normal may be a little higher in a hot climate. For example, if you're vacationing in Mexico and come down with diarrhea (Montrenzuma's revenge), a temperature slightly over 99 degrees may reflect the heat outdoors and not the bowel infection. To check that out, stay in your air-conditioned room (or toilet!) for a while, and see whether this "fever" clears up. (As for the diarrhea, that's discussed in Chapter Eight.)

Also allow for some increase in temperature after a hot bath, or after a vigorous workout. If you're a woman, you'll spike slightly the day or two after ovulation. The reading on your thermometer may alarm you after you gulp down a cup of hot coffee, while a bowl of ice cream may mask a real fever if you have one.

TAKING YOUR TEMPERATURE

You can take your temperature three different ways —by inserting a thermometer into your mouth, into your armpit or into your rectum. Whichever method you choose, be sure to shake the mercury column down first. If you're using an "old-fashioned" mercury thermometer, allow three minutes. The newer electronic digital units tell you when the time is up.

When taking an *oral reading,* be sure to keep the thermometer in place with your lips tightly shut. Don't bite on it, especially if it's a glass mercury thermometer. Breathe through your nose if you can (that's not always easy if you have a cold and are congested). Some doctors have the annoying habit of popping the thermometer into your mouth and then asking you questions. Answer with your hands, not your mouth. A *rectal reading* is preferable for infants and anyone who is very sick. These readings are one degree Fahrenheit higher than oral temperatures, while those from the armpit are one degree lower.

WHEN YOU REALLY DO HAVE A FEVER

Now suppose you've done it right. You've felt sick and feverish, you took your oral temperature, and the reading is 99.8. It's kind of gratifying to know that nature is helping you prove to the world that you're really sick when you feel so lousy. (Without fever, who'd believe you?) But don't rush to lower your elevated temperature. Fever is not a disease, it's a symptom, and it's often a good thing—nature's way of dealing with a virus or bug that's affecting you. Most such organisms don't thrive in a hot environment. In fact, hyperthermia (raising the body temperature) is one method of treating cancer. If you bring your temperature down quickly, be it with aspirin, acetaminophen (Tylenol) or an alcohol sponge, without determining why it's high, you're not only obscuring the cause, you're depriving yourself of a natural defense mechanism.

Another piece of advice: If your child has fever because of a viral infection like the flu or chicken pox, *never use aspirin.* If you do, he or she may develop Reye's syndrome, a serious neurological disorder. But if the fever is above 103 degrees and the child is very uncomfortable or is having convulsions, then you *should* lower the temperature. You can do so with an alcohol sponge (which cools by evaporating quickly on the skin) or by giving acetaminophen.

Heatstroke, caused by prolonged exposure to very high temperatures with which the body's heat-regulating mechanism (sweating) simply cannot cope, is characterized by a dramatic high fever and a host of neurological symptoms ranging from convulsions to coma. If you encounter such a victim, call an ambulance immediately. In the meantime, do everything you can to lower the body temperature with cold water and wet sheets. Curiously, *heat exhaustion,* which is caused by the excessive loss of body fluids during periods of high temperature or vigorous exercise, is not usually associated with significant fever. The symptoms usually subside with rest and lots of fluids. One way to tell heatstroke from heat exhaustion is by feeling the skin, which is hot and dry in heatstroke, and moist and cool in heat exhaustion.

FINDING THE CAUSE

That's not as easy as it sometimes may seem. Unexplained fevers that continue for days or weeks are referred to by doctors as fevers of undetermined origin—FUOs. Most are due to a hidden infection. But there is also *drug fever.* Say, for example, you see your doctor for some problem, he prescribes a medication, and a few days later you develop a rise in temperature. Naturally you blame it on your illness. You may be right, but always bear in mind that it could be from the drugs you're taking. Fever can also accompany any condition in which body tissues are damaged—heart attacks, strokes, cancer and autoimmune diseases, or when the body's metabolism is revved up, as it is in hyperthyroidism.

Getting to the bottom of what's causing a fever often requires smart medical detective work in which you, the patient, can and should participate. Begin your sleuthing by recording your temperature at various times of the day and the night. If it's never below 100 degrees orally, and you have no other symptoms, review *all* the medications you're taking. *Any drug can suddenly cause fever out of the blue,* even one that you've been taking for years. The most frequent offenders are:

- *Antibiotics, including sulfa.* It's ironic that something one takes to eliminate infection and fever can itself cause temperature elevation.
- *Antihistamines.* You take an antihistamine to control an allergy, and you suddenly develop a fever. If you have no obvious infection and stop the drug, the temperature will usually return to normal.
- *Barbiturates.* These sedatives, most of which end in *al* (phenobarbital, Seconal, Nembutal, Tuinal) are very widely used for insomnia or to control epileptic seizures. Every once in a while they result in fever.
- *High-blood-pressure drugs.* Hydralazine (Apresoline), methyldopa (Aldomet) and thiazide diuretics (Hydrodiuril, Esidrix, Dyazide, Maxzide, Moduretic) are consumed by the hundreds of

thousands each day to control high blood pressure or to eliminate excessive body fluid. They can all induce fever.

Though these are the most common potentially fever-producing drugs, remember that *any* medicine can do so no matter how well you are tolerating it otherwise.

Another important cause of chronic, unexplained fever is *subacute bacterial endocarditis (SBE),* an infection of a vulnerable heart valve. By "vulnerable" I mean one that was either deformed at birth or damaged later in life, usually by rheumatic fever. Such valves can become infected as a result of something as innocent as a teeth cleaning, squeezing an infected pimple or pulling a hair from an inflamed follicle in the skin. Any of these maneuvers releases bacteria into the bloodstream, which then settle down on the valve, ultimately destroying it. Before antibiotics were available, SBE was often fatal.

A low-grade fever, sometimes lasting for months, may be the only symptom of subacute bacterial endocarditis. If you run such a fever and know that you have a heart murmur, try to remember when you were last at the dentist's. And have you recently squeezed a boil or pulled out an ingrown hair? Have you been to the urologist or the gynecologist, and were you catheterized for some urinary problem? Did any of these happen *before* the fever started? If so, SBE is a real possibility.

Here are some other clues to the causes of fever:

• If you have fever most of the day, but it returns to normal at least once every twenty-four hours, the source may be an *abscess,* a walled-off collection of pus, hidden somewhere in the sinuses, the gums, the liver, behind the teeth, in the kidney, the lungs, the abdomen, under the diaphragm—in fact, anywhere in the body. But cancer can also give you such an intermittent fever.

• Have you been to a Third World or tropical country in the past six months? If so, you may have contracted amebiasis or malaria.

• *Where you live* may provide an important clue to the source of your FUO. In the United States, there are five infections in particular which often cause mysterious temperature elevations. Each is indigenous to a specific geographic area: coccidioidomycosis (valley fever), a fungus infection prevalent in the Southwest; Rocky Mountain spotted fever, a tick-borne infection in the West, the Northeast and the Middle Atlantic states; blastomycosis, a fungus infection in the Mississippi Valley; histoplasmosis, a fungus infection in the East and the Midwest; and, most recently, Lyme disease, a tick-borne infection in the Northeast. A friend of mine was virtually written off as incurable some years ago. He was serving in the Army, stationed in the southwestern United States, when he developed a persistent low-grade fever and began losing weight. He had every test under the sun, none of which provided the diagnosis. For several months he became sicker and sicker. Finally a repeat chest X ray revealed a "shadow" in his lungs. Skin testing and a biopsy proved it to be coccidioidomycosis. He was treated and cured.

• Your *occupation* or your *pastimes* may have a bearing on the diagnosis of your FUO. Workers in the plastics industry develop fever if they inhale fumes in their work environment; meat processors can contract *brucellosis,* a chronic infection from slaughtered animals, in which the patient has fever and diffuse aches and pains. There are countless facts of which only you are aware that can clinch the diagnosis or at least point the investigation in the right direction. For example, if you're a hunter and have had skin-to-skin contact with a wild animal, you may have picked up tularemia; if you're a falcon or bird fancier and inhaled the dust of decaying bird droppings, you may have contracted a lung disease called *psittacosis*. Have you been for a walk in the woods recently and been bitten by a tick? Perhaps you visited a farm and were persuaded to try some "delicious" unpasteurized milk or cheese to see how great it used to be before man tampered with it. It may have tasted great, but was it worth your brucellosis or listeriosis? And how about that little out-of-the-way Chinese restaurant you love so much? Did you think there was something wrong with your last order of Moo Shu pork, like maybe it wasn't completely cooked? Well, the fever you've now got may be due to *trichinosis*. I remember the embarrassment of one of my patients, a rabbi no less, who had an FUO for several weeks. The diagnosis resisted all reasonable investigation. He turned out to have trichinosis from eating what was advertised as a kosher eggroll. Who would ever have thought of looking for trichinosis in a rabbi?

If you're an IV drug abuser, this is no time to have secrets from your doctor, because you are particularly vulnerable to AIDS, abscesses and SBE. Most physicians examine the skin pretty carefully in patients with an FUO, looking not only for rashes but for telltale needle tracks. If your doctor missed yours, don't play games. Show him what he's looking for and tell him what he needs to know.

While your doctor continues to track down the origin of your fever, you can be of further help by reporting any of the following symptoms:

- *Shaking chills,* which point very strongly to some kind of bacterial infection—an abscess, SBE, a gallbladder attack or some trouble in the urinary tract.
- *Profuse sweats* during the night suggest tuberculosis. One doesn't hear much about TB these days, but don't for a moment think it's extinct. With more and more people suffering from impaired immunity, especially persons with AIDS, and with the growing number of poor and homeless in this country, TB is on the rise again and is especially prevalent among the elderly living in nursing homes. As opposed to its awful death toll fifty years ago, TB can now almost always be cured by antibiotics.
- If together with your fever you're also *losing weight,* a *malignancy* is a real possibility. However, you may have nothing more than a hidden and curable infection.
- The combination of fever and *diarrhea with pus or blood in the stool* raises the possibility of a parasitic bowel infection. It may take repeated stool analyses to find these invaders, so don't abandon the search after a single negative test. A malignancy or inflammatory bowel disease (ulcerative colitis, Crohn's disease) can produce similar symptoms.
- *Painful voiding,* a burning sensation during urination or the need to "go" every few minutes, almost certainly points to a urinary tract infection, especially if the fever is accompanied by shaking chills.
- *Enlarged glands* are another clue when they accompany fever. But don't jump to the conclusion that you have a glandular malignancy (lymphoma) just because some glands have enlarged. While this diagnosis is, of course, a possibility, so is a viral, or

indeed any, infection and drug-induced fever. As always, remember to check your medicine cabinet.

- Show any *skin eruption* to your doctor immediately. The rash may reflect a tick-bite fever such as Lyme disease or Rocky Mountain spotted fever, some other infection or a malignancy of the lymph glands.

- The one symptom shared by many of the *autoimmune disorders*—in which the body directs its defense mechanisms against its own healthy tissues —is *joint pain or arthritis*. A persistent low-grade fever along with tenderness, swelling, redness or pain in the joints is a strong indicator of an autoimmune disorder like polyarteritis, polymyalgia rheumatica, rheumatoid arthritis or systemic lupus erythematosus (SLE).

- Your *family history* is an important clue. Ask every member of your family you can find, even those with whom you don't have much contact, whether they are prone to recurrent episodes of low-grade fever and joint pain. There is a condition called *familial Mediterranean fever*, found mostly, as the name suggests, in families whose roots lie in countries surrounding the Mediterranean. The condition is characterized by attacks of abdominal pain, joint symptoms and low-grade fever lasting for weeks at a time.

- Persistent fever accompanied by *muscle pains* can mean any of the following: a viral infection; trichinosis, from eating improperly cooked or raw pork; toxoplasmosis, from raw meat (exposure to a cat's droppings can do it, too); infection with two organisms in particular, Listeria and Yersinia, in unpasteurized dairy products; Lyme disease from a tick bite; or an autoimmune disorder.

- When *back pain* accompanies fever, the first thing to consider is an infection either in the kidney or in a vertebra. Bacteria can penetrate these structures from the bloodstream and settle down in them.

- Tiny blood clots (*emboli*) to the lungs, usually from the legs or the pelvis, can cause *chest pain* and low-grade fever. This happens most commonly in women, especially those with varicose veins, who are on the Pill and smoke cigarettes, who have recently had a baby or who have a gynecological infection (pelvic inflammatory disease, or PID).

- When the *abdominal pain* accompanying an FUO is in the right upper quadrant and comes in waves, it's probably due to gallbladder disease (stones or infection). But this pain/fever combination can also be caused by a pelvic infection, a kidney abscess or a tumor.

- In addition to telling your doctor about these symptoms, take the initiative yourself and check those parts of your body accessible to you. For example:

- *Look very carefully at your skin, fingernails and toes.* SBE can produce tiny hemorrhages which look like splinters under your skin and under the nails of the fingers and the toes. Their presence virtually clinches this diagnosis. Make sure, of course, that they're not real splinters!

- *Feel for lumps* in your neck, under your arms, in your groin, in your belly and anywhere on your skin, especially *after* you've been to the doctor and he has found nothing. So often, telltale findings appear between visits.

- *Press on your breastbone.* If it feels tender, the presence of a bone malignancy must be considered.

Beyond a very careful physical exam, sophisticated tests may be necessary to track the origin of an FUO. To begin with, there will be a complete blood count and biochemical survey. The number and kinds of cells in your blood are key. For example, one variety called *eosinophils* are the hallmark of *allergy*. If your fever is due to a parasite, the number of these cells will increase dramatically. Total white-blood-cell count constitutes an important finding, too. If it's very high, a bacterial infection is a more likely cause of the fever than is a viral infection, in which the blood count may actually remain normal despite elevated temperatures.

Various malignancies, especially leukemias, are detectable in a routine blood smear. You'll be checked for anemia (fever and anemia in combination point to a chronic and serious process). Your blood will be sent to a laboratory for tests to identify the presence of an autoimmune disorder. It will also be cultured—that is, incubated under strictly sterile conditions—to see whether any organisms grow out of it (normal blood is sterile). Your doctor will go beyond your blood and take anything he or she can get from your body—stool, urine, sputum—and send it off to the lab to be checked for everything from bacteria to cancer cells.

If the answer is still not forthcoming, additional tests may include:

- CAT scans of the head, chest, belly or spine, depending on the area under suspicion.
- If you have bone pain, your doctor is sure to ask for a scan of your bones to identify infection, arthritis or the presence of a tumor.
- A lung scan will be ordered if clots to the lungs are suspected.
- A gallium scan of the body will identify the location of a hidden abscess.
- A needle may be inserted into the bone marrow to aspirate some of its cells in a search for malig-

nancy. This procedure sounds terrible, but it's actually quite painless when done by an experienced hematologist.

As a final word of reassurance, don't let all of this scare you. The fact is, 90 percent of the time the cause of your FUO will be identified and treated. In the rest, the fever clears up on its own.

Points to Remember

Symptom: Fever.

What It May Mean	What to Do About It
1. Make sure it's abnormal. There is some variation in temperature in healthy persons.	
2. A beneficial bodily response to infection.	Don't rush to lower it unless it causes extreme discomfort or convulsions in a child. Never give a feverish child aspirin; use acetaminophen.
3. Heatstroke.	Medical emergency.
4. Medication side effects.	Change the medication.
5. Subacute bacterial endocarditis.	Antibiotic therapy.
6. Abscess.	Locate and drain.
7. Any infection—bacterial, fungal or parasitic.	Appropriate therapy.
8. Malignancy.	Appropriate treatment.

9. Autoimmune disorders.	Cortisone and other medications.
10. Emboli to lungs.	Anticoagulants.
11. Allergic response.	Antihistamines, steroids; avoid exposure.

CHAPTER 5

IT'S ALL IN YOUR MIND—OR IS IT?

I remember my first lesson in human biology in grade school. I must have been all of nine or ten years old. My teacher's first words in that course were "Think of your body as a car. Your heart is the engine, your backbone is the axle and the suspension, your muscles are the transmission, and your arms and legs are the wheels." And she left it at that. "But what about the brain?" I asked. "Ah, that's where the analogy breaks down," she said. "A car lacks one vital component to make it go—the driver. The body, however, has its driver built in. We call it the brain and the nervous system." I've loved automobiles and the secrets of the human body ever since.

This chapter is about your nervous system and the symptoms that point to its malfunction—in other words, what happens when the "driver" starts making mistakes.

SEIZURES

A brain seizure is very frightening to behold. In a classic attack, an arm or leg suddenly starts jerking uncontrollably, the neck may go rigid, the eyes roll back and the mouth foams. Throughout it all, the victim may either lose consciousness or remain wide-awake. But seizures are not always so dramatic. They may be quite subtle, consisting of only a brief "loss of contact," or a few moments of what looks like daydreaming. There can also be strange visual, auditory or odor hallucinations (seeing, hearing or smelling things that aren't there), or some inappropriate behavior lasting only a few minutes.

But every seizure, whether violent or mild, is due to sudden abnormal function of the brain—and there are many different possible causes for such malfunction. A *blow on the head* will do it; so will a *stroke* (in which a portion of the brain is temporarily deprived of oxygen), a *brain tumor,* a very *high fever* (especially in children) and a *heart attack* that may have left the cardiac muscles too weak to pump enough blood to the brain or beating too rapidly or too slowly. There may also be *malfunction of the liver or the kidney,* so that toxic substances normally cleared by these organs accumulate in the body and irritate the brain, producing a fit. In short, anything that upsets the delicate environment in which the brain functions can cause a seizure. The most common among the many possible causes are tumor, infection and damage to the brain.

Although no two seizures are ever identical, there are some generalizations that are helpful in sorting out the underlying cause. For example, seizures that begin in adult life are most likely due to a brain tumor (30 to 40 percent of patients with brain tumors experience a seizure at some time or other in the course of their illness). Head injuries at any age are responsible for almost 40 percent of seizures. There's usually an interval of months between the accident and the first attack. Interestingly enough, while strokes too can result in seizures, they do so relatively infrequently as compared to injury, infection and tumor. And where does *epilepsy* "fit" in? Doctors define an epileptic as someone whose seizures recur in a predictable pattern. There is a very characteristic change in the encephalogram (brain-wave test) taken during these attacks, so if there is any question about the diagnosis it can be settled then and there. Epilepsy begins anywhere between the ages of three and fourteen years and continues indefinitely thereafter. Happily, these seizures can now be effectively controlled by medication.

If you should happen to witness a seizure, try to remember what you saw. The information you pass on to the doctor can help him or her figure out what kind of fit it was. Note which limbs were twitching during the attack, and on which side. Did the head twist, the neck go rigid, the eyes turn or roll? Was there drooling, foaming at the mouth, a chewing motion or smacking of the lips? Was there any alteration of consciousness? Perhaps there was no twitching at all, just a sudden "not being with it," like a faint. Indeed, it may have been a faint if the victim recovered promptly after lying down. In an epileptic seizure, it usually takes minutes or hours to recover.

If you yourself have suffered a seizure, do you remember what happened just before the attack? In some epileptics, seizures are triggered by something in the environment—bright sunshine, flickering lights, loud sounds, a big swig of alcohol, even adjusting the TV set. In fact, one rock-music video consisting of a series of strobelike images was banned from broadcast in Britain for fear it might trigger such seizures in vulnerable individuals.

Here are a few helpful clues to the interpretation of some of these observations:

- If your child has a high fever and suddenly loses consciousness, and the extremities twitch and jerk in a random fashion, it's a febrile convulsion. It usually occurs when the body temperature is higher than 104 degrees Fahrenheit.
- Does the seizure involve the whole body or does it

affect only one limb? In epilepsy and febrile convulsions, there is loss of consciousness first, followed by the abnormal movement of several groups of muscles. When only an arm or a leg twitches, and the rest of the body is not involved, a tumor, a stroke or some other process affecting a specific area of the brain is the likely cause.

- When there is slurring of speech or weakness of some part of the body, followed by a seizure, it's probably due to a stroke.

- Is the subject *diabetic*? Anything that impairs the nutrition of the brain can cause a seizure. When an artery is blocked, the supply of oxygen to the brain is cut off and the result is a stroke. But sugar is also a vital fuel. When a diabetic takes too much insulin so that the blood-sugar level drops sharply, he or she will have a seizure. Such insulin attacks are sometimes misread as strokes or, what's even worse, as evidence of alcoholism. It's a good idea to wear a bracelet or a necklace identifying you as a diabetic and subject to such attacks.

- In patients with advanced kidney disease, the poisons that should be excreted accumulate to toxic levels and irritate the brain. This condition, called *uremia,* is often accompanied by seizures.

- Are you taking any *medications*? Several can cause seizures, especially amphetamines ("speed," formerly prescribed legally as an appetite suppressant and now used sometimes as an antidepressant) and tranquilizers, notably the mood-elevating agents imipramine (Tofranil) and amitriptyline (Elavil). A drug against tuberculosis, isoniazide, can cause fits, too. So can certain antiasthma preparations, as well as penicillin in someone who's allergic to it.

- Have you recently kicked a drug or alcohol habit? Quitting cold turkey can produce seizures (DTs).

The clues I have listed will steer you in the right direction. Whatever you make of them, report all seizures to your doctor. This is not a trivial symptom. Even when the cause seems apparent, as in a child with a high fever, it's always wise to check it out. The temperature elevation may be coincidental to some other underlying disorder which is producing the convulsions.

Points to Remember

Symptom: A seizure.

What It May Mean	What to Do About It
1. Head injury.	Thorough evaluation, antiseizure medication, possible surgery.
2. Stroke.	Supportive therapy.
3. Brain tumor.	Surgery, radiation, chemotherapy.
4. High fever, heatstroke.	Lower the body temperature quickly.
5. Cardiac-rhythm disturbances.	Medication, pacemaker implant.
6. Heart attack.	Supportive treatment.
7. Liver failure.	Supportive treatment, diet.
8. Kidney failure.	Diet, drugs, dialysis.
9. Epilepsy.	Medication.
10. Diabetes (when the sugar level is too low).	Glucose.
11. Medication side effects.	Substitute other medications or reduce the dosage.

FAINTNESS AND FAINTING: DON'T DO SOMETHING, JUST STAND THERE!

Does the following scenario sound familiar? You're in a restaurant. It's warm and stuffy, with lots of cigarette smoke around (before the days when tobacco addicts were segregated). You're nursing a drink but haven't yet eaten anything. You either are sitting up straight or have just stood up on your way to the washroom. Suddenly you feel very weak, giddy, light-headed, as if you've just taken a whiff of nitrous oxide at your dentist's; your vision becomes blurred or dimmed; you begin to feel nauseated; you sense that if you don't hold on to your chair, you're going to pass out. You instinctively lie down, and in a few minutes you begin to feel better. If you delay in assuming the horizontal position, you may actually faint.

An observer of this chain of events would have seen you turn pale, break out into a cold sweat and slump to the ground. Now, if you were lucky enough to have been left alone, you would have "come to" spontaneously in a couple of minutes. If you were unlucky, you would have been "helped" by a Good Samaritan. He would have been absolutely convinced you had had a heart attack, and he would have leaped into action. Although he had never learned how to do CPR, he had seen it demonstrated often enough in TV hospital dramas to be confident. He would have straddled you and begun to pound your chest and breathe mouth to mouth. Before the ambulance arrives, you wake up, alive and well, except for mammoth bruises and a couple of cracked ribs. The Good Samaritan can't believe it—he has finally actually saved someone's life!

The truth is, your life didn't need saving and you

would have been spared the bruises and cracked ribs if you had simply been left alone.

A little knowledge can be very dangerous under these circumstances. If you're really set on saving a life, take an accredited CPR course. Don't depend on what you've seen in the movies or on TV. In addition to teaching you how to resuscitate someone who really needs it, a CPR course will spell out the differences between a simple fainting spell and a cardiac arrest. Unless and until you've taken such a course, when you see somebody suddenly slump to the floor, please don't immediately start cracking ribs. Give nature a chance for a couple of minutes. Have the person lie down and make him comfortable. If you feel you *must* do something, elevate the legs to increase the blood flow to the brain. Nine times out of ten, your "patient" will probably wake up on his own in a few moments. Here's the bottom line. Most "faints" are not cardiac arrests, but if there is *any* question in your mind as to what caused the one you witnessed, the very first thing to do *immediately* is call an ambulance. Then, after the victim has been lying down thirty seconds or so and still has not come to, you may apply CPR—*but only if you know how to do it.* (Before starting, however, be sure you are unable to feel a pulse and/or the victim isn't breathing.) Don't learn on the job! Find out if anyone present *has* been trained in CPR. If you take charge, someone who really knows how may not step forward, on the assumption that you're qualified —when you're not!

Fainting is the result of a sudden reduction in blood supply to the brain, usually brought about by a sharp, rapid drop in blood pressure. There are a number of ways that can happen. Remember that blood pressure is kept stable by several complex mechanisms acting together—some raise it, others lower it. In a simple faint, the latter win out. The attack I described in the restaurant is called a *vasovagal faint,* and is usually triggered by putting alcohol into an empty stomach in a hot, stuffy environment. But pain, injury or fright can also do it. From time to time patients will pass out while having their blood drawn if they're in the sitting position.

Here are some other situations in which vasovagal fainting can occur: vigorous coughing, straining at stool and emptying the bladder, especially when an enlarged prostate makes it difficult to do so. If your prostate is enlarged, get into the habit, whenever you can, of sitting down while you urinate. When standing at a urinal in a men's room, take your time and don't force it, no matter how long the line behind you happens to be. Standing up too quickly from the recumbent position can also result in fainting, because of a sudden drop in blood pressure. This is most apt to occur in older people, especially those who are on blood-pressure-lowering medication.

There is a sensitive area in the neck called the *carotid sinus.* You can easily find its pulse if you feel for it on the upper right, just below the jawbone. Doctors massage it when a patient has a very rapid heart rate that must be slowed. In older individuals, even turning the head can compress the carotid sinus, slow the heart rate, drop the blood pressure and make them faint. In fact, pressure on the carotid sinus by any mechanism may result in your passing out.

You've probably heard this story: From time to time, with no warning, this man we will call John would suddenly lose consciousness. It was frightening—and dangerous. So he was thoroughly evaluated with a battery of sophisticated and expensive tests. Nothing abnormal was found. He was finally told that he had a "condition," with which he would have to live, and that his long-term outlook was uncertain.

So, on the assumption that his life span was limited, John indulged himself in pleasures he had previously forgone. He invaded his capital without any qualms whatsoever. What the hell, he might as well enjoy it while he could. He traveled to exotic lands, dined out in the finest restaurants, gave his wife expensive jewelry and bought himself an elegant new wardrobe. For this last, when asked by the salesclerk what his collar size was he replied, "Sixteen." The salesclerk looked surprised—he was pretty good at sizing people with his eyes—and asked John when was the last time he had bought a shirt. "Eight years ago," was the reply. The clerk then measured his neck just to be sure and informed John that his collar size was actually seventeen. "Sixteen is way too small for you, sir," he said. "In fact, if you wear a sixteen, you're going to faint a lot."

Sudden decrease in blood pressure and reduction of blood flow to the brain, both inducing a faint, can also result from *medication*. Virtually any tranquilizer, many heart drugs and almost every preparation that is used to treat high blood pressure can bring you to your knees, especially if you're elderly. One drug, in particular, is very tricky that way: nitroglycerin, the classic agent used to relieve angina pectoris. Slip it under the tongue when you feel that deadly pressure behind the breastbone, and your symptoms will disappear in less than a minute. Nitroglycerin works by dilating arteries everywhere, including the coronaries in the heart. This relieves the spasms in these vessels so that blood is once more able to flow freely through them. But when the arteries in the general circulation are also widened, the blood pressure within them falls. This drop can be quite substantial, especially if the patient is standing at the time—and the result is a faint. The overall picture looks very much like the innocent vasovagal faint. In both instances, lying flat restores the blood pressure and ends the crisis. Even though it may turn out to have been unnecessary, play it safe anyway and do go to a nearby emergency room where an ECG can be recorded. If you have angina and need nitroglycerin from time to time, remember to sit down or recline a bit before taking it.

You may also lose consciousness when the heart abruptly beats *very slowly,* and by that I don't mean forty-five or fifty times a minute. In some athletes, the usual pulse rate is even lower than that. No, I'm talking about a drop all the way down to below thirty. Certain drugs in combination, for example beta blockers like Inderal especially when taken with digitalis, can do that. So can a condition called "heart block." Whatever the cause, at that rate your brain isn't getting the blood it needs and you may lose consciousness.

Also, you may faint if your heart is beating too *quickly.* Again, I'm not referring to the 150 beats per minute you generate after a hard-fought racquetball game. But when your ventricles are pumping two hundred times a minute or more while you're just sitting around, your heart doesn't have the time to recover after each beat. It starts shooting blanks, hardly ejecting any blood at all with each contraction. The result is loss of consciousness. The cause of such rapid arrhythmias is not always understood, but it frequently occurs in persons with underlying heart disease.

Here's one way you can tell a simple vasovagal faint from one caused by something more serious. A

simple faint is rarely preceded by pain, pressure, constriction in the chest or shortness of breath—just by
weakness, giddiness and nausea. Also, when the
cause is a disorder of heart rhythm, the "faint" occurs regardless of the subject's position. A vasovagal
attack will happen only when the person is upright.
So, if you're lying in bed and suddenly lose consciousness, it's not a harmless event.

Anxiety and hysteria may cause lightheadedness
that occasionally ends in a faint when the individual
hyperventilates. This type of breathing consists of
deep, rapid respiration, which all of us do from time
to time when we're under stress. In some persons,
however, it becomes a habit. Hyperventilators feel as
if they're not getting enough air and so they breathe
more deeply. In so doing, they blow off too much
carbon dioxide, and that's what gives them their
symptoms. To see for yourself, take a few very deep
breaths (remember, just a few). Your hands and feet
will soon tingle and your head will begin to swim. If
you continue long enough, you'll faint. Don't.

There are, of course, several more serious causes
of loss of consciousness: diseases of the nervous system, massive blood loss, valvular disorders of the
heart, emphysema, blood clots to the lung, heart attacks, strokes, and in diabetes when the blood sugar
falls too low (*hypoglycemia*) because of excessive insulin.

Here are some additional clues to help you determine why you "fainted":

• Do the faints occur frequently, perhaps even several times a day? If so, you may have some underlying cardiac problem or be an epileptic.
• Did you recover rapidly after fainting? That's
  characteristic of a vasovagal episode or a drop in
  blood pressure for whatever reason. But if you

were "out of it" for any length of time, say as long
as an hour, think about having had low blood
sugar (if you're a diabetic) or a cardiac or neurological condition.

- Do you feel faint or actually pass out when you
  lean over forward, as you might do tying a shoe-
  lace? A rare benign tumor (atrial myxoma) within
  the heart may be the cause.
- If you faint while exerting yourself, there are a
  number of possibilities, most of which relate to
  heart or lung disease.
- If lying down flat when you feel faint restores your
  strength, your blood pressure is too low.
- When a fainting spell is accompanied by a seizure,
  it's due either to a heart problem, a neurological
  disorder or epilepsy.
- If you fainted and later noticed that your stools are
  black or tarlike, you have had an internal *hemorrhage* and are severely anemic.

Among the key things to remember in this chapter
are the following: Whenever you come across someone who has fainted, before beginning heroic resusci-
tation measures let the person lie there for a few
moments, but call an ambulance. Chances are he or
she will recover. That is not to say that you shouldn't
help someone in distress. You should, but only if you
know what you're doing. Learn CPR. And, if you
have angina pectoris, remember how nitroglycerin
works. Make sure to sit down *before* putting the pill
under the tongue.

Points to Remember

Symptom: Loss of consciousness.

What It May Mean	What to Do About It
1. Simple faint (vasovagal faint).	Lie flat until recovery. Investigate the underlying cause.
2. Pressure on the carotid sinus.	Relieve it.
3. Tranquilizers and high-blood-pressure medication.	Reduce the dosage or avoid them.
4. Nitroglycerin in cardiac patients.	Always sit down before taking nitro, when possible.
5. Too slow a heart rate.	If due to drugs, adjust the dosage. In heart block, pacemaker implant.
6. Too rapid a heart rate.	Medication.
7. Hyperventilation.	If it's a habit, try to correct it.
8. Stroke.	Supportive care.
9. Heart attack or vascular problem.	Appropriate treatment.
10. Hypoglycemia.	Avoid insulin reaction if you're diabetic; low-sugar, high-protein diet.
11. Hemorrhage.	Stop the bleeding, replace blood.

FACIAL PARALYSIS: STROKE OR JUST A VIRUS?

Patients sometimes call to say that one side of their face is paralyzed or has become distorted and that they're sure they either suffered a stroke or have a brain tumor. But there is another cause of facial asymmetry that has nothing to do with either of these two ominous conditions: *Bell's palsy*, which is probably caused by a virus. Strokes and brain tumors are life-threatening, while the consequences of Bell's palsy are largely cosmetic. Although the facial distortion it produces usually improves with time, there's often some permanent deformity. But that's a far cry from the implications of a stroke or a brain tumor.

You can often tell what's going on by the characteristic symptoms. Those due to a brain tumor develop gradually, while Bell's palsy and stroke usually come on abruptly. A brain tumor is often accompanied by headache, seizure or even blindness, rarely seen in strokes and never in Bell's. When facial paralysis is due to a stroke, an arm or a leg may also become weak or paralyzed. Not so in Bell's palsy. But here is the real clincher: In facial paralysis due to a stroke, you can close the eye on the affected side and wrinkle your forehead. That's not possible in Bell's palsy. So if you wake up one morning and find your face distorted, you can immediately set your mind at ease that you haven't had a stroke by trying to close your eye. If you can't, and it rolls up instead, you should be very happy! You'll also notice other symptoms in Bell's palsy: For example, the angle of the mouth droops, saliva will dribble from the mouth, and when you try to puff out your cheeks the paralyzed side balloons out more than normal. But the key to it is the eye.

Points to Remember

Symptom: Facial paralysis.

What It May Mean	What to Do About It
1. Tumor—when accompanied by headache, seizures or blindness.	Surgery, radiation, medication (steroids).
2. Stroke—when the muscles in the body are involved, and you can shut the affected eye and wrinkle your forehead.	Anticoagulants; control the blood pressure; supportive care.
3. Bell's palsy—no other neurological abnormalities are present, and you cannot wrinkle your forehead or close your eye.	No specific therapy.

TREMOR: THE KIND OF HAND "SHAKE" YOU CAN DO WITHOUT

Your hands may shake briefly at some time or other when you are very tired, stressed, anxious or enraged. ("I was so mad, I was shaking!") That's clearly nothing to worry or wonder about. But there are tremors which are neither so transient nor so benign, and which involve not only the hands but other parts of the body too, especially the tongue and the head. Here are some of the more common ones and what causes them:

The first concern of anyone who develops a

tremor is *Parkinson's disease.* And quite properly so, because this neurological disorder is serious, incurable and often crippling.

No one knows why some people develop Parkinson's, or how to prevent it, but we do know what happens in the brain of those who suffer from it. They have a deficiency of a chemical called *dopamine.* Modern therapy focuses on trying to replace some of the missing dopamine and neutralizing the effects of its absence.

The following paragraphs contain the clues that will help you distinguish one tremor from another.

You can develop a tremor from the *toxic action of a chemical or a drug.* Too much coffee ("I just can't get by on less than ten cups a day") and excessive alcohol are classic examples. Medications taken by asthmatics to relax their constricted air passages (theophylline) and by epileptics to control their seizures (Dilantin) may also induce tremors. Compazine, an excellent tranquilizer and antinauseant, will every now and then produce tremor and head-bobbing, especially in older people—symptoms frighteningly similar to those of Parkinson's disease. Simple withdrawal of the drug eliminates the shaking.

Then there is the *"essential" tremor,* an often hereditary condition in which one or both hands shake. This causes panic when mistaken for Parkinson's disease, and it shouldn't. The tremor in Parkinson's is constant at rest and improves when the subject reaches out for something. By contrast, an essential tremor is rarely present when the hands are not being used, and becomes most apparent when you try to do something like reaching for an object or writing. Emotional stress makes matters even worse. But most important, persons with an essential tremor have none of the other symptoms of Parkinson's disease—no drooling, no muscle rigidity, and they walk normally. In short, they are not and never do become sick from their "condition."

Like Parkinson's disease, essential tremor is most common in older people (there is a 15 percent incidence in those over seventy-five years of age—which is why it is also referred to as "senile" tremor), but I have seen it in thirty-five- and forty-year-olds too. And even though essential tremor is not a manifestation of disease, it does have one unfortunate consequence in particular: A couple of drinks make the shaking much less evident, so individuals with such a tremor come to rely on alcohol to tide them over embarrassing situations. In time, they can develop a drinking problem.

Tremor can accompany a variety of diseases, including advanced *liver trouble, kidney malfunction* and an *overactive thyroid.* Any brain disorder, whether it's Parkinson's, *multiple sclerosis,* a head injury with concussion or a *stroke,* can also cause the shakes. But in all these conditions, the tremor is usually the least of the problems and not the singular telltale or clinching symptom. For example, in the case of an overactive thyroid, there's usually a constellation of other symptoms: nervousness, palpitations, warm skin, rapid pulse, bulging eyes, fine hair and quivering of the extended tongue. If you suspect that's what you have, extend your hands palm down, spread the fingers and put a piece of thin tissue paper over the backs of the hands. A fine vibration is typical of hyperthyroidism. The Parkinson's tremor is quite characteristic, too. As I mentioned earlier, it's at its worst at rest and least apparent during intentional movements. It also disappears during sleep.

If your hands begin to shake, here is what to look for:

- Is there a new drug in your medicine cabinet? Check specifically for Compazine, Dilantin or barbiturates (phenobarbital), any of which can be the culprit. I have one patient, a man in his seventies, who always enjoyed excellent health. One winter, he went on a Caribbean cruise. After his first day at sea, he became deathly sick from the ship's motion. The only relief he obtained was from Compazine. Three or four days later, he developed "Parkinson's disease." He telephoned ship to shore to arrange a neurological appointment back home in New York. After the ship docked, he no longer needed the Compazine. By the time he got home, his "Parkinson's disease" had disappeared!
- If you take cocaine or other "recreational" drugs and your hands begin to shake, the reason is pretty obvious.
- If you're otherwise well but have a fine tremor in the fingers of one hand, perhaps accompanied by some involuntary movement of the head, both of which are worse when you're nervous, you have benign, or "essential," tremor. This condition is often present in several family members. It can start early in life and then clear up, or it can get worse with age. *It does not reflect an underlying disease.* Be sure not to become dependent on alcohol to help you through important business or social occasions.
- If you're *seventy or older,* otherwise in good health and have noticed a little shaking of your hands and possibly the lower jaw as well, it's just a minor inconvenience that's sometimes present in some persons as they get older. Don't worry—it's not going to lead to anything else.
- *Alcoholism* is one of the most common causes of tremor. If you find that a drink in the morning is "absolutely necessary in order to start the day off

right," you've got the answer to your tremor right there—and a big problem.

- If you're *diabetic* and have taken too much insulin, low blood sugar may give you the shakes. But then you'll also feel weak and sweaty. Everything will clear up promptly after you take some sugar or orange juice.
- Tremor due to an overactive thyroid also involves the tongue, which has a fine quiver when protruded.

Remember, tremor is not a disease, but a symptom which may be present in otherwise healthy persons as well as in those with a wide variety of medical disorders.

Points to Remember

Symptom: Tremor.

What It May Mean	What to Do About It
1. Stress.	Relax.
2. Parkinson's disease—when the shakes are worst at rest, and least intensive when you reach for something.	Medication, brain surgery (still experimental).
3. Reaction to drugs.	Avoid, reduce the dosage or switch.
4. "Essential," "familial" or "senile" tremor.	Not a disease. Relax, but avoid dependence on alcohol.
5. Liver disease.	Medication, diet.
6. Kidney disease.	Diet, dialysis.
7. Overactive thyroid.	Drugs, surgery, radiation.

8. Multiple sclerosis.	No treatment at present.
9. Stroke.	Supportive care.
10. Normal aging.	No treatment necessary.
11. Alcohol.	Avoid.
12. Diabetes.	Avoid insulin reactions.

WHEN YOU'RE NUMB AND TINGLING—HERE, THERE AND EVERYWHERE

Suppose someone accidentally touches your arm with the burning end of a cigarette. The nerves right there immediately conduct a message which travels to and up the spinal cord and ends in the appropriate part of the brain. If the brain is normal, it interprets the stimulus (in this case, excessive heat) and sends back a signal which tells you to get your arm the hell away from the cigarette! You do so instantly, reflexively. The round trip from burn to withdrawal and "ouch" takes no time at all.

In order for you to feel any sensation on the surface of the skin—pain, heat, cold, tingling, crawling or itching—those connections to the brain must be intact. When an area of the skin is *numb* so that you are not aware that the burning cigarette is touching it, something is wrong with the nerves in the skin itself, or there is some foul-up along their path to the brain, or the brain itself has been damaged so that it cannot interpret the message properly.

Local nerve malfunction is usually due to *injury* and/or the formation of scar tissue in the area. If you've ever had an operation, you know that even though the scar itself is healing nicely, the skin around it is numb. That's because the nerves have been cut and are no longer able to transmit impulses to the brain—and they probably never will.

Interference with the transmission of the nerve impulse along the pathway between the skin and the brain is most often due to *spinal-cord* injury or to some disease or tumor within the spinal cord, the trunk line to and from the brain.

When the problem lies within the brain itself, it's usually due to damage following a *stroke* of some kind.

When you feel a *tingling* anywhere, there must have been some damage or irritation to the nerves serving the area involved, either locally, along their pathway or in the brain. Unlike numbness, however, the nerve is not completely dead or severed—just injured or being *pressed upon*. Tingling, then, is a sort of middle ground between the extremes of pain and numbness. As the disorder, whatever it is, gets worse, you may experience all three sensations: first the tingling, then pain and finally complete loss of sensation, and numbness. That's the usual sequence of events, as, for example, when you have a disc somewhere in your spine pressing on a nerve. In this latter example, not only is sensation lost, but muscle power diminishes, too, as the "motor" nerves also become impinged upon.

Nerves are vulnerable to many different disorders: pressure from other structures adjacent to them (tumors, discs, swellings, arthritic bones, carpal tunnel syndrome); *toxic effects* of various poisons and drugs —lead, alcohol, tobacco; neurological problems ranging from stroke to tumors; *deficiency diseases* like pernicious anemia; *chemical abnormalities* such as diabetes. In most cases of numbness, tingling or pain, the cause is obvious. If it is not, you may have to undergo a thorough evaluation to determine its origin.

Points to Remember

Symptom: Numbness and tingling.

What It May Mean	What to Do About It
1. Local injury to the nerves in the skin.	No specific treatment.
2. Spinal-cord injury or disease.	May require surgery.
3. Brain damage, e.g., stroke.	Treat the neurological disorder.
4. Pressure on nerves (discs, tumors, abscesses, arthritic bones).	Relieve the pressure.
5. Toxic action on nerves (lead, alcohol, tobacco).	Remove the underlying cause.
6. Pernicious anemia and other deficiency diseases.	Correct the deficiency.
7. Diabetes and other chemical abnormalities.	Appropriate medical management.

LOST YOUR SENSE OF SMELL OR TASTE?

How would you like to be flying on an airplane at 35,000 feet with an eighty-year-old pilot at the controls? I wouldn't! Would you shun a delicate operation by a very experienced eighty-five-year-old surgeon? I would! For no matter how much we *know,* as we get older we don't see as well, we don't hear as we used to and we inevitably lose some coordination. That's why there aren't any practicing eighty-year-old commercial pilots or eighty-five-year-old brain surgeons. But we are so preoccupied with sight, hearing and coordination that we don't think much about what happens to our sense of smell and taste. So we're puzzled when someone close by complains of an offensive odor of which we are not aware, and we may not realize for years that our food just doesn't taste as it should—or used to—through no fault of the chef.

Loss of acuity in sense and taste as one gets older is due to an impairment somewhere in the nervous system and is usually a gradual process. In most cases, there's no obvious or immediate cause, other than the calendar—and there's no treatment either. But if it happens to you when you're younger, or the symptoms come on abruptly, you may be able to trace them to a recent "heavy cold" or other *viral infection,* in which case they may improve slowly after weeks or months. Make sure, too, that you don't have *nasal polyps.* You're likely to if you're allergic. They certainly affect the sense of smell. So will the chronic use of *decongestant sprays,* which shrivel your nasal lining and can permanently destroy your sense of smell. Not uncommonly, too, loss of taste and/or smell is due to a *brain tumor.* So if you've noticed a sudden and continuing impairment in either or both of these faculties, tell your doctor about it—even if you suspect it's all a matter of age. You may be wrong.

While your main consideration with these symptoms is your inability to smell the American Beauty roses you've slaved over in your garden, or the fact that your legendary chili has lost its fire, there are also some very important health and safety considerations. For example, you may not be able to detect the smoke of a fire in your home. That can be disastrous if you're living alone. So make sure you have lots of smoke detectors around. The failure to detect escaping gas is another hazard. Equip your home with gas-leak alarms as well. Loss of taste can influence the diet you select. I remember one elderly lady with worsening heart failure. She had lost her sense of taste and in order to make her food palatable would smother it with salt. This increased sodium load was too much for her weakened circulation and caused her lungs to fill with water.

Remember, then: at any age, but especially if you are sixty-five or older, it is very important to recognize a diminished sense of taste and smell, not only for what it may imply medically but because it also leaves you vulnerable to environmental dangers.

Points to Remember

Symptom: Diminished sense of taste and smell.

What It May Mean	What to Do About It
1. Natural aging process.	Make sure your home is equipped with fire, smoke and gas detectors.
2. Recent viral upper respiratory infection.	Some doctors prescribe zinc supplements. Symptoms often improve on their own.
3. Nasal polyps.	Surgery or medication.
4. Nasal decongestants.	Avoid chronic use.
5. Brain tumor—an important cause.	Surgery, radiation, chemotherapy.

INCONTINENCE: WETTING YOURSELF AT ANY AGE

It's one thing to laugh so hard that tears roll down your face, but it's not so funny when you wet your pants in the process. Neither is it a joke to find your bed damp in the morning. Involuntary loss of urine can affect anyone at any age—children, young women and the elderly of both sexes. When it's provoked by coughing, sneezing or laughing in women, we call it "stress incontinence"; in your child, it's referred to as "bed-wetting"; in middle-aged and older men, it's labeled "incontinence" and is often due to an enlarged prostate gland. Frequently the problem is only temporary and clears up on its own. More often, it requires treatment of some kind. When that fails, the individual may have to wear a diaperlike garment to soak up the consequences of the unpredictable "accident."

What causes incontinence? Even though voiding only when you want to seems simple, it's actually a complicated process that involves several different organs and nerve pathways. It all begins when the urine made in the kidneys flows down into the urinary bladder and distends it. When the bladder wall has been sufficiently stretched, nerves located within it send a message up the spinal cord to the brain saying in effect, "Let's go!" Those nerves may be diseased and unable to either receive or transmit the "full bladder" signal to the brain. And even if they do, the pathway to the brain may be interrupted by tumor, infection or injury of the spinal cord. After the message is received by the brain, it must be properly interpreted. A variety of neurological conditions, ranging from a brain tumor to Alzheimer's to stroke, can interfere with the brain's ability to do this. Nor is that all. After the signal has been received and correctly evaluated, there must be an intact and unobstructed nerve pathway going in the other direction back to the various muscles (called sphincters), instructing them to relax (and thus allow the exit of urine) and then to close (preventing incontinence). Finally, in addition to all the physical interactions among nerves, muscles and brain, there is yet a higher psychological component; just ask any man who is shy, anxious or modest what happens when he stands in front of a urinal in Yankee Stadium with a long line of beer-filled patrons behind him, even if his prostate gland is not enlarged!

So there are a host of possible explanations for incontinence. Let's look at bed-wetting first.

Your *child* may be perfectly normal in every way, perhaps even toilet-trained during the day, but, come morning, the bed sheets are soaking wet. If he or she isn't retarded and doesn't have epilepsy or some other neurological disorder, the condition will clear up on its own. Your pediatrician won't worry about the problem unless it continues beyond six years of age. Before that, chances are that the cause is psychological, not physical. The toilet-training process may have backfired and the bed-wetting may represent rebellion against parental authority. If, however, bed-wetting persists beyond age six, one is obligated to have some special tests, looking for a diagnosis that may range from neurological dysfunction to chronic infection of the urinary tract.

The most frequent cause of stress incontinence in *women* is weakness or malfunction of the urinary sphincter, a muscle which normally permits you to retain all your urine until it's convenient for you to pass it. A poorly functioning sphincter in females is usually the result of multiple pregnancies which have stretched the pelvic muscles and weakened them. This allows both the bladder and the uterus to drop (prolapse). When symptoms are bad enough, either a pessary to hold the organs up or an operation to "tighten" the muscles may become necessary. A recent report suggests that phenylpropanolamine (PPA), the drug used to control appetite, may help people with stress incontinence. Some women become incontinent after a vaginal hysterectomy, commonly done because of uncontrollable bleeding or very large, painful fibroids. (The uterus is removed through the vagina, without an abdominal incision.)

Incontinence in *males* is almost always due to an enlarged prostate. It happens this way: Normally, after a certain amount of urine accumulates in the bladder, you get the signal to void, and, if there's nothing blocking the outflow, you do so freely. But an enlarged prostate gland presses on and blocks the duct through which the urine leaves the body (the urethra), so that more and more urine accumulates in the bladder and dilates it. Even though the bladder is distended to capacity and cannot accommodate even another drop of urine, the kidney keeps making more and sending it down. This literally forces the urine out of the bladder and the urethra in small amounts, or "dribbles." Such "overflow" incontinence is something over which a man has no control.

If your prostate has been removed, the nerves controlling the urinary sphincter may have been *damaged*. That will leave you incontinent. If the gland was malignant and was treated with *radiation,* that too can interfere with the voiding mechanism.

Older persons of either sex may develop urinary incontinence for neurological, not muscular, reasons —as, for example, after a *stroke* or a spinal-cord injury. Such individuals lose urine without provocation or stress. Also in the elderly, the urinary sphincter may be weak but controllable in most circumstances. But a *diuretic* prescribed for heart failure or high blood pressure may be the proverbial straw that breaks the camel's back, leaving the individual incontinent.

Anxiety, tension and nervousness can affect your control over voiding, too, as will any inflammation or infection of the urinary tract.

So if you are incontinent, here are some ways to tell why:

- You're a man, and along with your incontinence, you have trouble emptying your bladder; when you void, the stream is thin and often split; you have to get up several times a night to urinate; it takes longer than usual to start, and when you finally do, it seems to go on endlessly; you have to strain to begin and you continue to dribble after you think you're done; a few minutes after you've left the bathroom, you feel like going again. If you have any combination of these symptoms, it's your enlarged prostate that's making you incontinent. Don't wait too long before consulting your urologist. If you do, you may damage your kidneys or you might find yourself in urinary retention—an emergency situation in which you are unable to get enough urine out of your bladder. This requires urgent catheterization. That's not always possible if it happens on an airliner or in stalled bridge or tunnel traffic.

- Have you become incontinent after a prostate operation? You expected the surgery to end your countless trips to the toilet during the night. It may have, except that you are now unable to hold your urine. The muscles controlling the sphincter that holds the urine back and releases it when convenient were damaged during the procedure. This complication is difficult to correct.

- You're incontinent, and when you urinate it feels as if you're passing hot water; your urine has a strong odor regardless of what you've been eating (you're not taking any vitamins either). You probably have a *urinary tract infection*. If your incontinence is accompanied by pain or discomfort in the lower part of the belly, the infection is in the bladder.

- You're incontinent and have rectal pain. It always feels as if you're sitting on a golf ball. The most likely diagnosis is an inflamed or infected prostate gland (*prostatitis*).
- If you're under forty years of age, male or female, and have noticed that along with your incontinence you've become somewhat clumsy, that you tend to drop things, and have trouble walking, you may have *multiple sclerosis* (a neurological disorder of unknown cause). At any age, if you need to press on your abdomen to get your urine flow started, your incontinence is due to an overextended bladder. *Diabetes* and stroke are prime culprits in this setting.
- Suppose you have low back pain and sciatica (pain shooting down the back of your hip into your leg). X rays have revealed a *bulging disc* pressing against the nerve. If one day you wake up to find your bed wet, it's probably because the disc is now also pressing on the nerves supplying your bladder.
- You've had four or five children; your last pregnancy was some years ago. You're fine except that when you cough, strain, sneeze or laugh very hard you lose some urine. The muscles made lax by childbirth have interfered with the urinary voiding mechanism.
- If you've had a stroke, your incontinence is due to damage to the area of the brain that controls urination.
- If you've had pelvic surgery followed by radiation for a tumor in the uterus, the ovary or the prostate, and several weeks or even months later you become incontinent, the nerves in the area have been injured by the radiation.

The bottom line? Any disease or disorder of the nerves or muscles, ranging from syphilis or diabetes (diabetic neuropathy) to multiple sclerosis or some other trouble within the brain can cause you to lose control of your urine. How long the problem persists and what to do about it depends on what underlying condition is eventually discovered. But generally speaking, involuntary loss of urine is usually not an emergency.

Points to Remember

Symptom: Urinary incontinence.

What It May Mean	What to Do About It
1. Bed-wetting in children: due to psychological or physical problem.	Not of concern before age six in the absence of obvious neurological disease.
2. Stress incontinence in women who've had children.	Pessary, surgical repair for lax pelvic muscles, or phenylpropanolamine.
3. In middle-aged or older men: enlarged prostate.	Surgery, drugs.
4. After prostate surgery or pelvic radiation: nerve or muscle damage.	Difficult to correct.
5. Result of a stroke.	Bladder retraining; medication.
6. Use of diuretics in the elderly.	Try to avoid.
7. Urinary tract or prostate infection.	Antibiotics.
8. Neurological disease like multiple sclerosis or Alzheimer's.	Medication or intermittent catheterization may help. Supportive care.

| 9. Diabetes, with nerve involvement. | No treatment. Self-catheterization may be appropriate. |
| 10. Disc disease. | Physiotherapy, surgery. |

WHEN PEOPLE ACT "FUNNY": NO LAUGHING MATTER

It seems to me that more people these days worry about their memory than ever before, not only the elderly but those in their forties and fifties too. They usually express their anxiety with "Doctor, I can't remember names anymore. I'll meet someone who has been part of my life for years. Her name is on the tip of my tongue, but I just can't recall it. It's happening more and more. I'm as sharp as ever in every other way. Does this memory loss mean I'm getting Alzheimer's disease?"

This concern is so real that these individuals often ask for a thorough neurological work-up. When that fails to reveal any abnormality, as is usually the case, I reassure them although I have neither an explanation nor any treatment to offer. "Senile dementia" is, however, a major problem in America today, because people *are* living longer than ever before. Still, the diagnosis of Alzheimer's is made far too often. We are too quick to apply the "senile" label to someone simply because he or she is old. Here are some other reasons an elderly individual may be acting "out of sorts":

Whenever anyone at any age begins to get "mixed up," first make sure, with a neurology consultation, that the cause is not a *brain tumor,* a *stroke* or some other neurological disease. Once these have been ruled out, there are five common nonneurological conditions to consider which mimic Alzheimer's: malnutrition, medication, depression, unrecognized head injury and chronic exposure to cold (hypothermia). These are all treatable and often reversible.

Nutrition in the elderly is often poor even in this, the most affluent nation in the world. Old persons living alone may not have the money, the energy, the motivation, the adequate eyesight or, in the case of many widowers, the know-how to prepare a decent meal. The condition of their remaining teeth may be such that chewing is a problem, and so the selection of food they can eat is narrowed further. Also, in so many urban areas, the elderly fear to leave their apartments even in broad daylight, and so don't shop often enough to buy fresh fruits and vegetables. They then become deficient in the water-soluble vitamins, especially the B group, which are so important for normal brain function. It has been shown time and again that many older individuals who are mentally "slow" bounce right back when given a healthy diet. In my view, every senior citizen, especially those living alone, should take a multivitamin supplement just to be sure. One can argue about the need for such supplementation in the general population, but when it comes to the elderly, why not play it safe? Of course, no supplement is a substitute for a nutritious diet, but it will reduce the likelihood of critical vitamin and mineral deficiencies which can cause both physical disease and mental aberrations.

Another frequently overlooked cause of mental change in the elderly is *medication*. We are a nation of pill poppers—taking "uppers" and "downers" by the millions to manage our moods, and appetite stimulants and suppressants to control weight. Many of the drugs we depend on are necessary to treat disease. But virtually every medicine, whether prescribed by a doctor or purchased directly over the counter, can affect the ability to think when taken in the wrong amount or at the wrong time, forgotten, suddenly withdrawn or combined with other drugs. Older people whose cognitive senses, especially memory and coordination, may be somewhat compromised to begin with are especially vulnerable.

Alcohol, in excess, can affect anyone's behavior, particularly the elderly. When you abruptly go on the wagon, you may develop DTs (delirium tremens), with its confusion, depression, hallucinations and physical pain. Suddenly stopping *any* "psychoactive agent" can produce similar withdrawal symptoms.

Stimulants can also affect behavior. The street term for amphetamines is "speed" and it's an appropriate one, for they do speed you up. The slang designation for coming off amphetamines, "crashing," is also accurate, because it is often accompanied by depression and confusion.

There's a whole list of *drugs* used in the treatment of psychiatric disorders that can work wonders for the patient, but that also interfere with thought processes—lithium, barbiturates, the tricyclic antidepressants and bromides. So can medications prescribed for "physical" diseases—antispasm drugs, atropine, cortisone preparations and digitalis. So whenever you witness altered behavior in anyone, think diet and drugs first.

Emotional problems can also induce or mimic dementia. I saw a brilliant lawyer a while back, a man not yet in his eighties. He had had a sterling career, was still in full possession of his faculties and yet was terribly depressed. His law firm had merged with another and he'd been "kicked upstairs," given a token title and a job that left him nothing to do. He had never developed any hobbies or interests in his life other than his work. His children had grown up and moved away. His wife had died several years earlier. He was alone and simply could not adjust to not being needed. His ego couldn't handle the fact that while there were issues and cases to which he could contribute, no one was asking his advice anymore. He became withdrawn and, in the typical vicious circle, was abandoned by his friends, who no longer found his company scintillating.

A minor cardiac problem had brought this man to my office, but it was his depression and lethargy that impressed me most. It would have been easy to attribute it all to aging. Instead, we had several long and frank discussions about his life situation. It did not really require a psychologist to understand what was going on. After developing some insight into his depression, and with the temporary aid of a mood-elevating medication, he perked up. As he began to explore new vistas for his talents, his "senile dementia" disappeared. So did his need for the "happy" pills!

It's not always easy for those who are younger and working, who are without serious financial or health problems, who aren't constantly reminded of death by virtue of their age and who have companionship, to identify and empathize with an elderly person who appears to be undergoing a personality change. Yet, if you take the time to do so, you may find that they are in fact sad, not mad.

A seemingly trivial *head injury,* one that's often not even remembered, can result in behavioral changes. The undersurface of the skull and the coverings of the brain are laced with a network of small blood vessels which become more rigid and fragile with age. Bopping your head on a cupboard door is all it takes to make them bleed. The blood forms a pocket, creating pressure on the surface of the brain. The first symptom may be a run-of-the-mill headache. You may later, however, develop several neurological symptoms, including an overall mental deterioration. Unless the possibility of trauma is considered, the proper diagnosis may never be made. And the unfortunate subject is relegated to the Alzheimer's category. I have seen this happen more than once.

I'm sure that within the nursing-home population there are those whose behavioral changes are actually due to an undiagnosed subdural hematoma (the medical term for what I've just described; "hematoma" means an accumulation of blood, "subdural" refers to its location in the skull). All it takes to detect it is a CAT scan and a high index of suspicion. The treatment is simple: cortisone (which causes the reabsorption of the blood) or sucking out the hematoma with a needle. The results are dramatic.

Another frequently overlooked cause of mental change in the elderly is *hypothermia*, chronic exposure to low temperatures. In some animals, cold weather so slows their metabolism that they hibernate, or sleep away the winter months. Well, living in an underheated apartment can also slow the metabolism and the mental function of older people. In my own practice I have occasionally discovered that the reason for a patient's personality change was a stingy landlord! Turning up the thermostat and a good hot meal worked wonders.

Certain *diseases* may be responsible for changes in mental state at any age. Youngsters with high fever may exhibit wild behavioral swings. Pneumonia is a classic cause of confusion in the elderly. If the heart or the lungs aren't working right, the brain may not receive the oxygen it needs and so the individual becomes sleepy, confused, irrational or hard to rouse. Liver trouble, kidney disease, industrial poisoning— especially with lead (it may have been lead poisoning that caused van Gogh's dementia and suicide), mercury and manganese—all can damage the brain and produce behavioral changes.

There are two special circumstances of temporary mental alterations in hospitalized patients that are a source of great anxiety to those who witness them: the *"sundowning effect"* and the disorientation after *cardiac surgery*.

A patient admitted to the hospital with a heart attack is treated with a wide variety of medications, among them powerful painkillers and sedatives. In the setting of decreased oxygen to the brain because of the injured heart, the result is confusion, disorientation, even paranoia. These symptoms are more pronounced at night, hence the term "sundowning." Many people who visit coronary patients are concerned when they see a friend or relative in this state. I can assure you that in most cases the patient will snap back once the brain recuperates from the oxygen deprivation, when the painkillers and sedatives are no longer needed, and when he or she is moved from the austere isolation of the intensive-care unit to the comfort of a regular room with more liberal visiting hours.

A similar situation occurs after heart surgery. I remember one man in his sixties who underwent a quadruple bypass. Prior to this operation he was very "well balanced," a solid individual and a distinguished educator. The surgical resident taking care of him was extremely kind and attentive. One evening, while I was visiting the patient on my rounds, he sat up, totally alert, and said, "I don't know why Dr. Jones is trying to poison me. I overheard him say he wouldn't be satisfied until I was dead."

Unlike the evening and nighttime delusions of the sundowning effect, this talk went on round the clock. His wife and family were naturally very worried about him, especially when he threatened to ask the

Police Commissioner and the Mayor of the City of New York to have the doctor charged with attempted murder. This paranoid state lasted about two weeks and then cleared completely. These patients usually don't recall their temporary derangement, but this man did. Weeks later I asked him why he had picked on that particular doctor and not, say, on a nurse, and why he had thought he was about to be murdered. He told me that many years ago in his native country he had been a member of an underground movement. He was captured by the police and imprisoned. In protest he began a hunger strike. Because of his prominence, his death would have been embarrassing to the occupying power, and so he was restrained and force-fed by doctors. Since then he has been suspicious of *all* medical personnel. He assures me, however, that I am an exception.

Here, then, specifically, are some questions to think about if you observe a mental or behavioral change in someone:

- Has it been developing over a period of months or years? If so, *Alzheimer's disease* is a possibility, but check out chronic drug use or abuse and even pernicious anemia (a deficiency of vitamin B_{12}).
- If the impairment has been gradual and protracted, but with intervals of lucidity, think of some fluctuating disorder such as liver or kidney disease, as well as a subdural hematoma.
- If the abnormal behavior waxes and wanes, a series of small strokes may be doing it. A complete neurological evaluation, including a CAT scan, will usually confirm that diagnosis.
- Has there been a recent blow to the head, however minor? Suspect a subdural hematoma.
- Was the person recently given painkillers postoper-

atively? He or she may be suffering from with-drawal.

- Are there any mood-altering drugs in the medicine cabinet?
- Can you detect alcohol on the breath in the morn-ing, slurred speech, bloodshot eyes and loss of ap-petite? Older people who continue to drink their "usual" amount may no longer be able to handle it. Two martinis at age seventy-five pack a much stronger wallop than they did at age forty-five.
- Was there a period of fever and chills before the mental changes set in? An infection anywhere may be responsible.
- Have there been complaints of headaches? Any process within the brain such as a tumor, an infec-tion or a leaking aneurysm may all produce head-aches along with the behavioral changes.
- Is the memory loss most apparent for events in the immediate past—what was eaten for breakfast, where the car keys were put—combined with an intact memory for events many years earlier? That's typical of early Alzheimer's. In advanced cases, the memory loss is only part of the picture. There's also confusion, depression and loss of bladder and bowel control.
- If the person is between the ages of twenty and fifty, look for abnormal movements and strange postures, and ask whether any family member in the previous generation was diagnosed as having *Huntington's chorea*—a genetically transmitted defect which ultimately leads to a total neurologi-cal collapse.
- Is there anything in the individual's home or work *environment* exposing him or her to lead, man-ganese, mercury or carbon monoxide? Any of these, inhaled or ingested, can cause brain dam-age.

- Have you observed a general slowing down, a yellowish tint to the skin and a deepening voice? The problem may be due to *low thyroid function.*

Points to Remember

Symptom: Memory loss, confusion and behavioral changes.

What It May Mean	What to Do About It
(*Asterisks indicate causes which affect the elderly especially.*)	
1. Anxiety, emotional problems.	Reassurance and support.
2. Primary neurological problems, e.g., brain tumor, stroke, infection.	Treat the underlying brain disorder. For recurrent stroke, aspirin.
3. Malnutrition.*	Proper diet and vitamin supplements.
4. Medication.*	Adjust dosage, change, eliminate.
5. Alcohol in excess.*	Moderation or abstinence.
6. Amphetamines and antidepressants.	Discontinue them.
7. Emotional problems.*	Psychological counseling.
8. Head injury (subdural hematoma).*	Proper diagnosis and treatment.
9. Chronic exposure to cold (hypothermia).*	Adequate heat.
10. Nonneurological diseases, especially with fever (e.g., pneumonia).	Treat the underlying cause.

11. During a heart attack (sundowning effect) or after heart surgery.	Temporary. Reassure. Avoid prolonged use of sedatives and painkillers.
12. Alzheimer's disease.*	No treatment or prevention. Sympathetic care, occupational therapy, family support.
13. Huntington's chorea.	Supportive care.
14. Environmental causes.	Modify them.
15. Low thyroid function.	Replacement thyroid hormone.

CHAPTER 6

VISION:
When the Eyes Have It

A ny change or deterioration in eyesight, from blurring to blindness, generates great anxiety. Sadly, thousands of people lose their vision needlessly every year as a result of accidents or because they couldn't be bothered to take protective measures when their eyes were in jeopardy—as when chopping wood or engaging in contact sports. Blinding accidents, however, are not what this chapter is about.

THE AGING EYE: YOUR ARMS AREN'T TOO SHORT!

If you've noticed the need to hold the print farther and farther away from your eyes in order to see what you're reading, you are probably *farsighted*. New glasses will solve the problem. If your vision is blurring, you may be developing *cataracts*. A routine eye examination will confirm that, in which event you and your ophthalmologist will decide *together* on the timing of the surgery. Either way, you can be confident that you will not lose your eyesight.

Let's focus on those conditions which may not be so obvious and which, if left untreated, can result in blindness. They range from abnormalities within the eyes themselves to some disease process deep inside the brain, such as a stroke or a tumor. They may also stem from something that has nothing to do with either the eyes or the brain. But whenever you have *any* problem with your vision, you should see, in this order, (1) your doctor, (2) an ophthalmologist and then, if necessary, (3) a neurologist.

SPOTS, BLURRING, HALOS AND DOUBLE VISION

Here is a spectrum of symptoms that can affect your vision:

- Blurred vision.
- Spots before your eyes.
- A halo effect when you're looking at an illuminated object like a streetlamp or the headlights of an oncoming car.
- A loss of peripheral vision—that is, you can see straight ahead, but only narrowly, and not on the sides.
- Double vision.
- Flashes of light or zigzagging lines.
- Blind spots.
- Intolerance to bright light.
- Bad central vision—you see best on either side.

The causes of these symptoms—and many others —generally fall into one of the following categories:

1. A local disorder of one or both eyes.
2. Weakness of the muscles that control eye movement.
3. A neurological problem within the brain.
4. A disease that is in no way related to the eyes or the brain.
5. Reaction to a medication.
6. Trauma.

In sorting out the possibilities, first look into your medicine cabinet.

- Blurring, spots and halos can all be induced by *drugs*. Several, including antidepressants, cor-

tisone, antiagitation medication (Haldol), oral
contraceptives, certain cardiac medications and
those used in the treatment of Parkinson's disease,
impair vision by increasing the pressure within the
eyes. This can aggravate preexisting low-grade
glaucoma and will result in difficulty focusing, loss
of peripheral vision, a halo effect when you look at
lights and a general loss of visual acuity.

• If you have double vision (doctors call it diplopia),
it's important to know whether it affects one or
both eyes. (Incidentally, it *is* possible to see double
with just one eye.) To determine that, close one eye
at a time. If you continue to see double, the problem is a local one in the eye itself. However, if
double vision is present only when *both* eyes are
open, then something is affecting the muscles
which move the eyes, the commonest causes being
vascular disease within the brain—usually a stroke
—myasthenia gravis, hyperthyroidism, diabetes or
a brain tumor.

• If you're forty years of age or older and have begun to see spots or *floaters* before your eyes, do
not be concerned. This is a very common symptom
in perfectly healthy older people and is due to debris in the fluid of the eye. You're more likely to
see these spots if you're myopic (nearsighted).
With time, they'll bother you less and less. *If*, however, the spots are so numerous or so large that
they interfere with your vision, see your eye doctor
(although, frankly, I don't know what he or she is
going to be able to do for you).

• If suddenly it seems as though you are seeing
showers of sparks and have a curtain drawn across
your eye, you may have suffered a *detachment of
the retina*. This often occurs in older people who
have become nearsighted. As the lens in the eye
curves, the retina behind it curls up and detaches.

See your eye doctor immediately, because early treatment with lasers can work wonders with this previously untreatable disorder.

- Has bright light suddenly begun to bother you? Many fair-skinned people go through life unable to tolerate intense lighting. However, if this symptom is new to you, it may reflect *infection, inflammation* or *injury* to the eye. It also suggests *glaucoma* and certain types of cataracts. Check it out.

- If you suddenly notice a blind spot when you're looking straight ahead and it persists for a few days, see your doctor. You may have *bled* within the eye.

- If you see spots of light, halos or zigzag patterns or have lost your peripheral vision, followed by a bad headache, you've had a *migraine attack*. These visual abnormalities will soon disappear.

- If you've suddenly noticed either intermittent or fixed double vision and you're *diabetic,* your eye muscles have been weakened by the disease. That symptom is usually temporary.

- If you are in your sixties or seventies and have had double vision for a few minutes or hours, it is probably due to either a spasm (*transient ischemic attack,* or TIA) or a closure of one of the arteries in the brain (*stroke*), especially if you also have high blood pressure. See your doctor immediately.

- If you're under forty years of age, suddenly begin to see double or have blurred vision and, in addition, have noticed some imbalance walking, the most likely cause, at least statistically, is early multiple sclerosis. Although the victims of this disease may be symptom-free for long intervals, multiple sclerosis is generally progressive over the years.

- If you're a woman in your thirties, take the Pill, smoke cigarettes, and have developed blurred or double vision, you have a *vascular problem in the brain*. While the hormones in the Pill are partially responsible, most of the blame lies with the cigarettes.

- If you're *diabetic,* you may find that some days your glasses are fine and at other times your vision is blurred. These changes are due to fluctuations in blood-sugar levels. Don't spend your money on new glasses, because no prescription will be completely satisfactory until your blood-sugar level has stabilized.

- If you suddenly become blind in one eye and your sight is not restored promptly, chances are the *central retinal artery* behind the eye has been closed off either by a blood clot or by arteriosclerosis (hardening of the arteries). *This is a medical emergency*. The moment it happens, see your eye doctor. He may be able to save your vision if you get to him early enough.

Here are other scenarios to look out for:

- You're over age fifty, every muscle in your body has been aching and stiff for days, you've been running a low-grade fever, you have no appetite and you're feeling weak. Suddenly, as if that wasn't enough, you lose the sight of one eye. You almost certainly have *temporal arteritis,* inflammation of certain arteries of the head. The diagnosis requires a biopsy and, once established, immediate treatment with cortisone. The alternative is blindness!

- If you're sixty or older, have glaucoma, diabetes or high blood pressure and begin to notice a *gradual* onset of blindness in one eye, chances are that the *central retinal vein* (as opposed to the central retinal artery) is clogged. Again this is a medical emergency for which you should see a doctor as soon as possible.

- If you're a pre-menopausal woman on the Pill and have attacks of flashing lights followed by periods of temporary blindness, you have migraine.
- If you're in your sixties or older and are losing central vision, but see best on the side, you have senile, *macular degeneration*. This is part of the aging process, and there is neither prevention nor satisfactory treatment at this time.

Vision is a priceless gift whose loss is a tragedy. Every one of the symptoms described above mandates your seeing a physician immediately.

Points to Remember

Symptom: Change in vision.

What It May Mean	What to Do About It
1. The aging process.	Proper glasses.
2. Cataracts.	Surgery.
3. Reaction to medication.	Adjust the dosage or switch.
4. Stroke or transient ischemic attack (TIA).	Supportive care, anticoagulants, aspirin.
5. Brain tumor.	Surgery, radiation or chemotherapy.
6. Floaters.	Harmless. No treatment.
7. Retinal detachment.	Laser therapy or scleral buckling.
8. Eye infection, inflammation or injury.	Antibiotics or local treatment.
9. Glaucoma.	Medication or surgery.
10. Bleeding within the eye.	Determine the cause and stop the bleeding.

11. Migraine.	Vision clears up spontaneously.
12. Complication of diabetes.	Optimum sugar control.
13. Multiple sclerosis.	No treatment.
14. Vascular problem in the brain.	Medication, surgery.
15. Closure of the central retinal *artery*.	A medical emergency.
16. Temporal arteritis.	A medical emergency.
17. Clogging of the central retinal *vein*.	A medical emergency.
18. Macular degeneration.	Laser therapy may help.

WHEN YOUR EYE DROOPS—AND YOU'RE NOT WINKING

I don't think I've ever seen anyone whose two eyes were identical in size. Examine a photograph of yourself, or, better still, look in the mirror. You're apt to see a certain asymmetry in the size of your own eyes. That's perfectly normal. But there are circumstances in which one eyelid can't be opened fully (the medical term is *ptosis*). It's sometimes present at birth (the drooping may be severe enough to require surgical correction), but usually occurs in later years.

A fallen eyelid is most commonly due to *injury of the nerve* supplying the muscles that raise it. There are several different muscles that move the eye: one set pulls it to the right, another to the left, one raises it, and so on. When one or more nerves are injured, as, for example, by a virus or a small stroke, the result is paralysis of the eye muscles they supply. If the affected one raises and lowers the eyelid, that eye will remain closed. On the other hand, the nerve supply may be intact, but the *eye muscles* themselves may be diseased. The classic example of this condition is *myasthenia gravis,* in which a substance needed to make the muscles contract after the nerves have stimulated them is missing. Other muscles are also involved, mainly in the head, the neck and the chest. When Aristotle Onassis suffered from this disease, both his eyelids were affected, and he was unable to keep them elevated except with Scotch Tape. When the missing chemical in myasthenia is replaced in the form of oral medication, the eyelids usually perk right up.

One or both eyelids can also droop when they are injured, swollen or involved in an *allergic reaction.* They also sag when they are infected by the trachoma organism, which causes blindness.

So, a variety of conditions—neurological, infectious, allergic and muscular—can all cause one or both eyelids to droop. Here's how you can tell, with your one remaining open eye, why the other is closed:

- When one of your eyelids doesn't open as widely as the other, have someone look at the pupil in that eye. If it's smaller than the one in your other eye, and the eyeball looks a little sunken, and the skin is somewhat drier than on the opposite side, you have *Horner's syndrome,* a condition caused by a tumor in the lung or the chest, an enlarged lymph gland, or an extra rib (with which some people are born), pressing on a nerve supplying that side of your face.
- If, in addition to the drooping eyelid, you also have double vision and a whopping headache, it's probably due to *migraine.* Nevertheless, the combination of drooping eyelid and headaches should

send you to a doctor immediately because a work-up may reveal a *brain aneurysm* or *tumor*.

- When the drooping eyelid is accompanied by swelling around the eye and you have muscle aches and pains, you may have been infected by the worm found in raw or improperly cooked pork (*trichinosis*). However, tumors in the eyeball itself may also cause such drooping and swelling.
- When the drooping comes and goes, you've got either myasthenia gravis or migraine.

Now, here's a coincidence. The morning after writing this section on the drooping eyelid, I was visited by a sixty-five-year-old man who had noticed a very slight drooping of his right eye. It didn't bother him and he would have ignored it except that his son-in-law is a neurologist. The latter instructed the patient to undergo a long list of tests to exclude the possibility of myasthenia gravis, brain tumor or lung cancer—all serious and ominous conditions. After a battery of expensive, time-consuming and frightening examinations, the diagnosis turned out to be "levator dehiscence." Sounds bad, but it isn't! "Levator" is the name of the muscle that raises the eyelid, and "dehiscence" simply means weakness. This man simply had weak eye muscles, with no underlying heinous cause. As we get older, muscles anywhere from our toes to our eyelids tend to weaken somewhat. So if you have a slightly drooping eyelid, don't panic. Do report it to your doctor, but not to your neurologist son-in-law.

Points to Remember

Symptom: Drooping eyelids.

What It May Mean	What to Do About It
1. Normal individual variation.	Nothing.
2. Nerve injury.	Surgical correction.
3. Myasthenia gravis.	Medication, removal of the thymus gland.
4. Allergic reaction.	Antihistamines, steroids.
5. Horner's syndrome (pressure on a nerve by a gland, a tumor or an extra rib).	Treat the underlying cause.
6. With headache and double vision: migraine, brain aneurysm or brain tumor.	Treatment depends on the specific cause.
7. With muscle aches and swelling around the eye: trichinosis.	Medication.
8. Normal aging process.	No treatment necessary.

CHAPTER 7

HEARING PROBLEMS:
Deafness, Buzzing and Noises
in Your Ears

Older people often have trouble hearing clever repartee at the theater and small talk at noisy cocktail parties. The letter *s* sounds like *f* and vice versa, key words are missed—that sort of thing. Such hearing loss is called *"sensorineural,"* or, as it is better known, *nerve deafness*. By age fifty-five, one person in four no longer enjoys completely normal hearing. But don't panic. This condition rarely progresses to total deafness, and newer hearing aids can help greatly. The onset of nerve deafness is gradual, but in this section I will also discuss the disconcerting and frightening realization that you're not just hard of hearing but actually deaf—in one or both ears. In order for you to understand the implications of these symptoms, you must first appreciate how it is we hear.

Sound waves enter into your ear canal and hit the eardrum, making it vibrate. Attached to the inner side of the drum are three little bones that wiggle in response to this vibration. Their movement, in turn, stimulates tiny nerve receptors which send the information about the noise along the acoustic or auditory nerves to the brain. For hearing to be normal, the ear canal must be clear so that it can transmit sound waves. So the most common cause of deafness in adults is a buildup of wax in the canal. In children, it may be due to something they've stuck into their ear that's the right fit and stays there, like a small toy, a jelly bean or a peanut. In both adults and children, chronic disease and infection of the lining of the canal can cause it to swell and so impair hearing.

Next, things can go wrong with the eardrum itself. It may be *scarred,* or *perforated* by infection or an injury (as when you used a toothpick or a bobby pin to dig out wax) or after a sudden sharp pressure change when the ear hasn't first been "cleared" (as happens in a rapid airplane descent or a deep underwater dive). A drum that's scarred or punctured, for whatever reason, doesn't vibrate normally and so fails to transmit sound signals as well as it should.

There may also be a problem with the tiny bones behind the eardrum. In older persons, these become *fused* and unable to wiggle independently of one another, thus failing to stimulate the nerve endings.

But even when the ear canal, the drum and the tiny bones are all intact, the sound message won't get through to the brain if there is something wrong with the nerve-transmission mechanism. It may be damaged when the blood vessels that nourish it are hardened by *arteriosclerosis* (as happens in older people) or are blocked by a tumor. Finally, if everything else is okay, the brain itself may have been injured, leaving it incapable of interpreting the signal it receives.

There are also conditions unrelated to the hearing process which can result in some degree of deafness. Patients with *very low thyroid function* usually don't hear too well. Replacement thyroid hormone restores normal hearing. *Rheumatoid arthritis* may also be associated with hearing loss. As a rule we think of this disease only in terms of inflamed joints, crippling stiffness and pain, yet rheumatoid arthritis affects many other organ systems, including the hearing mechanism. So during an acute attack or flare-up of rheumatoid arthritis, you may experience a disturbing degree of hearing loss.

Diabetes is another "non-ear" disorder in which hearing is affected. Whereas normalizing an elevated sugar improves eyesight, tight sugar control does not always restore hearing acuity in the diabetic.

If your cholesterol and triglyceride levels are too high, and especially if you're overweight, your hearing may be affected. *Kidney trouble* can also cause deafness, as can heavy *smoking,* allergies, aspirin in large doses, certain antibiotics and sensitivity to other drugs.

Here are some symptoms into which the mechanisms described above are translated. Understanding them can help you pinpoint the cause of your deafness.

- Statistically, the most common cause of sudden, *painless* loss of hearing (in you or your child) is a blockage of the ear canal by either wax or a foreign object.
- What *medications* are you taking? Large doses of aspirin, antibiotics (especially streptomycin, gentamicin and kanamycin), diuretics (ethacrynic acid) and heart drugs like quinidine may impair hearing. One of my older patients complained of worsening hearing loss which I thought was due to hardening of the arteries—until I discovered that he loved tonic water. The quinine in tonic water can cause noises in the ears (doctors call it "tinnitus") and impaired hearing in those who are sensitive to it.
- If your ears hurt and you can't hear well, you probably have an infection, either in the canal itself or inside, beyond the drum.
- If you've got a head cold, your ears may feel stuffy and your hearing won't be as acute for a few days.

This will get worse if you're foolish enough to fly with that cold, because the *eustachian tubes*, which run from the back of the throat into your middle ear, become blocked. They normally serve to equalize the pressure difference between the ear and the outside environment. When the plane descends, the pressure on your eardrums increases. In most cases, you'll experience pain for a few days, and then, as your eustachian tubes slowly open up, your ears will clear and your hearing will return to normal (unless, of course, the eardrum ruptures as a result of the pressure differential).

- If you're troubled by noise in your ears, along with your deafness, you may have *Ménière's disease,* a disorder of the labyrinth, a structure in the inner ear which monitors the body's balance and equilibrium.
- Some persons with migraine hear noises and lose their hearing before, during or after an attack because of spasm of the auditory arteries within the ears. Similar symptoms in someone without the migraine reflect arteriosclerosis and/or high blood pressure.
- If you're progressively losing your hearing and at the same time have become aware of noise in *one* ear, see your doctor right away. You may have a tumor of the main hearing nerve (an *acoustic neuroma*). It's curable by surgery.
- If you're diabetic and experience sudden deafness in *one* ear, the diabetes has probably affected your auditory nerve.
- If you've had a head injury which has left you totally deaf, dizzy, with noises in your ears, your internal hearing mechanisms have been damaged.
- Many cases of hearing loss are occupational. If your work environment is *noisy,* either use ear protection or get a new job. Don't simply assume

your ears will get used to the din—they won't. Speaking of din, turn the volume down on your Walkman headphones and ration the number of nights spent at your favorite disco.
• Deafness, sudden or gradual in onset, is frightening. If you can spot the cause, it may be reversible, controllable, avoidable or curable.

Points to Remember

Symptom: Hearing loss.

What It May Mean	What to Do About It
1. Nerve deafness: age related.	Hearing aid.
2. Wax or a foreign body in the ear canal.	Have it removed.
3. Scarred or perforated eardrum.	Hearing aid.
4. Fusion of the ear bones.	Surgery.
5. Arteriosclerosis of the auditory arteries.	Low-fat diet.
6. Low thyroid function.	Thyroid hormone replacement.
7. Rheumatoid arthritis.	Anti-inflammatory drugs.
8. Diabetes.	Sugar control.
9. Kidney trouble.	Medication.
10. Heavy smoking.	Quit.
11. Reaction to medication.	Reduce dose or switch drugs.
12. Blocked eustachian tubes.	Nose drops.

13. Ménière's disease.	Difficult to treat.
14. Acoustic neuroma (tumor).	Surgery.
15. Damage from noise.	Avoid it. Prevention is more effective than the treatment.

CHAPTER 8

THE DIGESTIVE SYSTEM:
Problems with Intake and Output

The digestive system is responsible for extracting and absorbing nutrients from the food we eat and eliminating what's left. These *intake* and *output* mechanisms involve a series of complex steps, which sometimes break down. That's why so many people visit their doctors with complaints relating to the digestive system.

In this chapter we'll be looking at some of the more common and important symptoms associated with malfunction of the intestinal tract, everything from loss of appetite to bloating and belching, from constipation to diarrhea.

LOSS OF APPETITE

Any illness—from something as trivial as the common cold to a life-threatening condition like AIDS or cancer—can wipe out a previously hearty appetite. If what you've got is curable, your appetite will return when you're cured.

In addition to disease, *medication* used for its treatment can also eliminate your interest in food. Here are some of the more commonly prescribed drugs that frequently suppress appetite. In my experience as a cardiologist (every specialist has his or her own pet agents), digitalis, vitally important in the treatment of heart rhythm disorders and weakness of the cardiac muscle, heads the list. After you've taken it for any length of time, even exactly as prescribed, it can gradually and insidiously build up to toxic levels in the bloodstream, especially in older persons. When that happens, the appetite is totally squelched. I've seen countless patients over the years with "unexplained" weight loss who were sure they had cancer. In fact it was their morning digitalis pill that was killing their appetite.

Here are some other drugs that can diminish your interest in food:

- Virtually any antibiotic.
- "Cold" preparations containing phenylpropanolamine (PPA). If you take a decongestant with PPA in it for your stuffy or runny nose, you're not apt to look forward to your next meal. This is so predictable that pharmaceutical manufacturers now market PPA purely as an appetite suppressant.
- Codeine, morphine, Demerol, indeed any painkiller, even aspirin, can do away not only with your discomfort but with your appetite as well.

The bottom line? If you're on *any* medication, whether prescription or over-the-counter, and you don't much feel like eating anymore, suspect the drug as well as the disease for which it is being taken.

Emotional upset can do away with your interest in food—you're "too nervous" to eat, or you're so sad that you forgot about lunch and dinner. Loneliness, boredom, tension, anxiety, not to mention anorexia nervosa, can all leave you totally uninterested in even the most delicious food. Failure to appreciate this association between lack of appetite and your emotional state can result in an expensive weight-loss work-up looking for some other explanation that doesn't exist.

Another major cause of decreased appetite at mealtimes is more apparent than real. I have known many overweight persons who insist that they are gaining weight despite no great desire to eat. They even bring witnesses to the office to "testify" to me how little their obese friend actually consumes. The explanation, of course, is that the pastrami sandwich "snack" at 11 A.M. and the jumbo bag of potato chips with a tin of sour-cream dip at the 4 P.M. break are what's killing the appetite at mealtime.

WHEN YOU'RE SICK TO YOUR STOMACH

Nature's way of insuring that we don't continue to suffer from past miseries is to render memory capricious. We easily recall pleasant experiences ("the good old days" that get better as the years go by), but we tend to block out those that caused us grief—physical or emotional. But an episode of nausea that was persistent and unrelenting is hard to forget. If you've ever been seasick, you know what I mean—the horrible churning and the "wish I were dead" feeling that won't go away.

Everyone has experienced nausea at some time or other—during an acute anxiety attack, food poisoning, pregnancy, hepatitis. The sickening feeling results from a very complicated interaction of signals that originate in several parts of the body. Sometimes the nausea progresses to vomiting, at other times it doesn't.

If you're nauseated, you usually know why. It may be *something you ate,* or the *chemotherapy* you're receiving for cancer; you may develop *motion sickness* while on a boat or airplane being tossed about by turbulence, or while traveling in a car in hot weather without adequate air conditioning. In this section, however, let's look at the nausea that comes on for no apparent reason. Here are some clues that may pinpoint the cause in your particular case:

- If you develop nausea when you move your head or sit up after lying flat, you probably have a viral infection of the inner ear (*labyrinthitis*), some other disorder involving the balance mechanism or a ruptured eardrum.
- *Medication,* whether it's an over-the-counter product or one prescribed by your doctor, is a common and often unsuspected cause of nausea. That new potent vitamin your friend recommended, the one that's supposed to beef up your libido or, if you're a woman, put more hair on your head and less on your face, or make you live longer and look younger, or decrease your appetite—or whatever —might just be making you sick. In my own case, the mere odor of concentrated B complex nauseates me for hours. Fish-oil capsules, currently touted as a prevention for almost every ailment from heart disease to arthritis, can also cause nausea and vomiting, especially if the oil in the capsule has become rancid.

As mentioned above, digitalis, a commonly used cardiac drug, is notoriously responsible for nausea. It does so only after prolonged use, when its concentration has built up in your bloodstream. The first evidence of toxicity is an insidious revulsion to food. Most nausea comes on or worsens when you see or smell food, but when you're digitalis-toxic just thinking about it will make you retch. Unfortunately, some people on digitalis don't know they are taking it. A "doctor" may have sold them a "miracle pill" to suppress the appetite, one of whose "secret" ingredients is digitalis! As the drug accumulates in the body, it will eliminate your desire to eat and even possibly eliminate *you* by inducing a fatal cardiac arrhythmia.

Other drugs that commonly cause nausea are

those used in the treatment of asthma (theophylline), many antibiotics, salicylates (painkillers), potassium and zinc supplements in excessive amounts, several anticancer medications (as well as radiation therapy) and cough mixtures containing codeine.

So, consider any recently prescribed drug as the culprit whenever you develop unexplained nausea, but never abruptly stop any medication before discussing it with your doctor. If after you do so you're still sick to your stomach, consider these other possibilities:

- Nausea that has plagued you intermittently over the years is probably *emotional* in origin. (Were any physical disease responsible, it would have made itself apparent.) Just being nervous or apprehensive can make you feel sick. Even seasoned performers occasionally throw up before going onstage. If your overall appetite is good, but you become nauseated immediately after eating, that's further evidence that the problem is psychogenic in origin.

- If you're a woman of childbearing age and your nausea is of recent onset and worse in the morning, consider *pregnancy,* especially if your last period ended more than six weeks ago. However, morning nausea also occurs in chronic *smokers* and in individuals with a *postnasal drip.*

- Does your nausea come on about two hours after eating fatty foods? Think of *gallbladder disease,* particularly if you are a female, overweight, forty-ish (or younger and on the Pill), have had children, are plagued with more gas than you can handle, and if your mother also had trouble with her gallbladder.

- If the nausea is associated with vomiting and severe chronic headaches, it's probably due to *mi-*

graine. A brain tumor can also cause the same symptoms but is statistically much less likely.

• If your nausea has become chronic, and is associated with pain or discomfort in your belly, you may have a peptic ulcer, a hiatus hernia, gallbladder disease or trouble in your pancreas.

• If your nausea is accompanied by vomiting and weight loss, that raises the question of either a tumor somewhere or drug intoxication (digitalis).

• The combination of acute nausea, sweating and chest pressure is typical of a heart attack in progress.

• Are you nauseated and do you have a slight fever? Have you also lost your taste for tobacco? Is there some discomfort in the right upper portion of your belly? You may have hepatitis. The jaundice, the light-colored stools and the urine that looks like tea all come later.

• When the kidneys stop working properly and toxic waste substances accumulate in the blood (uremia), chronic nausea is almost always present.

Points to Remember

Symptom: Appetite loss, nausea and vomiting.

What It May Mean	What to Do About It
1. Any illness, but especially hepatitis, cancer, kidney disease.	Treat the underlying disorder.
2. Medication.	Adjust the dosage or change the drug.
3. Emotional upset.	Supportive treatment.
4. Food poisoning.	Antinauseants.
5. Cancer therapy.	Marijuana (legally obtained) and other antinauseants.

6. Motion sickness.	Meclizine, scopolamine, Compazine.
7. Labyrinthitis.	Meclizine.
8. Pregnancy.	Self-limited.
9. Heavy smoking.	Quit.
10. Postnasal drip.	Treat the sinus infection.
11. Chronic gallbladder disease.	Low-fat diet, removal of the gallbladder.
12. Migraine.	Abort attacks with ergotamine, treat with Fiorinal.

GAINING WEIGHT FOR NO REASON

The never-ending list of new diet books and weight-reduction programs by countless "specialists" (many of whom are celebrities, not scientists) bears testimony to the widespread interest in controlling obesity and the fact that we've not yet been able to do so. Those who have trouble with their weight often insist, at least publicly, that they have no idea why, despite all their efforts to knock off a few pounds, they just can't do it. But secretly, deep down, they usually know the answer.

Part of their problem is that their weight goals are unrealistic, spawned by society's attitude toward fat people. In the Western world, thin is very much in. But not all of us can look like a model in a Diet Sprite ad no matter how hard we try. The fact is, every individual is born with unique physical characteristics, which cannot be changed no matter how hard he or she struggles to conform to Madison Avenue standards. Try to maintain a weight consistent with good health, not with a fashion model's appearance. You will find that objective much easier to achieve.

Men					Women			
Height Feet Inches	Small Frame	Medium Frame	Large Frame	Height Feet Inches	Small Frame	Medium Frame	Large Frame
5 2	128–134	131–141	138–150	4 10	102–111	109–121	118–131
5 3	130–136	133–143	140–153	4 11	103–113	111–123	120–134
5 4	132–138	135–145	142–156	5 0	104–115	113–126	122–137
5 5	134–140	137–148	144–160	5 1	106–118	115–129	125–140
5 6	136–142	139–151	146–164	5 2	108–121	118–132	128–143
5 7	138–145	142–154	149–168	5 3	111–124	121–135	131–147
5 8	140–148	145–157	152–172	5 4	114–127	124–138	134–151
5 9	142–151	148–160	155–176	5 5	117–130	127–141	137–155
5 10	144–154	151–163	158–180	5 6	120–133	130–144	140–159
5 11	146–157	154–166	161–184	5 7	123–136	133–147	143–163
6 0	149–160	157–170	164–188	5 8	126–139	136–150	146–167
6 1	152–164	160–174	168–192	5 9	129–142	139–153	149–170
6 2	155–168	164–178	172–197	5 10	132–145	142–156	152–173
6 3	158–172	167–182	176–202	5 11	135–148	145–159	155–176
6 4	162–176	171–187	181–207	6 0	138–151	148–162	158–179

Metropolitan Life Insurance Company.
Source of basic data: 1979 Build Study, Society of Actuaries and Association of Life Insurance Medical Directors of America, 1980.

You may think you're fat, but are you—really? Doctors make that judgment by measuring skinfold thickness on your back and above your elbow. Since that's something you're not likely to be doing yourself, you should refer to the latest height/weight table from the Metropolitan Life Insurance Company (above). If, according to that table, you weigh fifteen to twenty pounds more than you should for your age, height and frame, then you are indeed overweight.

Regardless of how or why it happened to you, being fat is an important risk factor for many diseases, including arthritis, high blood pressure, heart trouble, diabetes and possibly even cancer. The excess fat also makes you more vulnerable to fat embolism during an operation. Little globules of fat from tissues cut by the surgeon's scalpel get into your bloodstream and end up blocking a blood vessel in the lungs, the brain or elsewhere. That's one of the reasons I worry whenever one of my really obese patients needs an operation.

If you are in fact "hopelessly" fat, take a hard look at your lifestyle first: your *eating habits* and your level of *physical activity*. If those don't really account for it, here are some other possibilities:

• You may have *Cushing's syndrome or disease,* with too much cortisone in your body. Get some old pictures of yourself and see whether you've changed, and in what way. Cushing's produces a characteristic appearance. The weight gain is basically limited to the trunk, so that while the belly, the chest and the back are fat, the arms and the legs remain thin. This diagnosis is all the more likely if you're a woman and from time to time your menstrual flow is either sparse or absent.

• Have you gained weight and also noted a change

in your vision, or begun to have headaches? You may have a *tumor* in the area of the brain which controls appetite.

- Are you sensitive to cold, and constipated too? Has your menstrual flow become more profuse? Have you been losing your hair? These symptoms, combined with general sluggishness, point to an *underfunctioning thyroid gland*.

- Are there times during the day when you're uncontrollably hungry? Do you also have palpitations, tremors and sweating? You may have true *hypoglycemia*, a rare condition in which your pancreas is secreting too much insulin. That lowers your blood sugar and makes you hungry, so you eat more and gain weight.

- You are not only heavy but have swollen feet and shortness of breath as well. You are retaining fluid. If the swelling also involves your fingers, face and eyelids, the evidence points to *kidney trouble* as the cause. If you have difficulty lying flat in bed at night, then it's more likely to be a *cardiac* problem.

- Young women just starting on *the Pill* gain weight.

- Several commonly prescribed *tranquilizers* can put weight on you, too.

- If your doctor is old-fashioned and is treating your ulcer with lots of *milk,* which we now know is not at all good for you (because of the cholesterol) or the ulcer (because it causes the stomach to secrete even more acid), you may be putting on weight simply because of the extra calories in the milk.

- If you've stopped smoking, don't be surprised if you gain some weight in the next few weeks. But don't use this as an excuse to keep smoking. *It's much better to be fat than to smoke.* And the weight gain will soon stop. But you've got to be very careful about how much you eat—and get lots of exercise.

- Persons who are *depressed*, bereaved, sad, lonely or bored look for pleasure wherever they can find it. Food is often the solution for them. The never-ending snacking and gluttony put pounds on.

- Your *drinking habits* will also induce weight gain. One glass of beer contains 120 calories; a martini or a similar cocktail has 200 (before adding sugar, juices and soda).

- Retirees who suddenly find themselves low on funds and unable to spend as much on food as they once did now eat less expensive, *high-carbohydrate, high-calorie* meals which put on weight. This is the kind of menu they're apt to get if they live in nursing homes that are looking to cut operating costs.

I have focused, in the foregoing, on the reasons why you might suddenly or gradually be gaining weight. But then there is *constitutional obesity*—persons who have in fact been fat all their lives. In most cases, their attempts to trim down will be futile. The reason for such obesity probably lies in the genes, and although a significant and *permanent* change in lifestyle can improve matters somewhat, it rarely results in a svelte, modellike appearance. I don't believe it has anything to do with what one was fed as a child—or how much. It's probably much more likely a matter of the number and distribution of "fat cells" in the body, something beyond one's control. But if you think you're in that category, nihilistic abandonment is not the answer. You then must work even harder, in terms of dietary self-control, to prevent your obesity from getting totally out of hand.

In the final analysis, if you think you're overweight, you're not alone. By current statistics, about

40 percent of all Americans are. If it's only a matter of a few pounds, your cosmetic ambitions can usually be easily fulfilled. Any more than that may be more difficult to whittle away because of constitutional or genetic factors.

Points to Remember

Symptom: Weight gain.

What It May Mean	What to Do About It
1. Overeating.	Restraint, willpower.
2. High-carbohydrate, high-calorie diet.	Proper diet.
3. Lack of exercise.	Proper exercise.
4. Cushing's syndrome (excess cortisone production by the body).	Surgery.
5. Brain tumor (rare).	Surgery, radiation or chemotherapy.
6. Low thyroid function.	Thyroid replacement.
7. True hypoglycemia—over-secretion of insulin by the pancreas, causing hunger (rare).	Surgery.
8. Heart or kidney failure, with fluid retention.	Diuretics, other medications.
9. The Pill.	Other forms of contraception.
10. Tranquilizers.	Reduce the dosage or switch.
11. Milk diet.	Abandon it.

12. Kicking the cigarette habit.	Weight gain is temporary. Proper diet, lots of exercise.
13. Depression with compulsive eating.	Get professional help.
14. Alcohol.	Cut down.
15. Constitutional obesity.	Do the best you can.

TROUBLE IN SWALLOWING

Like breathing or blinking the eyes, we rarely give the swallowing mechanism a second thought. But in order to swallow comfortably and effectively, several very complicated mechanisms must be working perfectly and in concert. In healthy persons, the body automatically coordinates swallowing and breathing. Despite the common portal of entry, the mouth, what you swallow doesn't go to your lungs, and the air you inhale doesn't end up in the stomach. If they did, in the first instance you'd choke to death, while in the other you'd distend your stomach and burst it! Opening and closing the various pathways leading from the throat is effected by nerves and muscles. If you have trouble swallowing, the *nerves* may be damaged locally or by a neurological disease in the brain (e.g., a stroke). The *muscles* can become weak, as, for example, in myasthenia gravis. Then, too, the food pipe may be blocked by cancer or infected by a fungus, making it both painful and difficult to swallow. An autoimmune disease called *scleroderma* leaves the esophagus stiff and inflexible so that it doesn't propel the food down to the stomach as it normally does. When organs adjacent to the food pipe become enlarged, they may press on and narrow it from without. Finally, the most obvious and common cause of swallowing difficulty stems from any severe *throat infection* in which pain and swelling make it hard to swallow.

So there are many physical conditions that can interfere with your ability to swallow, some of which are potentially serious. *This symptom demands immediate medical attention.* To pinpoint the cause, your doctor may require special X rays and tests, but you can help him or her make the diagnosis sooner if you are on the lookout for and report any of the following:

- If your trouble is at the very *beginning* of the swallow, the problem lies in the pharynx (the area extending from behind your tongue down to the beginning of the food pipe). You may have a severe strep throat, tonsillitis, an abscess or a fungal infection, but nerve damage from a stroke or polio will also do it. Abnormal muscle function, as for example in myasthenia gravis, may make the initiation of swallowing very difficult, too. So can an enlarged thyroid gland pressing on your food pipe.

- If you begin to swallow normally, but then find it hard to get the food all the way down, then there's something wrong with the esophagus. It may be (a) narrowed by a tumor within it, (b) compressed by one from the outside or by enlarged glands or a dilated aorta (the main arterial trunk leaving the heart) or (c) simply not propelling the food properly.

- If you have trouble swallowing both liquids *and* solids, there's usually a major *infection* or a tumor within the esophagus. However, a neurological disorder or a loss of tone in the esophagus can produce similar symptoms.

- If you can handle solid food easily, but have trouble with liquids, the difficulty is not in the food pipe but in the nerves or muscles of the throat. If some of the liquid you try to swallow runs out of the nose, you have paralysis of the swallowing mechanism, most likely from a stroke.

- If getting solid food down gives you grief, and liquids are okay, then the esophagus itself or the area around it is mechanically blocked.

- If your throat tightens up when you're nervous or upset and you find it hard to swallow, or if you always seem to have a "lump in the throat," and a complete work-up has not provided an answer, you have an emotional disorder called *globus hystericus*. This occurs much more commonly in women than in men.

- The longer it takes, after you've swallowed, for the difficulty or discomfort to begin, the lower down the problem is. For example, if you're fine for the first fifteen seconds, but then develop a sense of obstruction, either there's some blockage in the lower part of your esophagus, near the stomach, or you may have a *hiatus hernia*, in which food regurgitates back from the stomach into the esophagus.

- If your swallowing has gotten progressively worse for weeks or months, cancer of the esophagus is a strong possibility.

- If the swallowing difficulty comes and goes, a nervous disorder or spasm is most likely. By contrast, physical blockage tends to be persistent and progressive.

- If swallowing is easier when your head is tilted back, the problem is in your pharynx, not your esophagus. Try it and see.

- When not only is it hard to swallow, but it hurts too, there may be either some reflux of acid from the stomach into the esophagus (esophagitis), a spasm, an ulcer or a scratch in the back of the throat. You may also have swallowed a chicken or

fish bone which hurt the lining of the food pipe as
it passed down.

- Do you regurgitate your food minutes or hours
after eating, especially while lying down? You have
either a loss of tone in the esophagus or a *diverticulum*—that is, a sac in its wall. The food you swallow fills the diverticulum so that you must
regurgitate in order to obtain relief. If that's your
problem, your breath may be bad because of the
decaying food in the sac.
- If you became hoarse weeks or months before the
onset of the swallowing difficulty, then the trouble
involves the vocal cords. But if it was the other
way around, that is, the hoarseness *followed* the
swallowing difficulty, that's strong evidence of a
cancer of the esophagus pressing on the nerve that
controls the vocal cords. Enlargement of the aorta
in the chest can produce similar symptoms.
- Have you a problem walking as well as swallowing? That suggests a generalized condition such as
amyotrophic lateral sclerosis (ALS, or Lou
Gehrig's disease), myasthenia gravis or some disorder in the brain.
- If you've got a swelling in your neck, an enlarged
thyroid may be pressing on the food pipe.
- If your fingers become painful when exposed to
cold and you also have difficulty swallowing, the
autoimmune disease *scleroderma* should be considered.

There are many symptoms in this book which you
may find alarming but which are actually trivial. The
swallowing disorder is not one of them. It requires a
careful work-up as soon as it is recognized.

Points to Remember

Symptom: Difficulty in swallowing.

What It May Mean	What to Do About It
1. Throat infection, tonsillitis, abscess, injury.	Antibiotics for the infections. Treat the symptoms caused by injury.
2. Nerve damage (polio, stroke, tumor).	Rehabilitation therapy.
3. Muscle disorder (myasthenia gravis).	Medical therapy.
4. Scleroderma (an autoimmune disorder).	Medical therapy.
5. Pressure on the esophagus by adjacent structures (glands, tumor, enlarged aorta).	Appropriate treatment, including surgery.
6. Disease of the esophagus (infection, tumor).	Surgery or medication.
7. Emotional disorder (globus hystericus).	Psychiatric treatment.
8. Spasm, hiatus hernia.	Medication.
9. Diverticulum.	Surgery.

JAUNDICE: YELLOW IS NOT NECESSARILY CHICKEN

Your skin has been looking a bit pasty recently. At first you pass it off because you know that skin color is a matter of how much time one spends out-of-doors and not necessarily a reflection of health status. You're further reassured by the fact that you

do go to work early in the morning and come home
late at night. Anyway, your vacation is coming up
soon, and a week in the sun will take care of the
pallor. But this morning you notice you're not just
pale or pasty-looking—you're actually yellow!

All right, so you're yellow. Does that necessarily
mean you are jaundiced? Look at the whites of your
eyes. If they are in fact yellow, you do have jaundice.
But if they are white while the rest of you is yellow-
orange, especially your palms and the soles of your
feet—then you have *carotenemia*, not jaundice. This
discoloration is common in healthy individuals with
a passion for oranges, carrots and leafy green vegetables. The pigment, carotene, in these foods discolors
the skin, making it look very much like jaundice. Although carotenemia is also present in persons with
low thyroid function, it is not in itself a disease and is
nothing to worry about.

Jaundice is the result of the staining of tissues by
bilirubin, a yellow pigment found in the red blood
cells, whose job it is to deliver oxygen to every part
of the body. Oxygen in these cells is carried by hemoglobin, which is made up of bilirubin and iron. Red
blood cells normally survive for about 120 days, after which they are destroyed by the spleen (located in
the upper left portion of your belly). This organ un-
cannily weeds out those red cells that are 120 days
old. When it does so, the hemoglobin molecule is
broken down into its two components, bile pigment
and iron, which then recirculate in the bloodstream.
The bile pigment goes to the liver, where it is pro-
cessed so that it can be used again, and it ends up
reuniting with the iron in the bone marrow, where
new red blood cells are made. Nothing is wasted.
Everything is recycled.

This perfect mechanism can be thrown out of
whack in two ways, both of which result in *too much*

bilirubin hanging around in the blood. In the first, the blood cells are destroyed sooner than every 120 days. So now there's a lot of extra bilirubin and iron in the circulation. Or something goes wrong with the liver so that it can't handle even the normal amount of bilirubin presented to it for reprocessing.

When red blood cells break up prematurely, the condition is called *hemolytic anemia*. It can be due to drugs, severe infections, allergy, autoimmune disorders (the immune system goes haywire and views the red blood cells as invaders, attacking and destroying them) and malaria (the parasite causing the disease actually gets into the red blood cells and breaks them up). Someone with hemolytic anemia has too much bilirubin in the circulation even for a healthy liver to process. The excess seeps out of the blood and into the tissues, including the skin and the eyes, staining them yellow.

When the *liver* is damaged—by drugs, tumors, viruses or other infections, or by chemical injury—it is unable to deal with even normal amounts of bilirubin in the bloodstream. So the pigment, with nowhere to go, accumulates in the blood and, again, leaks out into the tissues to cause jaundice.

Finally, the liver may be perfectly capable of processing all the bilirubin delivered to it, but the ducts through which it leaves the liver are blocked by gallstones or a cancer in the area (usually the pancreas).

So the main causes of jaundice are (a) abnormal breakdown of hemoglobin, (b) liver disease and (c) blocked bile ducts. The correct diagnosis, in any case, is made on the basis of the physical exam, blood tests, X rays and what you tell your doctor. You can get a pretty good idea yourself of what's causing your jaundice by making the following pertinent observations:

- Check your medicine cabinet. *Drugs* can induce jaundice in several ways: they can impair the liver's ability to process bilirubin; they can cause the bile ducts to swell and become obstructed; they can sensitize red blood cells so that the spleen destroys them earlier. The list of potential offenders is long and includes such antibiotics as erythromycin and sulfa drugs, several antidepressants, anticancer drugs, Aldomet (used in the treatment of high blood pressure), the anti-TB drug rifampin, steroids, antidiabetic drugs (chlorpropamide, tolbutamide), oral contraceptives, testosterone (the male hormone) and propylthiouracil (for the control of an overactive thyroid gland).
- Have you done your floors recently? The cleaning fluid carbon tetrachloride can produce liver damage if its fumes are inhaled in an unventilated space or if, heaven forbid, it is swallowed.
- The combination of *sudden* onset of both jaundice and anemia suggests either hemolytic anemia, viral hepatitis, gallstones obstructing the ducts or some chemical injury to the liver. If, on the other hand, the yellowish discoloration came on very gradually and is getting deeper all the time, there may be a tumor in the area (usually of the pancreas), cirrhosis (scarring of the liver in alcoholics or those who have had severe hepatitis) or a variety of other liver diseases.
- Do you have fever, chills and colicky pain in the right upper portion of your belly? Then the jaundice is due to a gallstone lodged in or passing through a liver duct.
- Have you recently eaten raw mussels, oysters or other shellfish, or have you been traveling in a country where the sanitation leaves something to be desired? You probably have contracted hepatitis A—the benign type that almost always clears up

without causing any serious permanent liver damage, but which will leave you jaundiced for some days.

- Are you an *intravenous drug user,* have you been tattooed or had any kind of injection using nondisposable needles whose cleanliness was in question? If so, and especially if you also have aching joints, then you probably have hepatitis B, the serious form of viral injury to the liver.
- Have you had a *blood transfusion* in the past few weeks or months? You may have contracted "non-A non-B" hepatitis, virtually the only kind you can now get from transfused blood.

Beyond these questions, there are some simple observations you can make at that point to the mechanism causing your jaundice:

- If the intensity of your jaundice fluctuates from day to day, there is intermittent obstruction from gallstones.
- If your urine is of normal color, chances are you have hemolytic anemia, but if it is the color of tea or mahogany, think of liver disease or obstructive jaundice.
- Stools that are very light in color or almost white indicate obstructive jaundice (because the normal brown color of the stool is due to bilirubin, which now cannot get out of the liver and into the gut).
- Are you nauseated and have you lost your taste for cigarettes? Normally I would applaud anything that got you to quit smoking, but an aversion to tobacco along with jaundice indicates viral hepatitis.
- Have you lost several pounds in the last few weeks? That's bad news when associated with jaundice, for it may reflect an underlying malig-

nancy, in either the liver, the pancreas or adjacent organs.

• Is your belly swollen? The presence of fluid in the abdomen suggests the diagnosis of cirrhosis of the liver, especially if you're an alcoholic or have previously had hepatitis B.

The diagnosis of what's causing jaundice is not always easy to make. Nevertheless, most cases fall into one of the categories I've listed above, and the questions and observations I have suggested can help you narrow the cause down to one category or another.

Points to Remember

Symptom: Jaundice.

What It May Mean	What to Do About It
1. Hemolytic anemia (destruction of red blood cells due to infection, allergy, autoimmune disease, drugs, malaria).	Cause must be determined and treated.
2. Liver disease (infection, chemical injury, tumor, drugs).	Diagnose and treat.
3. Obstruction of bile ducts by infection, tumor, gallstones.	Usually surgery, occasionally antibiotics. Depends on cause.
4. IV drug use.	No treatment.
5. Recent blood transfusion.	No treatment.

CONSTIPATION: WHEN THE GOING GETS HARD

At best it's a love affair, at worst a preoccupation—Americans and their bowels. When I ask patients, "Tell me about your bowels," I receive answers like "Beautiful," "Marvelous," "Fantastic" and "Wonderful." These people are obsessed with and love to discuss the frequency, quality and color of their stools with anyone who'll listen, even during lunch! At the other end of the spectrum is a minority that won't so much as glance at what's in the toilet bowl.

Regardless of the category into which you may fall, there are times when you will wonder and worry about being constipated. Of course, the perception of what constitutes constipation also runs a broad spectrum—from those who are panicked if they miss a single movement to others who pay no attention to their elimination for days on end.

Here are some guidelines for those who are not bowel "mavens." First off, the *daily* bowel movement is not a rule written in stone. Patterns vary from person to person, depending on what you eat, how much, when you eat it, your metabolism, elimination habits established in childhood, the amount of water you drink and what medications you may be taking. Some healthy people evacuate regularly and "normally" every two days, others twice a day and the majority probably once a day.

So when I refer in these pages to constipation, I mean a *change* in your usual pattern. For example, for years you've gone like clockwork every morning after breakfast, and suddenly things are different. Now you sometimes wait for a couple of days and then your stools are like pellets, or hard, or have lost their normal diameter and look like ribbons. At that point you're entitled to say you're constipated.

In order to appreciate the significance of constipation, you must understand the process of elimination. Food you swallow goes from your esophagus (food pipe) into the stomach. Here some of the nutrients your body needs are extracted and absorbed into the bloodstream. What's left then enters the small intestine, where the digestive process continues. The residue—that which your body cannot use —enters the large bowel, where water is added (from the wall of the bowel) to give the waste material a smoother ride down and out. The final staging point before departure is the rectum. When the stool reaches this lowest part of the colon, it distends it. That sends nerve signals to your brain telling you it's time to sit down and eliminate.

Any alteration in bowel movements results from a breakdown, either temporary and trivial or permanent and serious, in this orderly sequence. For example, your bowel can be made sluggish by disease (such as *underactive thyroid*) or some medicine you're taking (the *codeine* in your cough syrup). The waste material then has a slower trip down and out, and the net result is enough delay to cancel that day's movement. If you're *dehydrated*, the stool will likely be dry, fragmented and evacuated in pellets, because the bowel lacks the water with which to soften it. A *growth* in the large bowel obstructing the pathway will constipate you and also narrow the caliber of the stool. If, like so many people, you continually ignore your rectum's signal to "sit down," you're asking for trouble. The nerves in your rectum will become "lazy" and require more and more distention before sending the evacuation message to the brain.

Those are the basic things you should think about when you're constipated. Here are some additional clues to help you determine the nature and significance of your problem:

- Is your constipation associated with alternating attacks of diarrhea? If it is, tell your doctor about it. He will want to look for some obstruction—a *polyp* or a *tumor*—in the colon. Although this combination of constipation and diarrhea is usually an ominous sign, it sometimes occurs in diabetics as well as in persons with *irritable bowel syndrome*.

- Have you been able to pass gas that day? If not, your bowel may be completely obstructed and you may have a surgical emergency on your hands. But under those circumstances, you'll experience considerable belly pain and distention.

- If your constipation is an old and recurring story, probably because of a *low-fiber diet* and inadequate fluid intake, then you have a chronic disorder like a "laxative colon"—one that has been whipped by increasing amounts of laxatives. You may also, of course, have irritable bowel syndrome.

- Here are some prime suspects among medications that induce constipation: those that contain morphine and codeine; verapamil (a calcium channel blocker used in the treatment of high blood pressure, angina and cardiac-rhythm disorders); any of the beta blockers (usually prescribed for the same reasons as calcium channel blockers, but they can also cause diarrhea); various sedatives and tranquilizers; calcium supplements, especially the carbonate variety (to prevent osteoporosis); and several different antacids.

- Do you have the urge to go, but when you try you give forth no more than a little gas? You're probably guilty of having neglected the "call to action" too frequently in the past and now your rectum, although distended, needs more stool within it to effect evacuation.

- In addition to your being constipated, have your stools changed in shape and diameter? If their width is persistently narrow so that they look like ribbons, there may be an obstruction low down in the bowel. One always hears that "ribbonlike" stools indicate cancer. Let me assure you that they also occur when the bowel is simply irritable, in which case their width fluctuates.
- If you're constipated, look at the color of your stool. Blood streaks on the outside usually point to hemorrhoids or a fissure in the anus (but a cancer can sometimes fool you that way); a mucus cover without blood suggests an irritable colon; if the stool has blood mixed throughout it, then a tumor is suspect. Stools black as night and tarlike in consistency indicate the presence of bleeding high up in the intestinal tract (such as might occur from an ulcer or from erosion of the stomach lining by alcohol, excessive aspirin or related drugs).
- If it hurts when you move your bowels, chances are you've got large hemorrhoids around the anus or a tear in the surrounding skin.
- When you finally do move your bowels, do you feel that there's some left behind? Although that's often the case in chronic constipation or irritable bowel, you may be sensing a tumor low down in the bowel or the rectum.
- When constipation is accompanied by weight gain, suspect underfunction of the thyroid gland. The lowered metabolism slows the propelling contractions of the bowel and is also responsible for the extra pounds.
- If you are constipated and *losing* weight, think of a tumor first. But don't panic. Tension or anxiety may account for a change in bowel habits, too, and can also interfere with appetite.
- Have you been experimenting with a new diet? If

you suddenly revolutionize your eating habits—
and especially if you cut down your intake of fiber
—you may end up constipated. One of my patients
decided to try to reduce by eliminating breakfast in
the morning. She lost three or four pounds within
two weeks and was delighted. But then she became
constipated. For years, breakfast, which always included some bran, had triggered her bowel movements each morning. Now the signal came later in
the day, after lunch. But her busy routine as a
teacher made it difficult for her to accommodate
the urge at that time, and so she attended to it
when it was convenient. As a result, she became
constipated.

- Lack of *exercise* or confinement to bed for whatever reason can also cause constipation. If you're
  laid up, it's perfectly reasonable for you to take a
  stool softener (like Colace) until you're back on
  your feet.
- If your constipation is accompanied by more frequent urination, a growth in the rectum may be
  pressing against your urinary bladder (which is
  nearby), making you feel that you have to empty
  it, even when you don't.
- If your constipation is accompanied by a *decrease*
  in the number of times you void, you may have a
  disorder of the *spinal cord* affecting both your
  bowel function and your bladder contractions.

Let's stop here. There are many possible causes of
constipation, but the possibilities listed above account for about 95 percent of cases. The bottom line:
Don't become preoccupied with your bowel habits,
but don't ignore an obvious and persistent change
either.

Points to Remember

Symptom: Constipation.

What It May Mean	What to Do About It
1. Poor bowel habits.	Heed the call of nature.
2. Inadequate fiber and water intake.	Eat 30 grams of fiber and drink 8 glasses of water daily.
3. Medication (codeine).	Use nonconstipating medications whenever possible.
4. Sluggish thyroid function.	Thyroid hormone replacement.
5. Dehydration.	Water and other fluids.
6. Colon polyp or tumor.	Surgery.
7. Irritable or inflamed bowel.	Medication, antispasmodics.
8. Lack of exercise.	Start up again.
9. Spinal-cord malfunction.	Treat the cause.

DIARRHEA: WHEN RUNNING IS NOT GOOD FOR YOUR HEALTH

Chronic diarrhea is a way of life for many people because of an "irritable" bowel over which they have no control; enzyme deficiencies interfering with the digestive process; they may be diabetic, have food allergies or intolerance, an overactive thyroid or disorders of the pancreas; inflammatory bowel disease (either ulcerative colitis or Crohn's disease); a portion of the intestine may have been surgically removed; or the lining of the gut may be diseased so that absorption of food is impaired. You can tell what your diarrhea is due to by the following characteristics:

- When an infant has persistent diarrhea because the food goes right through the bowel and out, he or she is probably suffering from some disorder of absorption like celiac disease, in which the intestinal lining is abnormal and does not accept the nutrients delivered to it.

- If the diarrhea is chronic but intermittent—some days the stools are normal and at other times they're loose and watery—the diagnosis is an irritable colon, inflammatory bowel disease or intolerance to some food.

- If the diarrhea alternates with bouts of constipation (and assuming you're not a laxative junky), then a tumor of the colon must be considered—and soon! But remember, irritable colon and long-standing diabetes can also cause this diarrhea/constipation cycle.

- If the diarrhea never relents and you rarely have a firm movement, your thyroid gland may be overactive. In that case, there will be some other evidence of this disorder—nervousness, irritability, rapid pulse, insomnia, palpitations, intolerance to heat and excessive sweating. But such chronic diarrhea in a teenager is most often due to inflammatory bowel disease, infection or malabsorption.

- You may be lactase deficient—a very common disorder in which otherwise healthy individuals lack the enzyme lactase, needed to digest the lactose in milk and milk products. When they consume lactose in any form and in sufficient amounts, they end up bloated with gas and diarrhea. A change in diet miraculously effects a "cure."

- If the diarrheic stool looks greasy, is foul-smelling and floats, it almost certainly contains excessive fat —the result of its poor absorption in the small bowel.
- Clear mucus mixed with the stool reflects an irritable colon. In ulcerative colitis, there is actual pus. The presence of blood with or without mucus is an indication of anything from an irritable bowel and inflammatory bowel disease to chronic dysentery, cancer, polyps and diverticulitis.
- If the diarrheic stool contains neither pus nor blood, you may simply have an irritable bowel. The number of movements is important, too. Fewer than six a day suggests that the problem is originating higher up in your gut, perhaps because of poor absorption in the small intestine; more than six points to trouble lower down, somewhere in the large bowel or the rectum, especially if you have to go urgently each time.
- When loose movements occur mostly in the morning, an irritable or nervous bowel is likely. If you're awakened at night, an overactive thyroid, diabetes, ulcerative colitis or Crohn's disease should be considered.
- Your weight is a significant indicator of what's going on. If you've had diarrhea for a while and your weight is stable, you probably have lactase deficiency or a food allergy. But if you've lost weight, then cancer, an overactive thyroid gland and inflammatory bowel disease are possibilities, especially if you began to do so before the onset of the diarrhea.
- Chronic diarrhea may reflect a disease that doesn't primarily affect the bowel. For example, there is a tumor called "carcinoid" which secretes a hormone that causes cough, diarrhea and intermittent

flushing of the skin. Such tumors must be removed because of their potential to spread.

• Persons with chronic lung disease and cystic fibrosis may also have diarrhea.

Obviously, if you've had normal bowel function all your life and *suddenly* get the "runs," there are other possibilities. It doesn't take a medical Sherlock Holmes to make the association between these symptoms and a recent trip to Asia, Africa, Latin America —indeed, almost anywhere away from home. Or if, along with the diarrhea, you vomit too and develop aches and pains all over, a viral infection or acute food poisoning is probably the cause.

Many drugs can trigger diarrhea. The most common are laxatives, antibiotics (which kill off the normal bacterial inhabitants of the bowel and result in an overgrowth of contaminant bacteria—and diarrhea), digitalis, quinidine, oral agents for reducing blood sugar, antacids, high-blood-pressure medications, cholesterol-lowering drugs, anticancer agents, colchicine (therapy for acute attacks of gout) and radiation treatment to the bowel.

If there's still any question concerning the category into which you fall, here are some additional clues:

• If the diarrhea appeared almost immediately after eating, tainted food probably made you sick. You've been poisoned not by the bacteria themselves, but by the noxious material they've released into the spoiled food. If you were dining out with friends, check with them to see whether they were also affected. But if the symptoms did not begin for at least twelve hours after you ate that custard or cream pastry, chances are you've got bacterial food poisoning.

• If you can't make any association between what

you ate and your intestinal symptoms, then chances are you've got a viral gastroenteritis. This is usually short-lived and will clear up within a couple of days regardless of what you do about it.

- Was it something you drank? I have several patients who develop diarrhea after consuming certain kinds of alcohol or wine.
- Do you habitually eat undercooked pork? Trichinosis can cause diarrhea.

The appearance of the stools may provide additional clues to the cause. For example:

- If there is mucus with or without blood, some infection of the gut is possible.
- If the stool is watery, the cause is likely to be either a virus or infection by "giardia"—a bug made famous a few years ago when it contaminated the Leningrad water supply. It has since appeared in other cities and rural communities throughout the world.
- If there's a greenish hue to the loose stool, you're probably dealing with salmonella contamination (but giardia can also result in a greenish tinge). Salmonella infection has become a real problem in this country because of the antibiotics given to livestock to help promote their growth. After prolonged treatment, the harmless bacteria normally present in these animals become resistant to antibiotics. When they get into the human digestive system, they cause diarrhea which is difficult to treat.
- Fever accompanying diarrhea usually indicates infection. When nervous persons get diarrhea, they do not have fever.

If you develop diarrhea which doesn't clear up, don't just keep treating yourself with Lomotil, Imodium, Kaopectate or any of the other antidiarrheal preparations with the hope that it will go away. Tell your doctor about it. Diarrhea continuing for more than two or three weeks may be due to a variety of causes. Topping the list are inflammatory bowel disease, bacterial infection, some medication you're taking, or a worm, an amoeba or another parasite you've picked up. Once the critter is found (and it may take repeated stool cultures to identify it), appropriate treatment will clear your symptoms.

When the rest of you is okay and diarrhea is the only complaint, the cause is usually among the clues I've listed above. But after all is said and done, the most frequent reasons for diarrhea in our society are stress and laxative abuse.

Points to Remember

Symptom: Diarrhea.

What It May Mean	What to Do About It
1. Anxiety, stress, irritable bowel syndrome.	Emotional adjustment with professional help, if necessary. Antispasmodics, dietary manipulation.
2. Inflammatory bowel disease.	Medication (antispasmodics, Azulfidine, steroids), surgery.
3. Malabsorption syndrome.	Diet or enzyme replacement.
4. Removal of a portion of bowel.	Diet.
5. Food allergies.	Identify and avoid.
6. Hyperthyroidism.	Treat the thyroid disorder with radioactive iodine, medication or surgery.

7. Disorders of the pancreas.	Appropriate treatment, enzyme replacement.
8. Cancer of the bowel.	Surgery.
9. Medication.	Avoid, change or reduce the dosage.
10. Infection (dysentery, parasites).	Medication; antibiotics in some cases.
11. Diabetes.	Supportive care, blood-sugar control (not always successful).
12. Lactase deficiency.	A change in diet; lactase supplements.
13. Cystic fibrosis.	Medication, enzymes.
14. Food poisoning.	Symptomatic treatment.

CHAPTER 9

THE RESPIRATORY SYSTEM:
Is Breathing a Problem?

The movement of air in and out of the lungs, how easily you breathe, what happens to the oxygen you inspire once it reaches the lungs, how well the vocal cords work—all this and more relates to the respiratory system. And we hardly give it a second thought, unless something goes wrong.

In this chapter we're going to consider a potpourri of respiratory phenomena and what they may mean —not only how you breathe and why you cough, but also the kind of snoring you do and what may be wrong when you lose your voice.

CHRONIC COUGH: CIGARETTES, A COLD OR CANCER?

Coughing is the body's way of getting rid of "stuff" that has accumulated in your air passages. The respiratory tract starts high up in your windpipe and ends in your lungs. Every day a small amount of mucus is produced by the cells that line this tract. This mucus keeps the airways moist and traps any particles you have inhaled before they get into your lungs. Even though mucus is being made constantly, it doesn't normally accumulate, because it's continually swallowed in small amounts during the day. But when an excessive amount is produced in response to an infection or an irritation, you expel it by coughing. The appearance of what you spit up is important: white phlegm indicates simple irritation; a yellow or green color suggests infection; and red, of course, means blood.

You'll also cough if you inhale some substance or object. Ever had a piece of food "go down the wrong way"? You start coughing in an instant, reflexively. Most reflexes can't be controlled. When your doctor taps your knee with a reflex hammer, just try to hold back the kick! The sneezing reflex is partially controllable—you can often delay or abort it; but a cough is almost always manageable, at least for a while. The only time it can't be stopped is when your lungs are exposed to an immediate danger such as when you swallow something "the wrong way" or inhale irritant fumes.

A cough may last for just a few days if you have a cold, or continue indefinitely if you suffer from *chronic bronchitis*. (The main air passages going to your lungs are called "bronchi"; "itis" is a generic suffix meaning irritation or infection. So bronchitis is an irritation or infection of the bronchi.) When a cough persists for more than four weeks in anyone at any age, it *must* be evaluated. While periodic coughing is normal, a chronic cough is not, unless it is due to a nervous habit. It can mean something as ominous as *lung cancer*.

In the past year or two, several of my patients developed a persistent dry, nonproductive cough—that is, one in which they spit nothing up. They had no fever, they weren't smokers, their sinuses were okay—yet they coughed. They all, however, were taking a fairly new medication called an *ACE (angiotensin-converting enzyme) inhibitor*. The four brands now on the market in the U.S. are captopril (Capoten), enalapril (Vasotec) and lisinopril (Zestril, Prinivil). ACE inhibitors are effective in the treatment of high blood pressure and chronic heart failure, but in some patients they do cause a dry cough.

Unless you and your doctor are aware of this peculiar side effect, you may hack for weeks on end without relief.

There are some people who cough when they're under *stress.* You can tell it's psychological, because it disappears when they sleep. Chronic cough due to most other causes persists or even worsens at night.

A chronic cough may also be due to an *enlarged uvula.* That's the little tonguelike structure hanging in the midline in the back of your throat. When food or liquid comes into contact with the uvula, it triggers a muscular contraction which propels the substance toward the esophagus. But when the uvula becomes too big and stays that way (sometimes it swells briefly during an allergic reaction), it can repeatedly trigger a cough and require surgical removal.

If you have allergic or infectious *asthma,* in which the major airways go into spasm periodically, you will cough and wheeze.

Another cause of cough is *cardiac failure.* If your heart is too weak to pump out all the blood that is returned to it, the excess backs up into the lungs, filling them with "fluid." You're then unable to lie flat without coughing or shortness of breath.

Here are some useful pointers to help you determine why you are coughing, but be sure to see your doctor anyway. This symptom is too important to ignore or self-diagnose.

- If you've been coughing for three or four days and have fever, it's probably due to an acute *respiratory tract infection.* If it persists beyond two or three weeks, it is, by definition, chronic. You must then consider the possibility of a lung tumor, especially if you're a smoker.
- Years ago *tuberculosis* was much more common

than it is today. With the advent of specific antibiotics, its incidence has dropped dramatically. Now for a variety of reasons—an older population with impaired immunity, AIDS, crowded living conditions—TB is on the rise again. So whenever a cough persists or appears in an older person living in a nursing home, the diagnosis of tuberculosis must be considered.

- When somebody has been coughing on and off for several years and lung cancer and TB have been ruled out, then smoker's cough, chronic bronchitis and a disease called *bronchiectasis* must be considered. This last is a weakening of the walls of the air passages complicated by severe infection within the lung, triggering an ongoing production of foul-smelling sputum mixed with blood.

- Did the cough come on suddenly? Is it dry, that is, you don't spit anything up? While any acute process ranging from a cold to viral pneumonia can start that way, in a child you must consider the possibility that he or she has inhaled some small object like a peanut, a jelly bean or a piece of a toy, partially obstructing the air passages.

- If you started coughing suddenly, have some pain in your chest and varicose veins in your legs, and your calves are tender, the cough may be due to a *blood clot* to your lung. This is especially likely if the cough is accompanied by a slight fever and your sputum is tinged with blood.

- If you've been coughing up varying amounts of colored phlegm for several months, you've probably got chronic bronchitis. If it's as much as half a cup of greenish foul-smelling sputum, then you may have a *lung abscess* (a chronic infection within the lung that has become walled off and cannot easily be reached by antibiotics). If the stuff you cough up is clear or white, the cause is more likely to be due to irritation from pollution, a virus or even cancer, rather than bronchitis or another infection.

- A cough that produces frothy pink-tinged sputum and is accompanied by a marked shortness of breath (you feel as though you're drowning) signals pulmonary edema, which occurs when your lungs fill with fluid due to heart failure.
- Sputum that is rust- or coffee-colored and jellylike in consistency is classic evidence of pneumococcal *pneumonia*. You'll also have pain in the chest, as well as fever.
- *A cough that produces blood in any form should be treated as an emergency.* Just so you know, however, strenuous coughing can rupture small vessels in the back of your throat and cause bleeding. That's not serious, but you have to check it out anyway.
- A chronic cough without sputum suggests a tumor, heart disease or a nervous habit, or is a side effect of one of the new ACE-inhibitor drugs.
- A dry cough accompanied by pain in the center of your chest probably means acute laryngitis or tracheal bronchitis. Conversely, a deep loose cough is originating in your lower respiratory passages or lung (often an infection and a cough will begin high up in the throat and then spread down into the lungs).
- If you hurt when you take a deep breath, and you're coughing, you have *pleurisy*. The pleura which form an envelope that surrounds the lungs can become affected in the early stages of pneumonia, by lung cancer or by a virus.
- The combination of cough and profuse night sweats suggests tuberculosis.
- Weight loss and cough raise the specter of cancer of the lung. These same symptoms, along with se-

vere shortness of breath, are also characteristic of the fatal opportunistic lung infection that affects AIDS patients.

- Cough and hoarseness together are a bad combination and point to the possibility of a tumor.
- If you wheeze when you cough, you probably have chronic bronchitis and/or asthma.
- Loss of consciousness induced by coughing sometimes occurs in those patients with chronic bronchitis who are overweight, big smokers and heavy drinkers.
- What kind of work do you do? If you're a coal miner with a cough, the connection is obvious, but chronic exposure to any *dust* can give you an occupational hack.
- Do you have a pet bird, or do pigeons roost on your windowsill? You may have *psittacosis,* a lung infection spread by birds. Fungus infections of the lungs also cause coughing.
- Do you have a new cat or dog, or have you recently moved into an apartment, or bought new bedding, new clothes or a new rug? You may well be *allergic* to any one of these. Or you may have an allergic reaction to airborne pollen ("hay fever"), dust, mold, mites or somebody else's tobacco smoke.

Remember this: Every cough must be explained, especially if it lasts longer than three or four days. It's dangerous to assume that it is simply due to your pack-a-day habit and let it go at that.

Points to Remember

Symptom: Chronic cough.

What It May Mean	What to Do About It
1. The tail end of a cold.	Patience, and cough syrup.
2. Chronic bronchitis, laryngitis or tracheitis.	Antibiotics, stop smoking.
3. Lung cancer.	Surgery, medication, radiation.
4. ACE inhibitors (taken for heart failure or hypertension).	Switch to another medication.
5. Stress.	Learn to deal with it.
6. Enlarged uvula.	Antihistamines, surgical removal.
7. Asthma.	Bronchodilators, steroids.
8. Heart failure.	Diuretics, low-salt diet, digitalis.
9. Respiratory infection (viral, bacterial, TB).	Appropriate antibiotics.
10. Bronchiectasis.	Antibiotics, drainage.
11. Foreign object (especially in children).	Remove.
12. Blood clot to the lung.	Anticoagulants.
13. Lung abscess.	Antibiotics.
14. Pneumonia.	Antibiotics.
15. Pleurisy.	Treatment depends on the cause.
16. Opportunistic fungus infection due to AIDS.	A variety of experimental drugs.

17. Chronic exposure to dust.	Protective masks.
18. Psittacosis.	Medication.
19. Allergy.	Modify the environment; antihistamines.

SHORTNESS OF BREATH: OUT OF OXYGEN OR JUST PLAIN NERVOUS?

As you sit in your chair comfortably reading this book, your body is going through a myriad of biological and chemical processes of which you are unaware: your heart is beating, your eyes are blinking and, of course, you're breathing. Although breathing can be controlled voluntarily, we just let our body take care of it for us most of the time. Imagine having to remember to breathe fifteen or sixteen times a minute! But occasionally, you may feel the *need* to breathe—to take conscious control of your respirations because it doesn't seem as if you're getting enough air. In other words, you feel "short of breath." That's most likely to happen after a workout. It's perfectly normal to be breathless just after you've swum several lengths or climbed six flights of stairs. Shortness of breath can also accompany anxiety, stress, tension or depression.

Hyperventilation is a nervous habit which leaves you feeling as if you're short of breath. You find yourself breathing deeper and deeper in an attempt to be satisfied. But you never are, and it becomes a vicious cycle. This "air hunger" upsets the normal balance of oxygen and carbon dioxide in your blood, which results in generalized tingling, lightheadedness and even fainting. The tendency to hyperventilate is related to stressful life situations and is usually short-lived, or is improved after explanation, reassurance or tranquilizers. However, you can experience relief by breathing in and out of a paper bag. Rebreathing in this way replaces the missing carbon dioxide and helps restore the proper chemical balance in the blood.

But shortness of breath can be more than a normal response to exertion or a manifestation of anxiety. It may also signal a real lack of oxygen. In order for the body to receive adequate oxygen, there must, of course, be enough of it in the air you breathe. If you were suddenly transported to the summit of Mount Everest (actually, any peak over sixteen thousand feet or so will do) or if the pressurization in the plane you were traveling in broke down, you'd have a hard time catching your breath.

When sufficient oxygen is available, you've got to be able to get it into your lungs. If there is some obstruction in the air passages, you'll be short of breath. Even when enough oxygen does make it to the lungs, it may not get into the blood, its ultimate destination, because too much *lung tissue* is diseased (by emphysema, for example), infected (by pneumonia) or damaged (by a large blood clot) or has been surgically removed (because of a tumor). Under these circumstances, there is not enough pulmonary tissue to interface with the blood vessels waiting to receive the inspired oxygen.

Now, if there is lots of oxygen around, and your lungs are fine, you may still be short of breath if your *heart* isn't working properly. For although the oxygen can reach the bloodstream from the lungs, the cardiac muscle lacks the strength to pump enough oxygen-rich blood to the rest of the body. That can happen suddenly in an acute heart attack, or gradually as a damaged heart gets weaker and weaker. Or your heart may be fine, but if you are severely *anemic* and lacking in red blood cells which carry and discharge the oxygen, you will be short of breath. Also, the number of *red blood cells* may be sufficient, but there's something wrong with them so that they do not bind or release the oxygen normally. Certain chemicals and pollutants, even medications prescribed by your doctor, can injure the red blood cells in this way.

Even if every mechanism I've mentioned thus far is perfectly in order and normal concentrations of oxygen do reach your tissues, you'll still be short of breath if you have some condition which requires an abnormally large amount of oxygen. This happens with *high fevers*, a rapidly growing *cancer* and an *overactive thyroid*—any disorder in which your metabolism is accelerated. In that case, you have to breathe faster and faster to get more and more oxygen to your oxygen-hungry tissues.

Certain *medications* may also stimulate the respiratory center in your brain so that you breathe harder and are short of breath. Amphetamines ("speed") have that effect. And, finally, have you ever watched a very *obese* person climbing stairs? The huffing, puffing and difficulty in breathing are usually due to the fact that excessive fat prevents the chest from moving enough to permit the lungs to expand normally.

Whatever the cause—poor physical shape, nervousness, heart disease, lung trouble, a blood disorder—any persistent, inappropriate shortness of breath needs to be explained. On your way to the doctor, there are a few simple questions you can ask yourself that may provide the clues to *your* breathlessness:

• If you've been under a lot of stress, have difficulty getting a satisfying breath and feel lightheaded or dizzy, with tingling in your hands and feet, but you can lie flat in bed and do not have a cough, chances are you're hyperventilating. Your shortness of breath has no physical, or what doctors call "organic," basis.

- If you're overweight, rarely exercise and, to make matters worse, also *smoke,* and find yourself winded after only mild physical exertion, there's nothing your doctor can do for you. You're on your own. You've got to lose weight, start exercising and *stop smoking!* If you can do all of that, your shortness of breath will disappear.

- If you have heart trouble—angina, or a heart attack sometime in the past, rheumatic valve disease, long-standing high blood pressure which was never effectively treated—and your legs are swollen at the end of the day, and you don't feel comfortable lying flat in bed, then your breathlessness is likely due to heart failure. Your lungs are congested by blood, reducing their capacity to send the oxygen you breathe into the circulation. The same symptoms, with the exception of the swollen legs, can develop as a result of an acute heart attack too.

- Do you experience shortness of breath when walking up hills in cold weather? Does it clear soon after you stop walking? You probably have angina pectoris. For some people, angina manifests itself not as pain or pressure in the chest but as shortness of breath on exertion.

- If your child has been playing outdoors perfectly happily and then starts wheezing and is out of breath, but does not have asthma, he or she may have inhaled some *foreign object* like a piece of a toy or a peanut. Get to the doctor fast.

- If you're a cigarette smoker and have always had a dry cough, but now you've begun to feel short of breath too and are losing weight, lung cancer is a real possibility.

- Smoker or not, if you've had recurrent attacks of asthma or wheezing along with a chronic cough, and your fingers and toenails are "clubbed"—convex, like a spoon—your shortness of breath is probably due to emphysema or lung cancer.
- If you awaken in the night short of breath, foaming a frothy pink liquid, you're in pulmonary edema—a major medical emergency often due to a fresh heart attack. A sudden weakness of the heart muscle has caused blood to back up into the lungs.
- *Dust* can infiltrate your lungs and reduce their oxygen-delivering capacity. Coal miners who started work before the newer protective devices came into use are especially prone to this type of damage, but anyone who spends time in a dust-laden environment is vulnerable. Various fungal infections of the lung also lead to shortness of breath.
- If you have varicose veins and suddenly become short of breath—with or without a cough—and spit up bright red blood, you may have a *blood clot* to your lungs. It likely originated in a deep vein in your legs or in your pelvis, whence a piece broke off and traveled to your lungs. This is most apt to happen after prolonged bed rest, long airplane flights, pregnancy or surgery of any kind.
- You're a young man or woman and suddenly without apparent cause you become short of breath. You may or may not also have chest pain and a cough. Chances are you have had a *spontaneous pneumothorax,* the collapse of all or part of the lung. Some individuals have little blisters on their lungs which normally produce no symptoms until they burst, allowing air to escape into the chest—which, in turn, collapses the lung. In patients with emphysema, the excess air in the lungs causes sev-

eral of these blisters to form. When one bursts, the lung collapses.

- You've just been served a "funny" alcohol drink, contents unknown. ("Try it, you'll like it!") It doesn't taste quite right, and immediately after emptying your glass you become short of breath and begin breathing rapidly. Some complete fool has given you rubbing alcohol, not at all the same as the alcohol made for drinking. The alcohol in scotch may impair your ability to drive; rubbing alcohol blocks the red blood cells from carrying oxygen. If this happens, get to a doctor fast and then have the "bartender" drawn and quartered.

Shortness of breath, whether sudden or chronic, should always be taken seriously. Although many cases do boil down to harmless, obvious and correctable situations, this symptom requires a thorough medical evaluation.

Points to Remember

Symptom: Shortness of breath.

What It May Mean	What to Do About It
1. Physical or psychological stress.	Normal.
2. Hyperventilation.	Deal with the psychological causes. For immediate relief, breathe into a paper bag for a few minutes.
3. Rapid ascent to high altitudes.	Supplemental oxygen.
4. Airway obstruction.	Remove the blockage.
5. Chronic lung disease.	Treat the pulmonary disorder.

6. Heart disease, acute or chronic.	Strengthen the heart with rest and medication.
7. Anemia.	Replace lost or deficient blood.
8. Disease of the red blood cells.	Correct the abnormality.
9. Increased body demand for oxygen (high fever, overactive thyroid, rapidly growing cancer).	Treat the underlying cause.
10. Medications.	Discontinue them.
11. Obesity.	Lose weight.
12. Cigarette smoking.	Stop it!
13. Inhaling a foreign object.	Remove it.
14. Dust-laden environment.	Proper ventilation, masks.
15. Blood clot to the lungs.	Anticoagulants.
16. Spontaneous pneumothorax.	Reinflate the collapsed lung.

SNORING: SOCIAL NUISANCE OR DISEASE?

Snoring is a big joke—unless you happen to sleep with someone who does it. The problem is not commonly raised in a doctor's office, because the snorer himself is often not aware of it, while the victim has abandoned all hope—or has moved to a separate bedroom. For the most part, whether it's a gentle purr just loud enough to keep you awake or the window-rattling variety that even the neighbors can hear, snoring is usually not a manifestation of disease. But it *can* be, which is the reason for this section.

First, *why* do people snore? And why, for example, don't we do it during the day as we go about our business? Imagine standing there snoring while you wait for the bus, or in line at the bank, or queuing up for your table at a restaurant. After all, if it's nothing more than a variation of normal breathing, and all of us breathe twenty-four hours a day, why does it happen only while we sleep? You might think it's the lying down that does it, but that's not true. If it were, then every time you reclined on the couch to watch TV or read a book, you'd start "sawing logs." No, the key ingredient to snoring is sleep.

When you take in a deep breath, the air that is destined to end in the lungs passes first through the airways in the head and the throat. These passages are kept open by the muscles surrounding them, so that the air flows through them unimpeded. When you sleep deeply, however, especially after a *nightcap* or a *sleeping pill,* the muscles that are supposed to keep the passages open relax, and the airways collapse. You must now breathe more forcefully to keep the air moving, because of the resistance to its flow. This increased respiratory effort sets up vibrations in the tissues surrounding the air passages, vibrations that constitute the snore. Its intensity, loudness, pitch and resonance all depend on how narrow the airways have become and how loose the tissues in the area are. The more lax they are, the more they "rattle in the breeze" and the louder the snore.

But all of the foregoing explains only the noise. What has that to do with disease? When the respiratory pathways become so constricted that they reduce the amount of air getting through, you are vulnerable to a condition called *obstructive sleep apnea.* This means that you're not getting enough oxygen into your lungs and so there's less in your blood. As a result, virtually every tissue in your body is to some extent oxygen-deprived. Young healthy individuals can usually tolerate this temporary reduction in available oxygen, but as we get older the heart and the brain react adversely to the impact of a diminished oxygen supply.

"Apnea" means cessation of breathing. If you share a room with someone who snores, check out his breathing pattern at the peak of a snoring session. (Incidentally, I'm not being sexist by referring to "his" snoring. Obstructive sleep apnea affects men twenty times more than it does women.) Now, if your roommate has obstructive sleep apnea, you'll find his breathing characteristic. First there's the familiar rhythmic snoring while air is flowing "under pressure" through the constricted passages, vibrating the surrounding tissues. At some point, the obstruction becomes so severe that air no longer moves through the passages. The chest continues to heave as if he were still breathing, but in fact there is no air flow in or out of the lungs—and there is no sound. This period of silence and respiratory "arrest" lasts anywhere from a few seconds to as long as two minutes. During this interval, the oxygen content of the blood drops. When it hits bottom, a chemical signal is sent to the respiratory centers in the brain which stimulate the breathing mechanisms. Air is then once more forced through the constricted passages. The period of apnea, or "respiratory arrest," ends with a particularly loud snort, followed by a succession of smaller ones. The cycle of snoring, silence, a loud snort, paroxysms of shorter ones, snoring and silence then repeats itself.

If you have obstructive sleep apnea, you're apt to be sleepy and tired during the day, because at the end of every cycle marked by the loud snort you awaken briefly, without either knowing or remembering it. Since this happens every few minutes, you are deprived of sustained, deep sleep. This catches up with you the next day, so that you fall asleep driving your car or working at your desk.

Sudden death is a possible consequence of obstructive sleep apnea. This is unlikely in young healthy people, but someone whose heart is already deprived of oxygen because of diseased coronary arteries is especially vulnerable to the further temporary reduction which occurs in obstructive sleep apnea. There is a high incidence of high blood pressure and stroke in persons with sleep apnea. Since hypertension doesn't usually cause symptoms, anyone with a sleep-related breathing disorder, especially middle-aged or older men, should have the blood pressure checked. Chances are one in three it will be elevated if you're a big-league snorer.

Obstructive sleep apnea is also associated with chronic lung disease, central nervous system disorders (such as a brain tumor or infection), impotence and obesity.

We tend to joke about snoring, but remember that it may be a marker of important medical consequences. If someone you know snores heavily, and especially if they go through the cycle described above, advise them to see a sleep specialist. Apnea can be treated and its dangers reduced or eliminated.

Points to Remember

Symptom: Snoring.

What It May Mean	What to Do About It
1. Normal during sleep.	No treatment.
2. Too much alcohol or sedation at bedtime.	Cut it down or out.

3. Obstructive sleep apnea.   If the breathing-snoring
                                pattern is characteristic,
                                arrange for a sleep study.

WHEN YOU LOSE YOUR VOICE

The laryngitis you have with a common cold clears
up in a few days if you simply rest your voice, inhale
some steam, soothe the swollen vocal cords with loz-
enges and go about your business. But if the hoarseness persists for longer than two weeks, whether or
not it was preceded by a cold, have a throat specialist
examine you.

Most cases of chronic vocal-cord malfunction are
due to *voice abuse*. But some are caused by polyps or
tumors. The following case histories illustrate the
spectrum of possibilities when you no longer sound
like Caruso in the shower!

Joel, a twenty-eight-year-old attorney, visited my
office for a complete checkup. In the course of the
examination, I thought his voice sounded a bit
husky, but since he was a new patient I couldn't be
sure. When I asked him whether this was his "normal" speaking voice, he said that it was not. He told
me that he had been hoarse for a few months following a rather severe upper-respiratory infection. He
hadn't seen a throat doctor because his girlfriend
found the timbre kind of sexy and so he wasn't in a
hurry to do anything about it.

Well, three months is a long time for one's voice to
remain hoarse after a cold, and I was concerned. Was
he a smoker? No. Did he drink? Just socially. (I
asked these questions because heavy smoking and
drinking, especially in combination, can irritate and
inflame vocal cords and cause chronic laryngitis.)
Did he use his voice much in the course of his work?

No; as a matter of fact, he considered himself to be somewhat shy and soft-spoken. Was he feeling tired, cold, sluggish? (A low-functioning thyroid can lower the pitch of the voice.) No, he felt just fine. Was he coughing? No, only when he'd had the cold.

I referred Joel to a throat doctor, who found a thickened nodule on one of the vocal cords. You'd expect that in a singer, a floor trader, an auctioneer or a politician, but not in a "shy, soft-spoken" individual. The nodule did not appear to be cancerous, so Joel was given a trial of speech therapy for a few weeks. When that proved ineffective, the specialist recommended removal of the nodule. A few weeks later Joel was speaking in his normal, not particularly sexy voice.

At this point I still didn't know what had caused the vocal-cord nodule to form in this patient. At a routine visit after the surgery, Joel solved the riddle for me. It turned out that he is a Yale grad and, like many Eli alumni, is passionately devoted to his football team, the Bulldogs. As anyone within a one-hundred-mile radius of either New Haven or Boston is well aware, *the* event of the year is the Harvard-Yale match. It is, in fact, known as The Game. It was a rather chilly Saturday that year and the contest was a particularly close one. Joel admitted that he had been standing that afternoon in the cold November air yelling at the top of his lungs for three solid hours. Four days later he came down with a cold, but that's not what gave him the persistent hoarseness and nodule. It was the shouting that did it. Even so casual and transient an insult to the vocal apparatus can have long-term consequences which, though neither dangerous nor life-threatening, will affect the quality of your voice.

There was another patient, Charles, sixty-four years old, who complained of a chronic cough and hoarseness for the previous four weeks. He was a stockbroker, married and a nonsmoker. He had always enjoyed good health, and his past medical history was unremarkable—except for one episode from his army days many years before when he had contracted syphilis overseas. It had been treated early and successfully.

During our interview he coughed several times. It was a dry cough, without phlegm, and it had a brassy, hollow ring to it. In my examination, I heard a faint heart murmur. A chest X ray provided the answer to the cough, the hoarseness and the murmur. The aorta, the large vessel that comes out of the heart and from which all other arteries in the body branch off, was markedly widened. We call such dilatation an *aneurysm*. The usual cause is high blood pressure, but syphilis contracted years earlier, and inadequately treated, can also do it. If the aneurysm is not removed in time, it eventually ruptures and causes death. Before it reaches that point, it expands and presses on nearby structures within the chest, one of which is the nerve that opens and shuts the vocal cords. Charles's hoarseness wasn't due to overenthusiasm at a football game, but to pressure on that nerve. The aneurysm was removed at surgery, and in about six months (that's how long it takes for nerve function to be restored) the cough stopped and the hoarseness disappeared.

My third case history is that of a fifty-year-old woman who was a heavy smoker. She knew all about the dangers of tobacco and had tried to quit time and time again, but without success. She was now worried about lung cancer because of her "morning cough." Recently, along with the cough, her voice had become husky, then hoarse. Assuming that this was just part of the "smoker's profile," and reassured by a normal chest X ray, she didn't think much about it. However, I referred her to a laryngologist (throat specialist), who found a cancer on one of her vocal cords. She required extensive surgery in which her entire voice box and some nearby glands were removed. Today she speaks through a microphone placed against her throat. The only symptom pointing to her cancer was the persistent hoarseness. The cause was, as you might have expected, tobacco.

The bottom line in all these accounts is that *persistent* hoarseness, not the kind you get for two or three days with a cold, but that which lingers for weeks or months, has a variety of causes. Some are more dangerous than others, but all must be kept in mind.

If there has been an ongoing change in the quality of your voice, you should see not only your own doctor but a laryngologist, who will look directly at your speaking apparatus, the vocal cords. That can be an unpleasant experience—especially for someone who gags easily. In order to see what's going on in your vocal cords, the doctor eases a heated mirror down the back of the throat and has you say "Eeeh," "Aaah" and make other funny noises. Although the examination lasts only a few moments, for me personally it always seems like a lifetime. If this examination is not satisfactory, that is, if the doctor can't really get a good look, a very thin tube about the width of a strand of spaghetti is passed through your nose and manipulated down to your vocal cords. There's nothing to it, believe me. It can be left there for as long as necessary—five, even ten minutes— while the doctor evaluates the function of the cords and photographs them, even makes a video if necessary, so that you too can see what they look like and how they work.

The histories described above illustrate three conditions that can result in chronic hoarseness: a benign *nodule on the vocal cord,* an *aortic aneurysm* and a *cancerous tumor.* Several other things can go wrong as well. You see, the vocal cords aren't really cords at all. They're more like curtains which open and shut to varying degrees to create different tones. These curtains must be able to open widely and shut tightly for you to have a normal-sounding voice. In order for them to do so, not only must they be physically intact themselves, but so must the nerves and muscles that make them move. There is a very long nerve called the vagus that leaves the bottom of the brain and travels down the throat to the chest. One of its branches supplies the vocal cords. Anything that interferes with that nerve or its branches will make you hoarse. In Charles's case it was an aortic aneurysm, but lymph glands in the area, enlarged by infection or cancer, can do so, too.

The cords themselves can be injured by *vapors,* some of which are found in industry, by *alcoholism* and, of course, by *smoking. Generalized weakness* due to other diseases, and muscular disorders like *myasthenia gravis* can all cause chronic hoarseness, too. So can *reflux* from the food pipe (esophagus).

So, never make a self-diagnosis—and don't accept one offered by family and friends—of "chronic laryngitis" until all the possibilities have been checked out. Only if the tests come back negative can you safely accept the "chronic laryngitis" label. In that event, vocal training can help a great deal.

Points to Remember

Symptom: Chronic hoarseness.

What It May Mean	What to Do About It
1. Voice abuse.	Moderation.
2. Vocal-cord nodule, polyp or cancer.	Remove it.
3. Pressure on the nerve supplying the vocal cords (by an aortic aneurysm or a tumor).	Surgery.
4. Toxic fumes.	Avoid.
5. Chronic alcoholism.	Temperance!
6. Generalized weakness.	Treat the underlying cause.
7. Myasthenia gravis.	Medication.
8. Reflux into the esophagus.	Small meals; antacids; raise the head of the bed.

HICCUPS

Have you ever had an attack of singultus? Of course you have, even if you've never heard the word before. It's medicalese for hiccups (hiccoughs). What causes them? Many, many years ago, in the days when I was a smoker (pipes were my vice), I'd hiccup after having inhaled the hot smoke for fifteen or twenty minutes. I don't dare tell my brother-in-law a really funny story because whenever he laughs very hard he gets the hiccups. Some people do so after drinking too much (alcohol or hot fluids), or eating spicy irritating foods. Very often, hiccups come on for no apparent reason. In all such cases, they usually disappear after a few minutes. But they can persist for days, weeks, months—and even indefinitely. I have one patient, a diabetic, whose hiccups stop when he falls asleep (as most do) but recur every day for varying intervals, and have done so for well over a year now.

The symptom itself is caused by a spasm of the diaphragm due to irritation of the nerves that supply it. This irritation can be local or can originate in a specific portion of the brain. So any condition that irritates the diaphragm or its nerve supply will cause hiccups—a heart attack, pleurisy of the lung or pneumonia (involving the diaphragm), inflammation of some intestinal structure (also irritating the diaphragm), surgery, pregnancy (when the elevated uterus pushes against the diaphragm), hepatitis (when the enlarged or inflamed liver is in contact with the diaphragm) and indeed a whole variety of conditions ranging from cancer to kidney failure. Damage to the area of the brain in which the hiccup center is located (by a stroke or a tumor) will leave you hiccuping, too. In my own specialty, cardiology, the most frequent incidence of hiccups is in patients who have had heart or lung surgery. These attacks often persist for days or weeks.

It's often easier to determine why you're hiccuping than to stop them. My wife first tries scaring me, suddenly and without warning. Then she has me hold my breath for as long as I can, or drink a glass of ice water very quickly. If none of these works, she pulls on my tongue or presses on my eyeballs. If I'm still hiccuping after that, she has me swallow a teaspoon of sugar or some breadcrumbs. Finally, I breathe deeply in and out of a paper bag (avoiding plastic ones, which can stick to the nostrils). By that time the hiccups have disappeared, and she's hurt when I tell her they would have done so even if I had just sat there doing nothing!

When the hiccups persist for days at a time in my patients, I massage the carotid sinus in the neck. That's what a tight collar presses on, and it may make you faint, so don't you try it yourself. If none of the above works, there are drugs like phenobarbital, chlorpromazine (Thorazine), scopolamine (the active ingredient in the skin patch that prevents motion sickness), metoclopramide (Reglan, used in the treatment of reflux from the stomach into the food pipe) and even hypnosis. These are just a few of the treatments that doctors use to stop stubborn hiccups. There are many others, which may or may not work. If they do not, it may become necessary to "freeze" the hiccup ("phrenic") nerve temporarily or even, on rare occasions, cut it.

Points to Remember

Symptom: Hiccups.

What It May Mean	What to Do About It
1. Noxious fumes, hot and spicy foods or liquids, or no obvious cause.	Will usually disappear on their own. But home remedies sometimes shorten the duration of the attack.
2. Any disease or disorder that irritates the nerves controlling the diaphragm (e.g., pleurisy, pneumonia, chest or abdominal operations, diseases or organs in contact with the diaphragm).	Treat the underlying cause. For relief of symptoms, a variety of medications, physical maneuvers performed by the doctor and even surgery may be necessary.

3. Stroke or tumor affecting the "hiccup" center in the brain.   Depends on the duration. May require drugs or surgical intervention.

CHAPTER 10

SEXUAL PROBLEMS

When I was a medical student, there were two subjects we were never really taught—nutrition and sex. As a result, many doctors of my generation still tell their patients to eat a balanced diet (loosely defined as "enough" fat, protein and carbohydrates) —and leave it at that. Today, nutrition is a major course in medical school, and most recent graduates know a great deal more about what food is good and what's bad for you and how much.

As for sex, my contemporaries learned about all its dire consequences (syphilis and gonorrhea were virtually the most important sexually transmitted diseases in those happy days); but "sexuality," things like foreplay, performance, desire, homosexuality— none of these was a proper subject for ladies and gentlemen, even though they were destined to be doctors. So there are still some old-timers around who haven't a clue about sex and couldn't care less. They're apt to refer you to Dr. Ruth's TV show if you ask them "embarrassing" questions. Today's graduates are, by contrast, well instructed in sexual behavior patterns, both normal and abnormal.

MALE IMPOTENCE—FEMALE "FRIGIDITY"

Nothing causes greater concern than some sign or symptom that all is not as it should be in one's sex life, whether it's the inability to perform the sexual act, to derive pleasure from it or to conceive. Because the human reproductive system and the enjoyment of the sexual act are dependent upon a complex of both physical and psychological factors, it is not always easy to resolve such concerns. But knowledge of how the system is supposed to work, and recognition of the symptoms that signal sexual dysfunctions, many of which can be successfully treated, will go a long way to allay unnecessary fears.

One of the most troublesome problems now openly discussed by patients with their doctors is impotence—the failure to achieve and maintain enough of an erection to permit penetration and pleasure. Impotence should not, however, be confused with male infertility. A man unable to maintain an erection may be perfectly normal in every other way and quite capable of fathering a child.

Barring injury or sudden illness, impotence develops gradually. After a long and satisfactory sex life, you begin to notice that your prowess is fading. Initially you don't panic. After all, no one is perfect. Failure to perform now and then is to be expected, isn't it? So you chalk up your lack of success now and then to fatigue, too much alcohol, depression or pressure at work. You're quite confident that things will be better "next time." But when the "next time" rolls around, you're still not "up" to it. At some point, you begin to worry, and as things get worse you finally realize that something is very wrong. In this section, we'll look into what it may be in your particular case.

For you to understand why you've become impotent, you must first appreciate all the complex signals to and from various parts of the body that make an erection possible. The brain is the key player, because that's where desire originates—whether real from an available partner, or fantasy from a book, a porno movie or the recesses of your own thoughts.

To have an erection you want to do something about (as opposed to the early-morning variety that often comes on briefly with a full bladder), you need a sexy stimulus which your brain must be able to interpret as such. Once you have perceived whatever it is as being erotic, a chain of events is set in motion. Someone who is severely depressed or grieving is less likely to respond to such a stimulus than is a young man who has just received a big raise (no pun intended). However, the ability of the brain to interpret the stimulus as erotic is more than just a state of mind. Certain hormonal requirements must also be met. For example, a twenty-five-year-old woman will not react the same way as a man the same age to the sight of an attractive female hitching up her skirt to fix her pantyhose or lying on a beach in a much-too-small bikini. In order for a male to be sexually stimulated, he must have enough testosterone, the male hormone, circulating in his body. Remove his testes, the source of that hormone (as is often done in cases of advanced prostate cancer) or give him large doses of *female* hormone, and *nothing* will arouse him sexually.

Hormonal imbalance is why most male alcoholics ultimately become impotent. Men produce *both* male and female hormones; so do women. The difference between the sexes is that men generate a much greater preponderance of testosterone and only tiny amounts of estrogen, the female hormone, while women generate far more estrogen than testosterone. The liver maintains this normal balance. In males who have been drinking too much too long, *the liver is damaged* by the toxic effect of the alcohol, so that many of its functions are impaired. As the booze continues to pour in and the liver gets sicker and sicker, it can no longer control the level of estrogens in the blood. More and more female hormone ac-

cumulates, eventually neutralizing the effect of the
testosterone. These men then lose their male characteristics: they no longer have to shave twice a day,
only every second or third day; their testes shrink
and their breasts become big; their sex drive diminishes and so does their ability to have an erection.

But alcoholism and liver damage aren't the only
mechanism by which testosterone levels are reduced.
The *pituitary gland* in the brain makes a hormone
which stimulates the testes to produce testosterone.
When the pituitary gland is poorly developed, as it is
in some adolescents, or diseased, perhaps by a tumor, it doesn't secrete enough of that hormone, and
so the affected male is rendered impotent.

On the other hand, the pituitary may be fine but
the testes themselves diseased, and no amount of
prodding by the pituitary will make them produce
the needed hormone in sufficient amounts to give an
erection.

But let's assume the brain is physically fine, all the
hormones are flowing as they should and you're being sexually stimulated. Will that guarantee an erection? Not necessarily, because messages *from* the
brain must be able to reach the penis, and that requires an intact nervous pathway. Any condition
that affects those nerves—a *spinal-cord injury,* alcoholism, long-standing diabetes, especially if untreated—can stop the brain-to-penis signal dead in
its tracks. That's the worst scenario, because, unlike
the alcoholic with too much estrogen and no sex
drive, this man is sexually aroused in his head but the
command for the penis to arise is not carried out
because it is not received where it counts.

Let's go one step further. Suppose the neurological
system is intact and the appropriate message does
reach the penis, but there's still no erection. Why
not? Because there is one final requirement—blood.

A flaccid penis becomes stiff only when it is flooded with blood. That requires, among other things, healthy, unobstructed arteries. So the brain may be ready and willing, the pituitary in fine shape, the testes working at full steam making testosterone and the nerves intact, but if the arteries supplying the penis are clogged by *arteriosclerosis,* it's all in vain.

Here, then, are the five basic components required for an erection:

1. A responsive emotional state.
2. A healthy brain, including a normally functioning pituitary.
3. Testes that can make enough testosterone.
4. Intact nervous pathways.
5. An adequate blood supply to the penis.

In the real world, despite the fact that we now recognize a great number of *physical* causes of impotence, there is no question that most cases are due to failure to satisfy requirement number one above—a responsive emotional state. Under these circumstances, the brain, not the penis, is the most important sexual organ. Psychogenic impotence is most often traceable to *boredom, fatigue, depression, anxiety, sadness,* fear or some deep-seated, complex *emotional problem.*

A couple came to see me not long ago because the wife had finally prevailed upon her husband to do something about his impotence. He had had a heart attack some months earlier and had not really performed effectively since. We discussed the various possibilities for about a half hour, after which I arranged for a formal hormonal, urological and vascular evaluation. We all agreed that this was the thing to do, and the couple left my office apparently satisfied. However, later in the day the husband called to ask if he could drop by for another appointment—

alone. There was something he had forgotten to tell me. When we met again he said, "Doctor, there's one thing you should know. I have absolutely no trouble with my erections away from home. If you don't believe me, ask my girlfriend in your waiting room."

I'm not suggesting that you try your luck elsewhere if you've become impotent, but a lessening of desire for a partner of many years is a real phenomenon. Depression, anxiety and stress may have a similar effect on sexual performance. So can *fear*. The panic over AIDS probably doesn't interfere with sexual performance in couples who are well informed about the epidemic and have been living together monogamously for years, but it does in singles of both sexes.

There are other sources of fear. I have often witnessed the devastating effect that angina or a heart attack can have on sexual activity. Male cardiacs are terrified by the possibility of "death in the saddle." Unless the patient is continuously reassured from the *very onset* of his heart trouble that sex can be safe and, in fact, desirable, he may well become impotent for the rest of his life. Female heart attack patients are frequently paralyzed by fear, too, and may lose *their* sexual desire unless properly counseled.

But never assume that your impotence is psychological until the following physical factors have been excluded. *Medication* is high on the list. My cardinal rule holds as true for impotence as it does for virtually every other symptom: *When you wonder what's causing it, look into your medicine cabinet first.* Except for antibiotics, almost any drug can render a man impotent. There are at least eighty medications doctors commonly prescribe that can cause impotence. These include:

Mood-altering drugs—uppers, downers, sedatives, stimulants, antianxiety preparations, antidepressants and sleeping pills; these are the prime offenders. The next major group are those prescribed *to treat high blood pressure and heart disease.* These include the beta blockers, diuretics, Aldomet and even digitalis. To date, in my experience, the only anti-high-blood-pressure medications that do not appear to have this unwanted side effect are the ACE inhibitors— captopril (Capoten), enalapril (Vasotec) and lisinopril (Zestril, Prinivil). Other drugs that may cause impotence include such antiulcer agents as Tagamet and Zantac.

Data promoting a drug must, by law, list all potential side effects that have ever been reported. I think that with regard to impotence they err on the low side, because most men are too macho to admit, even to their doctor, that they "can't" anymore, or they don't know enough to blame their problem on the medicine, or they're afraid to because they feel it is protecting them against some life-threatening disease and they don't want the doctor to take it away from them. So, ask your doctor about *any* effect on potency of *any* drug you're given, even if the incidence is "infinitesimal."

Once you've eliminated medication, consider other physical or organic causes of impotence. Any obvious neurological problem, like *Parkinson's disease,* a stroke or a brain tumor, can render you impotent. Liver damage isn't the only mechanism by which alcohol can have this effect; it can also damage the nerves (alcoholic neuropathy). Since nicotine is a nerve toxin, heavy cigarette *smokers* may be sexually impaired. *Diabetes* is a major cause of impotence, which, in fact, may be the first manifestation of that disease. Whenever a man complains to me about his sexual inadequacy, I routinely check the blood sugar. Diabetes makes for impotence in two ways: it affects the nerves so that the messages sent from the brain to the penis never get there, and/or it accelerates the process of arteriosclerosis, which, in turn, narrows the blood vessels and reduces the organ's blood supply.

High blood pressure promotes hardening of the arteries and so also contributes to impotence. Patients with hypertension often blame the medication they're taking to control it, when in fact the elevated pressure itself is the villain.

Does aging itself cause impotence? If so, when? Patients at almost any age are apt to say, "It's not like it was when I was twenty." While there is likely to be some decrease in the frequency of sexual activity as a man gets older, that's not the same as impotence. In a normal healthy male, some sexual activity can continue virtually indefinitely. It's not the years that make for impotence, but the definable, recognizable, often treatable chronic disorders that set in along the way. The vital parts don't just wear out.

If you're worried about impotence, here is what may be happening in your particular case:

- You're in your fifties and have generally enjoyed good health. But in the last two weeks you've been feeling tired, your memory seems a bit off, you've slowed down and you're impotent. It all began when your doctor told you your blood pressure was high and prescribed a beta blocker. Five will get you ten that your problem will be solved if the medication is switched. The same scenario can be repeated with virtually any other drug.
- You have been diabetic for five or ten years, during which time you haven't been very careful about controlling your blood sugar. You now experience a pain in the calf of one or both legs when you walk quickly. It disappears when you stop. You also have trouble obtaining and maintaining an

erection. Both these symptoms are the result of a single problem—decreased blood supply to the legs *and* to the penis due to arteriosclerosis of the local blood vessels.

- You've been a drinker all your life—some might say "heavy," you prefer "hard." You've always been able to handle alcohol "like a man." But you don't feel much like a real man anymore. You used to shave twice a day; now it's every two or three days. What's worse, your "manliness" has also diminished. You're not very interested in sex anymore, and when you are aroused you have trouble getting an erection. The explanation? You've got too much female hormone in your body and too little of the male hormone because your liver has been damaged by your heavy drinking over the years.

- You've just recovered from a heart attack. You'll never forget how it happened. You were walking up the hill behind your house, mildly winded, when your chest suddenly felt as though it were caught in a tight vise. It was terrifying—the pain, the wailing siren of the ambulance, the intensive-care unit, the panic in your wife's face which she couldn't hide whenever she visited you in the hospital. Thank goodness you came through, and now you're home and feeling fine. But you never want to experience any of that again, so you vow to take things easy from now on. A few weeks *after* your return from the hospital, your doctor finally gets around to discussing sex, something you yourself wondered and worried about but were shy or afraid to bring up. He tells you it's "okay"—that's all. You're happy to get the news, but a little nervous about it. You finally muster enough courage to try, but way back in your mind you're petrified about feeling that terrible heart pain again. You don't, because you can't "get it up." Your wife persuades you to call your doctor, and he assures you that none of the medications you're taking could possibly be responsible for your problem. Explanation: It's probably psychological—the terror that sexual arousal will cause another heart attack and even death.

- You're divorced and you're anxious to have an affair. On a business trip to another city you meet a very attractive woman with whom you have "chemistry." At the crucial moment, you fail to become erect. Chances are you have "performance anxiety," either because of fear of failing or because you're worried about getting AIDS.

Regardless of why it happens, impotence often has a profound effect on morale. Psychological causes are usually more difficult to treat than most physical ones. For example, drug-induced impotence is easily reversed, and vascular abnormalities can sometimes be surgically corrected; when the trouble lies in the nerves themselves, the prognosis is gloomy. But even if impotence is in fact irreversible for whatever reason, there's still hope. Penile implants now available in a variety of configurations can make a "man" out of almost anyone.

Premature ejaculation, when orgasm comes on too quickly to satisfy either partner, differs from impotence. Men with this problem are able to achieve erection and penetration, so the vascular, nervous or hormonal causes responsible for impotence are not considerations here. In most cases, the reasons for premature ejaculation are emotional or psychological. Although difficult to treat, this condition is more responsive to psychotherapy than is impotence. I am not aware of any medications or diseases responsible for premature ejaculation.

Women with lack of sexual desire and/or response are termed "frigid" by their partners. In many instances, the causes are physical and result from the fact that intercourse actually results in pain or discomfort. I have listed in the section on painful intercourse (pages 100–103) the various structural abnormalities of the vagina as well as the most common types of gynecologic infection and disease that can interfere with sexual pleasure in women. But I believe that "female sexual dysfunction" is usually psychological in origin. Anxiety, depression and feelings of guilt and shame about sex often play a part, as does the fear of pregnancy. Many women who never seem to enjoy making love and who rarely, if ever, reach an orgasm during intercourse may nevertheless derive intense satisfaction and climax from masturbation. But just as a man who has become impotent may miraculously regain his "manhood" when he changes partners, so may a "frigid" woman frequently become orgasmic in the arms of a new lover. Although appropriate arousal and emotional involvement are the keys to satisfying lovemaking in both sexes, they are usually more important for a woman.

The female climax has been the subject of conjecture and debate for eons. Clitoral versus vaginal orgasm, and which is more satisfying or "natural," remains unsettled among those specializing in this field. Many women who enjoy intercourse require clitoral stimulation in order to experience orgasm. Others do not. It's very much an individual matter.

I have often been asked about the "G spot," whether it in fact exists, and how an obliging lover is to find it. The G spot is named after a Dr. Graffenburg, a sex researcher and physiologist. He postulated the presence of a specific area in the vagina, situated high up and way back in a straight line from the clitoris. When stimulated during intercourse, it allegedly produces a discharge associated with orgasm. Researchers are divided as to whether the G spot really exists. In my opinion, it doesn't really matter as long as the partners derive mutual pleasure in the act of love.

Points to Remember

Symptom: Impotence.

What It May Mean	What to Do About It
1. Hormonal deficiency due to disease or injury.	Hormonal (testosterone) replacement.
2. Liver disease, usually due to alcoholism.	Testosterone supplement may be helpful.
3. Brain damage (involving the pituitary gland).	Hormone supplements.
4. Nerve injury.	Penile prostheses.
5. Vascular disease.	Surgery may be effective.
6. Depression, anxiety, fatigue, boredom, stress, fear of failure.	Therapy, rest, imagination—often effective.
7. Deep-seated psychological problems.	Counseling (not predictably effective). Penile prostheses as a last resort.
8. Fear of infection.	When in doubt, don't.
9. Fear of recurring heart problem.	Reassurance.
10. Mood-altering drugs, medications (practically any you can think of).	Better to switch than fight it.
11. Smoking.	Stop.

12. Other diseases (Parkinson's, diabetes, high blood pressure).	Treat the underlying cause.
13. Premature ejaculation.	Counseling may help.

Symptom: "Frigidity."

What It May Mean	What to Do About It
1. Deep-seated psychological problems.	Counseling.
2. Fear of pain, infection or pregnancy.	Counseling. Birth-control techniques.
3. Local gynecological disease.	Treat the underlying cause.
4. Unskilled or uncaring partner.	Counseling.

INFERTILITY: CAN YOU AND YOUR PARTNER DELIVER TWENTY MILLION SPERM AND ONE EGG?

It happens so often: A young healthy couple decide to have children. It never occurs to them after years of contraception and dedicated efforts to *prevent* pregnancy that they might ever have trouble making a baby. Yet one in five couples in this country is infertile. What can possibly be wrong? A whole lot!

For conception to occur, the man must be able to produce enough healthy sperm in the testes and then deliver them through the various conduits in the male genital tract into the female vagina, from which they must find the target—the female egg waiting in the fallopian tube. For her part, the aspiring mother must have the egg to send down from the ovary into the tube to meet the sperm. For the union to be successful, the timing of that rendezvous must be just right. Once it has occurred, the environment in which the fertilized egg is to be nurtured, the uterus, must also be receptive. Any break in this biological chain results in infertility.

So, let's assume a couple have tried and tried to have a baby, but with no luck. Whose "fault" is it? It's just as likely to be his as hers, a fact not always appreciated until fairly recently. Infertility used to be invariably blamed on the "barren" woman. A healthy dose of feminism and good science have destroyed that myth. Never conclude, however, that either of you is infertile until you've worked at it for at least a year. After that, begin step by step to solve the problem—starting with the male, because his work-up is less expensive and easier to perform.

One possible source of male infertility is the *pituitary gland* in the brain, which produces a hormone that stimulates the testes to make sperm. When the pituitary is diseased, levels of this hormone drop so that the testes do not receive this signal, and so sperm formation is inadequate. Or the *testes* themselves may be injured or diseased, as, for example, by an attack of mumps sometime after childhood, and cannot respond to the pituitary hormone. The minimum number of sperm needed in order to land one on target is about twenty million. This critical amount can be temporarily reduced by certain *medications* (Tagamet, for example, widely used in the treatment of hyperacidity and ulcers) as well as by *pollutants* in the environment.

Suppose the brain and the testes are healthy, and sperm is normal and plentiful. It must still be able to get out of the man and into the woman. If the *ducts* which carry it to the urethra from the testes have been scarred and blocked by previous infection, such as gonorrhea, chlamydia or some other sexually transmitted disease, it cannot reach the egg.

Prostate surgery and several drugs, particularly

those used in the treatment of high blood pressure (Aldomet, labetalol) may cause *retrograde ejaculation*. Instead of traveling from the testes into the penis and through the urethra, the ejaculate goes backward into the urinary bladder, making it unavailable for procreation.

If the male checks out on all counts, the search for the causes of infertility should shift to his partner. She also may have a problem with the *pituitary*, whose hormones not only stimulate the ovary to release its eggs, but are also responsible for creating an environment within the uterus conducive to nourishing one that has been fertilized. Any hormonal imbalance, including malfunction of the *thyroid gland*, can leave the female infertile.

The pituitary and the thyroid may be in fine shape, but the *ovaries* may not be able to release their eggs because of cysts or infection. And just as the sperm needs a clear path for its journey out of the male body, so does the egg require that the *fallopian tubes*, which link the ovaries to the uterus, be unobstructed. If these tubes have been scarred by chronic inflammation, abscesses or other conditions which render them impassable, fertilization is impossible.

After the sperm makes it into the vagina, it faces an important barrier—the *cervix* (the neck of the uterus which protrudes into the vagina). Infection, cancer, scarring from numerous childbirths or narrowing for any reason can make that barrier impenetrable. The cervix may also produce substances which are hostile to and immobilize the sperm. Malignancy and infection of the *uterus* itself will also result in infertility.

You should understand the female *menstrual cycle* if you're trying to have a family. No matter how hard you work at it, if it's the wrong time of the cycle and sperm is sent to meet an egg that isn't there, nothing is going to happen. Focus on the four or five days at midcycle. Timing is critical. Here is another "pearl" which may help you increase the chances of conception. Heat reduces the vigor of sperm. (That's why the testes are on the outside of the body—to keep the sperm within them cool.) If a man has a prolonged fever, it may sometimes take months before his sperm regain their normal vitality. By the same token, vigorous exercise or a hot bath before lovemaking may also critically decrease the level of sperm mobility.

Finally, remember that fertility and sexual performance are not one and the same. There is more to conception than achieving an erection. Ejaculation of healthy, abundant sperm, no matter how premature, is the key factor for a man. In women, the egg must be in the right place at the right time. A couple may be very much in love and most compatible sexually, yet still be infertile.

If you and your spouse appear to be infertile, here are some of the signs to look for that may help you pinpoint the cause of your problem:

• Are your periods sparse? Do you have small breasts, too little fat on your body and straggly pubic hair? Or, if you're a man, are your testes tiny? Is that five o'clock shadow coming on later and later, so that you are shaving less often than you used to? These characteristics in both sexes suggest that the pituitary gland is not functioning normally, and that the hormones needed from either sex for a successful pregnancy are insufficient. This is easily confirmed by measuring their blood level. When such pituitary failure or malfunction is due to a tumor, one is not only infertile but troubled by chronic headaches and progressive loss of peripheral vision as well. Since pituitary hormones also keep the thyroid gland going, their deficiency due to any cause will result in additional symptoms of low thyroid function—sluggish speech, cold, dry skin, loss of hair and so on.

- A history of recurrent sexually transmitted disease calls for tests of the patency of the ducts both in men and in women.
- If you have been taking the Pill for a long time, it may be a while before your hormonal balance is sufficiently restored for you to become pregnant. The same is true after removal of an IUD.
- Keep a record of your temperature to determine whether or not you're ovulating. If it isn't slightly elevated at midcycle and remain so until just a few days before the onset of your period, chances are your ovary is not releasing its eggs.

Your doctor also has a few tests up his sleeve to determine the cause of female infertility. First there is the careful pelvic exam. Then he'll test your blood for hormone levels; he'll send you for X rays to see whether or not the tubes are open; he may take a direct look inside with a laparoscope; a sonogram will detect tumors in the pelvis, and bacteriological studies can identify a chronic infection.

In a male fertility work-up, the sperm are carefully scrutinized under the microscope—where they're counted and their movement is observed. Is their shape abnormal, or do they clump (that occurs when the body produces antibodies to its own sperm)? A urologist or your own doctor will have to determine whether or not the ducts that carry the sperm are blocked. Varicose veins in the testes—a common and treatable cause of infertility—can be detected in such an exam. Finally, blood is taken to measure all pertinent hormone levels.

A thorough fertility evaluation doesn't always

identify the problem. In that event, simply keep trying. But you do have other alternatives. Many centers throughout the world are performing "in vitro" fertilization. This is no longer an experimental technique, since the success rate is as high as 25 percent. It's done in the following way. First of all, the ovaries are "superovulated"—that is, stimulated to release more eggs, by the administration of specific medications. Then one of the eggs is removed, mixed with the sperm, and reintroduced through the cervix into the uterus. Then both of you keep your fingers crossed. If that doesn't work, adopt a baby.

Points to Remember

Symptom: Infertility.

What It May Mean	What to Do About It
In the male:	
1. Hormonal deficiency due to disease of the pituitary gland (in the brain) or the testes.	Correct the underlying cause and/or replace the missing hormones.
2. Depression of sperm production by drugs or pollutants.	Remove the cause.
3. Scarring of the pathway through which the sperm travel.	Surgical correction.
4. Retrograde ejaculation (due to medication or prior prostatectomy).	Change drugs. No effective treatment if due to prostatectomy.
In the female:	
1. Hormonal imbalance due	Correct the underlying

to pituitary malfunction, abnormal thyroid gland (too much or too little), adrenal-gland disease.

abnormality.

2. Ovarian disorders—infection, cysts, cancer.

Appropriate treatment.

3. Blocked fallopian tubes.

Surgery.

4. Disease of the cervix and/or the uterus, pelvic infection, tumor.

Correct the underlying cause.

5. Abnormal menstrual cycle due to poor nutrition or excessive physical exercise.

Regularize the menses with hormones, if necessary. Good nutrition, exercise in moderation.

CHAPTER 11

WHEN SYMPTOMS ARE ONLY SKIN-DEEP

The skin is the largest organ in the body and a very complicated one at that. Not only is it vulnerable to diseases of its own, it also reflects trouble deep in the interior of the body. What looks like a "simple" rash may in fact be evidence of a disorder in the heart (subacute bacterial endocarditis), the kidney (renal failure), widespread allergies, syphilis, cancer and many other conditions. When you consult a skin doctor because of an itch, he may well send you back to your own general physician because the problem lies in your kidney, your liver, your blood, or because you're diabetic. So in this chapter I'll discuss some common skin symptoms and suggest to you what they may mean.

IS THERE ANYTHING WORSE THAN AN ITCH?

Do you remember the scene in Alfred Hitchcock's *Rear Window* in which James Stewart, laid up in his apartment with a broken leg, gets an itch somewhere beneath the cast? The audience usually squirms in sympathy because everybody knows how awful it is to have an itch that can't be reached. Even the kind that you *can* scratch but which just won't go away is pretty bad, too. Ask anyone who has been hiking in the woods and had a little run-in with poison ivy or poison oak. All the scratching in the world won't make that kind of itch go away—in fact, scratching aggravates it. In some respects, a tenacious itch can be worse than severe pain, which one can at least control with painkillers.

If you've spent the night in a none-too-clean motel room and you wake up with the urge to scratch, you've almost certainly been *bitten* by an insect. Whatever the nasty little creature that ate you happened to be—mosquito, body louse, bedbug—you're going to itch like the devil. The more you scratch, the worse it is. If you've been camping, then the itch may also be due to *contact dermatitis* from poison ivy or poison oak. You can differentiate between a bite and a dermatitis by carefully looking at your skin. Unless you've been scratching very vigorously, bites are discrete, individual points, while the rash of dermatitis involves larger areas of the body which were in contact with the offending substance. If it was poison oak or ivy, it may be on the arm or leg that brushed against it; a new laundry detergent will affect your chest if you used it to wash your shirt; perfumes and fabric dyes will also produce a dermatitis where they have touched the skin.

A total body itch, with or without visible welts ("hives"), is usually caused by an *allergic reaction* to anything—a food or a pill (antibiotics are notable culprits in the medication department), insect bites or something in contact with your skin.

Several *childhood diseases* cause itchy rashes. If your child wakes up one morning with a little fever, feeling sick and scratching a very obvious rash, he or she may have anything from chicken pox to measles. Each such infectious disease of childhood presents its own characteristic picture. For example, chicken pox, which is caused by a virus, forms little watery blisters, usually on the trunk. These eventually burst and crust over. Measles, also caused by a virus, results in a red rash on the head and the body. Shingles (the reactivation of the dormant chicken pox virus later in life) is often preceded by local itching, tingling or pain for days before the typical rash appears.

A rash of which you should be particularly aware these days reflects *Lyme disease* (named after the community in Connecticut where it was first diagnosed). It is caused by the bite of a deer tick, especially prevalent in the northeastern United States. The rash itself is initially "ringlike" in appearance, but then it spreads. You may have several distinct rashes in different parts of your body. In addition to the local itching and discomfort, Lyme disease causes a host of symptoms, depending on which organs in the body it happens to involve. The common denominators, however, are fever and painful, swollen joints. One of my patients with these symptoms had "heart block" as well. The cardiac electrical conduction system was affected, causing the heartbeat to slow down to rates that rendered him unconscious! The diagnosis of Lyme disease, if suspected from the clinical evidence—the deer tick, the bite marks, the rash, arthritis, fever and whatever else is observed— is confirmed by blood tests. The treatment is simple: the appropriate antibiotic, usually tetracycline.

So the first thing to do when you get an itch is look at the area of skin involved, and try to remember what you touched and what touched you. Search for bites, rashes and even ticks that are hanging on, review your allergy history and bear in mind the possibility that it's from that new medication you've been taking. In most cases, the cause of the itching will be obvious. Remember, however, not every rash itches. For example, the rash due to secondary syphilis rarely does itch, while one of the most troublesome skin diseases, psoriasis, may or may not.

But what about the itch that comes on suddenly for no apparent reason and is not accompanied by a rash or bite marks? Here are some possible causes:

- If you itch all over and your eyes and/or skin have taken on a yellowish hue, you're *jaundiced* and the trouble lies in or around your liver. When the ducts from the liver to the intestinal tract are blocked or swollen, the bile that normally flows within them backs up into the bloodstream and produces severe itching. That usually occurs in chronic liver disease or cancer of the pancreas.

- If you have a generalized itch, feel for enlarged lymph glands above your collarbone, in your armpits, in your groin and around your elbows. If you find any, you may have a malignancy of the white blood cells (*leukemia*). A similar condition of the red cells (*polycythemia*) is not as serious, doesn't cause glandular enlargement, but frequently does make you itch. In either event, the sooner treatment is started, the better, so let your doctor know you're itching, even (and especially) if there's nothing to see.

- *Kidney disease,* especially in its late stages, is often associated with generalized itching. Toxic substances which should be excreted by the kidneys are retained, circulate in the bloodstream and cause the itch. So if you have a history of kidney problems and notice that your feet, hands and eyes are puffy, the itch is renal in origin.

- If you're a woman, *diabetic,* and suddenly develop a vaginal itch, you're spilling large amounts of sugar into your urine. This makes your vaginal area a prime site for itchy yeast infections. Whether a woman is diabetic or not, a vaginal itch may be due to a sexually transmitted disease such as chlamydia, or to a yeast infection from the antibiotics she has been taking recently. However, any organism that irritates the vagina will cause it to itch.

- Rectal itching is a common, troublesome and embarrassing symptom, especially when you've got to do something about it in public. The cause is most likely to be a skin problem in the area, or internal *hemorrhoids*. In this event, you will also have noticed some blood on your toilet paper or can feel a small lump in the rectal area. A word of caution here. Never *assume* that rectal bleeding is always due to hemorrhoids, even if you have them. The blood on your toilet paper may be coming from a tumor or polyp higher up in the bowel.

- A dry skin that itches is very common among persons with *low thyroid function*. In that case, there are other symptoms: you may be constipated and feel sluggish, tired and cold when everyone else feels warm enough. But if you're seventy plus, your itching may simply be due to *loss of moisture* in the skin.

The art and science of diagnosing one type of skin lesion from another—the simple brown keratosis or benign nevus versus a malignancy, the rash of one infectious disease from another, a cold sore due to a virus from one caused by syphilis—require years of training and specialization. When I encounter such lesions among my patients, I often refer them to a dermatologist for his special expertise. Even then, a biopsy is often needed to be sure. So if you develop any rash or have an itch, consult a dermatologist, unless the cause is obvious. Get to the bottom of the problem—*and try not to scratch*.

Points to Remember

Symptom: Itching.

What It May Mean	What to Do About It
1. Insect bites.	Local treatment.
2. Contact dermatitis.	Remove and avoid the offending substance; local treatment.
3. Allergy to food or drugs.	Avoid them.
4. Rashes due to various infections, most commonly occurring in childhood.	Treat the disease. Topical applications to the skin.
5. Jaundice due to obstruction of the bile ducts (liver disease, cancer of the pancreas).	Treat underlying disorder.
6. Blood disorder (leukemia, polycythemia).	Prompt medical treatment.
7. Kidney disease.	Medical treatment.
8. Vaginal itching: diabetes.	Better blood-sugar control.
9. Rectal itching: hemorrhoids.	Remove them or treat locally with ointment, creams, suppositories.
10. Hypothyroidism.	Replacement thyroid.
11. Aging skin.	Moistening creams.

BECOMING BALD—AND YOU'RE NOT TELLY SAVALAS

Men in our society are terrified of losing their hair. They are suckers for ads selling all sorts of products guaranteed to halt the retreat of the hairline across the scalp, to restore hair or prevent its further loss. They buy toupees that look like patches cut out of the shag rug in your den. Countless millions of dollars are spent in what is usually a fruitless pursuit.

Although baldness can and does affect women too, it is primarily a male phenomenon, and often *hereditary*. Several men in a family are likely to have similar hair patterns, but baldness can skip generations. The picture on the front of this book is a case in point. You can see that I am endowed with a full head of hair, yet my three sons all have receding hairlines. The eldest was almost completely bald by age thirty. Like Telly Savalas and the late Yul Brynner, he loves it and insists that the degree of male baldness is in direct proportion to circulating levels of male hormone. He raises the morale of his less enthusiastic brothers by reminding them that in more enlightened cultures baldness is considered to be very sexy—a sign of virility. His Christmas present to them last year was a bumper sticker on their car which reads: "God made some heads perfect. He covered the rest with hair." My sons did not inherit their hair loss from me. Their *maternal* grandfather and uncle, however, were both bald. (That's the way it has always been in our family—all the bad genes came from the "other side.")

Male pattern baldness generally starts at the front of the scalp on either side, or as a circular area on top. If it begins in the teens, it is apt to be fairly extensive in later life and the only solutions are resignation, a well-designed wig, a hair transplant or, as in the case of my son, enthusiastic acceptance. Minoxidil (Rogaine), a hypertension medication, has the additional action, in some men with pattern baldness, of slowing the hairline's retreat and perhaps even stimulating new hair growth. I have seen a few cases in which it has made a difference.

In some women the hair may thin up front and on the sides as they get older, but they are not subject to familial or hereditary baldness, for which my daughter is very grateful.

Male or female, we all lose some of our hair as we get older. But *sudden* hair loss may reflect *hormonal changes,* an underlying disease of the skin of your scalp, a prolonged fever or a medication, or it may result from radiation therapy.

The hormonal disorder most frequently responsible for hair loss is *thyroid trouble,* when the gland is either overactive or sluggish. When the "hyper" gland is successfully treated (by radioactive iodine, surgery or medication), the hair loss stops and growth often resumes. By the same token, when a thyroid-hormone deficiency is replaced with thyroid pills, the balding process is arrested and reversed. Hormonal fluctuations and accompanying hair loss sometimes occur after pregnancy and in other glandular diseases, especially those involving the pituitary.

Any serious illness, especially one accompanied by a *fever,* may result in temporary hair loss from the entire body, not just the scalp. When the underlying condition is successfully treated, the hair grows back. Autoimmune diseases like lupus erythematosus are also frequently accompanied by hair loss.

There is a disorder, probably autoimmune in origin, called *alopecia areata,* in which small, well-defined patches of hair are lost from the scalp or the beard. In adults, it lasts for several months, after which growth resumes. But when alopecia areata begins in childhood, hair loss is usually permanent.

Many *drugs,* especially those used in cancer treatment, cause hair loss, as does too much vitamin A, either in your diet or in supplements. Hair loss from *radiation therapy* eventually grows back in most cases.

Clearly, if your hair has always been full and it starts falling out just as you contract a disease, especially one accompanied by high fever, the reason is apparent. It's also obvious if the baldness coincides with your taking a new potent drug. Here are some specific tips to help you figure out why you are losing your locks:

- If you're a male teenager with a family history of hair loss, and your scalp hair is beginning to thin, you've inherited male pattern baldness. In that case, hair elsewhere on the body is not affected. By contrast, if you've had a fever or evidence of hormonal imbalance, started a new medication or received radiation therapy, then hair in other parts of the body, in addition to the scalp, is also involved.

- If the scalp hair loss is patchy, you may be suffering from alopecia areata. But you may also have a *fungus.* The most common one is tinea capitis, the medical term for ringworm of the scalp. It is contagious, affects mostly children and spreads like wildfire in schools and homes.

- Hair loss often accompanies *aging.* I don't know why it doesn't happen to every senior citizen, and why it happens at all. Maybe it's due to the individual genetic cards we have been dealt by our ancestors, or to poor nutrition or perhaps to some undiagnosed hormonal change. Again, despite all the claims and commercials, when an older person loses hair for no discernible reason, it's usually permanent.

Finally, there are causes of hair loss that have nothing to do with what's going on in your body. Some *nervous* children are in the habit of pulling it out. Always check out that possibility first if your child starts losing hair. *Excessive shampooing and blow-drying,* whether at home or at the salon, can injure the hair and cause it to fall out in substantial amounts. So, before you worry about male pattern baldness or hormonal trouble, make sure your grooming techniques aren't to blame.

Points to Remember

Symptom: Baldness.

What It May Mean	What to Do About It
1. Male pattern baldness (hereditary).	Enjoy it. If you can't, get a hair transplant or wear a wig.
2. Hormonal changes (thyroid disease).	Treat the underlying cause.
3. Any serious illness.	Appropriate treatment.
4. Fever.	Hair will grow back.
5. Autoimmune disorder (alopecia areata).	Appropriate treatment.
6. Medication (cancer chemotherapy, too much vitamin A).	Will usually grow back after consumption stops.
7. Radiation therapy.	Will grow back.
8. Fungal infections.	Appropriate treatment.
9. Aging.	No effective treatment.

| 10. | Nervous habit. | Supportive care. |
| 11. | Excessive shampooing and blow-drying. | Proper grooming. |

TOO MUCH HAIR

Few men complain of having too much hair. But women often do when it is growing in the wrong places. At this point, I'm going to define three medical terms, all of which relate to hair growth. Their significance, and the differences among them, will help you understand the meaning of excessive hair in your own case.

"Hirsutism" is a word which, when applied to women, means the presence of hair where it wouldn't normally be, because of a hormonal abnormality. "Hypertrichosis" means simply too much hair anywhere and on anyone and has nothing to do with hormones. Male or female, how much hair you have is a personal characteristic, one which is influenced by your *racial and geographic origin*. For example, women of Mediterranean descent—Greek, Italian, Arabic, Jewish—are more apt to have hypertrichosis than are Scandinavians. Oriental women, on the other hand, are not. So while some subtle hair growth on the upper lip of an Italian woman is not uncommon, you'll *never* see it on the face of a Chinese woman. The term "virilization" when applied to a woman refers to a process of masculinization. When it occurs, her voice deepens, her muscular development becomes manlike and her scalp may become bald. The clitoris enlarges, too, and her sex drive also increases. She begins to grow facial hair as well. There is loss of typical female features (the breasts become smaller, the periods stop and the vagina shrinks and becomes dry). Here you can be sure that the hirsutism is due to a significant hormonal imbalance.

There are several conditions in which a woman manifests excessive hair growth, in terms of location and amount. Here are some of the more common ones:

- Many women develop some facial hair at the time of *menopause* because of the decreased amount of estrogen being made by their ovaries. The condition can be treated, if there is no reason not to do so, by estrogen replacement therapy.

- *An overactive adrenal gland* producing increased amounts of its hormones due to a benign or malignant tumor causes hirsutism and virilization. The diagnosis is made by blood analyses and a CAT scan of the adrenal area.

- *Cushing's syndrome,* also the result of an overproduction of steroid hormones from the adrenal gland, has a similar effect. In addition to hirsutism, such patients have a moon-shaped face, and fat accumulates on the body and on the back, where they may develop a "buffalo hump."

- Special kinds of *ovarian cysts* (and rarely tumors) can, believe it or not, actually produce the *male* hormone, testosterone. That's what confers the hair and the virilization.

- A *pituitary tumor* may cause enough hormonal derangement to upset the normal male-female balance. Such growths also result in acromegaly, or gigantism, a condition characterized by enlarged jawbone, hands and feet.

- *Medication* can "make a man" out of you. Testosterone is often prescribed for women (usually in combination with estrogens) for relief of menopausal symptoms, and for the "fatigue" syndrome. While some females do benefit from it, others develop hirsutism, most apparent as hair on the upper lip.

Minoxidil, used in the treatment of high blood pressure, was noted some years ago to cause hirsutism in women. Far from being dismayed at this side effect of one of their important drugs, resourceful scientists have parlayed it into a treatment for baldness! It is marketed as Rogaine in the United States and Canada. So if you've noticed hair growth where you don't want it, and are taking minoxidil for your hypertension, give what's left in the bottle to your bald husband, and take something else to lower your pressure.

Points to Remember

Symptom: Excessive hair growth.

What It May Mean	What to Do About It
1. A normal variant depending on racial and geographic origin.	Cosmetic treatment, if desired.
2. Menopause.	Estrogen replacement therapy.
3. Tumors of the adrenal and pituitary glands and of the ovaries, and Cushing's syndrome.	Appropriate treatment (medication, surgery or radiation).
4. Ovarian cysts.	Removal.
5. Medications (minoxidil, male hormones).	Stop them.

WHEN YOU FLUSH AND BLUSH AND
ARE RED ALL OVER

Do you turn bright red when you're embarrassed, angry, feeling guilty or experiencing some other strong emotion? Such psychologically induced flushing is usually limited to the head and the neck and is of fairly brief duration. It occurs when tiny blood vessels (capillaries) near the surface of the skin, which are under nervous system control, dilate in response to an emotional stimulus. Once the stimulus subsides, these capillaries return to normal and the skin assumes its usual hue. Blushing is a common phenomenon and nothing to worry about. Indeed, the only major disadvantage of being an easy blusher is that you can't tell a lie, even a little white one, without your beet-red face giving you away. In some persons, a small amount of beta blocker taken just before an expected blush may minimize it.

Flushing of limited duration, and again restricted to the face and neck, also occurs in menopausal women—the so-called *"hot flush."* Unlike the emotional blush, it comes on without provocation at any time of the day or night, and is due to a drop in estrogen levels.

If you have high *fever*, your face will be flushed. Not only do you feel as if you're burning up, you look it. That's because the skin capillaries have dilated in order to permit the loss of the body's excess heat via the skin. Persons with an *overactive thyroid* may also look a little flushed, because their biological engine is running too fast and too hot, to which the capillaries accommodate by dilating.

Capillaries may remain chronically dilated and leave you looking perpetually red in the face. The classic example is the *alcoholic* whose red face—and nose—are the badge of heavy drinking. But don't jump to any conclusions from appearances alone. There are other diseases, and drugs, that can produce the same picture. For example, one drink can cause a facial flush in someone who is not an alcoholic but is merely *intolerant* to the stuff. Some of these people have been able to imbibe all their lives, and then one day, for no apparent reason, they find that a single glass of wine or a cocktail results in severe, uncomfortable flushing. I've seen this quite often in diabetics taking a sugar-lowering *medication* called Diabenase.

Other substances have a similar effect. Niacin is one of the safest and most effective drugs for lowering cholesterol, but it will give you intense flushing all over the body—a feeling of burning up. On occasion, when I've neglected to warn patients to expect this reaction, panic has ensued. One woman called in the middle of the night to say she was on fire without smoke! Steroid hormones also dilate capillaries and cause a red face.

Two *tumors* in particular may produce telltale flushing. One is *Hodgkin's disease,* a malignancy of the lymph glands. When patients with this disorder take alcohol, their skin becomes red and their glands hurt. A *carcinoid,* a hormone-secreting tumor originating in the lungs or the intestines, causes the capillaries to dilate, too. When there is no other cause for sudden, unexplained flushing, Hodgkin's and carcinoid should be considered.

There are several other major disorders in which flushing is a prominent symptom. When the lungs have been damaged by chronic disease, the body compensates for the resulting *oxygen deprivation* by producing more red blood cells. This makes for the reddish, flushed appearance so often seen in individuals with chronic emphysema or bronchitis. In fact, chronic oxygen deprivation due to *any* cause may result in an overabundance of red blood cells and the consequent reddish appearance of the skin. Flushing is also present in a blood disorder called *polycythemia vera* in which the bone marrow produces an excessive number of red blood cells. This thickened blood flows more slowly through the capillaries and causes the flushed appearance.

Here's how you can tell what's making *you* flush:

- If your periods are beginning to taper off and you have paroxysms during which you feel very hot and flushed, it's *menopause*.
- If you've been taking a new high-potency vitamin and notice that your face has been looking kind of red, check out the ingredients. Chances are it contains *niacin* (also called nicotinic acid). Or if you've been taking "something" to lower your cholesterol and have begun to flush terribly, it's probably niacin.
- If your face flushes after you take a drink, and you feel pain in your armpit or your neck, look for lumps or swellings. You may have Hodgkin's disease.
- If you're a diabetic, are on oral medication to lower your blood sugar and have noticed that even one or two drinks make you flush, it's due to the interaction between the alcohol and the antidiabetic pill.
- If you love to drink and have always handled it well, but your friends now tell you you've gotten some "high color" (the last time you sat in the sun was six months ago), the booze is making your face red. If you stop now or cut down drastically, the flushing won't necessarily go away, because

the capillaries may have become permanently dilated, but at least it won't get any worse.

- Your face is flushed; your eyes have become a little prominent; you're nervous and jittery much of the time; your hands have a fine tremor, as does your tongue when you protrude it; you're losing weight. The cause? You have an overactive thyroid gland. These symptoms, with the exception of the prominent eyes, will disappear when the condition is treated.

- You've suddenly developed attacks of diarrhea for no apparent reason, and you've also been wheezing. To top it all off, your face is occasionally flushed, too, even when you're not embarrassed. Those three symptoms, facial flushing, diarrhea and wheezing, are characteristic of a carcinoid tumor, which is secreting a substance called serotonin into your system.

- What's this? The back of your neck has gotten a hump in it; you've noticed some reddish blue streaks on your belly; your blood pressure is suddenly high; your body is fat, but your legs and arms are thin; if you're a woman, perhaps the most disconcerting observation is the mustache on your upper lip; and, man or woman, your face is reddish in color. If you've got any combination of the above, put your money on *Cushing's syndrome;* your body is producing too much cortisone. But you can also get to look that way just from taking cortisone tablets for a long time.

Points to Remember

Symptom: Flushing.

What It May Mean	What to Do About It
1. Normal response to embarrassment or anger.	If it's really troublesome, you can take a beta blocker.
2. "Hot flush": menopause.	Estrogen replacement.
3. Fever.	Reduce the temperature.
4. Hyperthyroidism.	Treat with medication, surgery or radioactive iodine.
5. Alcoholism.	Temperance.
6. Sensitivity to alcohol.	Eliminate it.
7. Medication (antidiabetics, steroids, niacin).	Switch or quit.
8. Carcinoid tumor or Hodgkin's disease.	Appropriate surgery.
9. Chronic oxygen deprivation.	Appropriate treatment.
10. Polycythemia vera.	Medical treatment.
11. Cushing's syndrome.	Surgery or medication.

WHEN YOUR SKIN CHANGES COLOR—AND IT'S NOT A PIGMENT OF YOUR IMAGINATION

Your skin coloring was determined by your ancestors and whence they came. If they were natives of Senegal in West Africa, you're probably very dark brown.

On the other hand, if your family originated in County Cork in Ireland, you're probably freckled and of pink complexion. The degree of skin pigmentation determines not only your appearance, but to some extent the various dermatological diseases to which you may be vulnerable. The lighter your color, the greater your susceptibility to skin cancer, although excessive exposure to the sun constitutes a risk to everyone.

In addition to pigmentation, there are other skin conditions whose significance you should appreciate. *Any mole or other discrete growth, especially one that has changed color, size or appearance, must be shown to your dermatologist right away.* It may be a *malignant melanoma,* a killing cancer which can be cured if removed early enough. Any growth that has persisted for more than a couple of weeks, no matter what it looks like, should be checked out. Here are some common skin discolorations and what they mean:

Vitiligo is usually a congenital condition found in perfectly healthy people. It consists of patchy areas of skin that have lost their pigmentation. Although it may occasionally indicate diabetes, pernicious anemia or thyroid-gland malfunction, in the overwhelming majority of cases vitiligo is of no significance, except for its cosmetic impact. The only practical "treatment" is camouflage with makeup. Psoralens and ultraviolet light are sometimes prescribed, but I have rarely found the results worth the effort.

In contrast to vitiligo, skin pigmentation may become more intense. The most common cause of such *hyperpigmentation* is, of course, exposure to the sun. Never forget that *sunburned skin is damaged skin.* There's no such thing as a healthy tan. It may look good for the moment, but you will pay for it years later with premature wrinkling and loss of skin elasticity, which will leave you looking older than your years. What's even worse, dedicated, obsessed sun worshipers are vulnerable to all kinds of skin cancers.

Addison's disease is a frequent cause of increased pigmentation. In this disorder, from which President John F. Kennedy suffered, the adrenal glands, which produce cortisone, function poorly or hardly at all. The signature characteristic of Addison's disease is the appearance of brown pigment in the skin and the mouth. Disorders of the liver or the intestinal tract, arsenic poisoning, vitamin deficiencies and malnutrition can all pigment the skin, but they rarely involve the mouth.

If you have *varicose veins* and your legs are chronically swollen, chances are there is some brownish pigmentation around your ankles. That discoloration comes from blood that has leaked out of the veins and into the tissues.

If you've undergone *radiation therapy,* the skin through which the X rays were beamed may become pigmented weeks after the therapy is finished. I've also noticed pigmentation in women taking *the Pill.* When they stop it, the discoloration disappears.

There's a disorder called *familial polyposis* in which the intestinal tract is studded with polyps along its entire length, from the stomach to the end of the colon. Because these polyps are precancerous, large portions of the bowel are often removed as a preventive step. As its name implies, this condition runs in families. Individuals who have it can be identified by the presence of dark, almost black pigmentation in their gums.

A perfectly normal kind of pigmentation occurs during *pregnancy*. If you're expecting and you develop dark brown discoloration on the cheeks and the forehead, you've got the "mask of pregnancy." Don't worry about it—it will clear up. Until it does, avoid excessive sunlight, which will make it worse.

Certain foods and medicines can alter your dermatological hue. In fact, there are more than fifty different drugs of which I am aware that can result in either discoloration or a rash, especially when your skin is exposed to the sun. The most important is *tetracycline*—a widely used antibiotic—and its derivatives. I've also seen such a solar reaction from sleeping pills, oral antidiabetic agents, a host of tranquilizers, antianxiety drugs and oral contraceptives and the new antiarrhythmic drug amiodarone. So, as always, when you develop any symptom, in this case a rash, first consider the medication you're taking.

If you're on a *beta carotene* kick because you think (not unreasonably) that lots of leafy green vegetables and carrots may protect you against cancer (particularly of the lungs), don't be surprised if your skin assumes a yellow hue. This will be most noticeable on the palms and the soles. But before you rush off to your doctor convinced you're jaundiced due to hepatitis, take a look at the whites of your eyes. In true *jaundice*, they too turn yellow; in carotene staining, they do not. If you're taking Atabrine to get rid of the amoebae in your stool, it is also likely to leave you bright yellow all over.

There are several diseases that can affect the color of your skin. A lemon tint may mean that your *thyroid* gland is underfunctioning, or that you have *pernicious anemia*. Pernicious anemia results from an inability to absorb the vitamin B_{12} in the diet because of a deficiency of an enzyme in the stomach called "intrinsic factor."

Finally, as a general rule, any change in skin pigmentation that occurs without an obvious cause and persists should be brought to the attention of your doctor or a dermatologist.

Points to Remember

Symptom: Change in skin coloring.

What It May Mean	What to Do About It
1. Moles or other growths: skin cancer, including malignant melanoma.	Medical evaluation and appropriate treatment.
2. Vitiligo (absence of pigmentation).	Usually of no significance. Cover the depigmented areas with makeup.
3. Addison's disease (look for brown pigment in the mouth).	Replacement of deficient steroid hormones.
4. Varicose veins (brown pigmentation in legs).	No treatment for the pigmentation.
5. Pigmentation from radiation therapy.	Eventually disappears.
6. Discoloration from using the Pill.	No therapy.
7. Pigmentation in gums caused by familial polyposis.	Appropriate treatment.
8. "Mask of pregnancy."	Pigmentation is temporary— avoid exposure to sun.
9. Reaction to foods and drugs (antibiotics, beta carotene).	Substitutes, avoid exposure to sun with certain medications.
10. Jaundice.	Treat underlying cause.

11. Hypothyroidism.	Thyroid supplements.
12. Pernicious anemia.	Monthly B_{12} injections.

ARE YOU REALLY PALE—OR DO YOU JUST LOOK THAT WAY?

There's a subculture of self-styled health experts in our society who have no special training or qualifications but who go about offering unsolicited health evaluations. Such "gurus" will quite gratuitously comment, "Gosh, you look pale. Are you feeling all right?"

When people do remark on your pallor, they may, of course, be right. If you really are pale, the most likely cause is anemia—for any one of many reasons ranging from malnutrition to cancer to blood loss. However, pale-looking skin doesn't necessarily mean you're anemic. Your skin color may be very light because your ancestors hailed from Scandinavia. Or you're not exposed to the sun very much. The office worker who gets into a car early in the morning, drives to work, spends all day indoors and then drives home after dark is not likely to have a rosy hue. A construction worker, on the other hand, always has a ruddy complexion because he's exposed to the elements all day, every day.

The bottom line: Unless your pale skin is accompanied by pale lips, tongue, palms of the hands, inside of the mouth and lining of the eyes, ignore any comments about how "pale" you look. If you're worried, check your stool for the presence of blood even if it's not visible to the naked eye. Also, be on the lookout for heart palpitations or recent shortness of breath—both additional signs of significant anemia.

I remember hearing a story that sums up how un-reliable a casual look at someone's skin can be, and why it's generally best to ignore unsolicited health observations. An elderly gentleman died in Florida while on a winter vacation. At the wake, one of his friends looked at the bier and commented, "What a tan. Doesn't he look great!"

Points to Remember

Symptom: Looking pale.

What It May Mean	What to Do About It
1. Normal color for you.	Nothing.
2. Lack of exposure to the elements.	You're better off pale than tanned.
3. Anemia (blood loss, poor nutrition, serious underlying disease).	Treat the underlying condition.

EXCESSIVE PERSPIRATION: HORMONES, HEAT OR ANXIETY?

To sweat is perfectly natural, something one doesn't wonder or worry about when it's appropriate. After a couple of sets of tennis or jogging in warm weather, you expect to perspire. And it's a good thing you do, because that's the body's way of eliminating excess heat produced by increased activity. As the perspiration evaporates, it cools the skin surface. Emotional stress may also cause you to perspire, since it results in an overproduction of adrenaline that triggers the sweat glands.

Excessive perspiration occurs in those parts of the body that contain most of the sweat glands—the palms, the soles, the armpits and the genital area. Normal perspiration has a characteristic odor, due to the action of bacteria present on the skin. It is particularly noticeable in the armpits. While it is generally considered offensive in our society, this odor is viewed as erotic in other cultures and the use of deodorants is thought to be absurd. When sweaty feet begin to smell—as they often do in younger persons—it's not the aroma of the sweat that offends, but the skin debris being decomposed by bacteria.

There is a rare psychological disorder in which the individual is convinced that his or her body is foul-smelling, even though it's not. This forces them into a hermitlike existence because they're afraid of being embarrassed or reviled due to their bad odor. If, however, your sweat truly does have an offensive odor, check out your diet. Onions and garlic in particular seem to come right out of the pores and into the noses of bystanders.

The *emotional* link to sweating is pretty obvious. If you break out into profuse perspiration when you're embarrassed, angry, nervous, afraid or anxious, you don't need a complicated diagnostic workup to tell you why. However, such emotion-induced sweating is usually limited to the hands, the feet, the face and, to a lesser degree, the armpits. When the entire body is enveloped in sweat, you should consider the physical causes discussed below.

Fever, whatever its cause, results in sweating because that's how the body cools itself off. Whatever the cause of the fever, whether it's cancer, pneumonia, some other infection or rheumatic fever, patients find themselves perspiring a good part of the day regardless of the ambient temperature. Some infections have characteristic sweating patterns. For example, when the sweating is most noticeable during the night, suspect pulmonary tuberculosis.

When the body's metabolic motor is revved up by an *overactive thyroid,* not only does your skin become moist and *warm* (this in contrast to the cold wet palms and soles of nervous individuals) but the hands shake, the hair thins, the skin is smooth and the pulse is rapid.

Hormonal imbalance can cause paroxysmal sweating in which the skin is dry one moment and soaking the next (in contrast to sweating due to an overactive thyroid gland, which is virtually constant). Classically, this intermittent perspiration occurs in *menopausal* women who are awakened at night by a hot flush and sweating in the absence of any external temperature change. This also occurs in men with *prostate cancer* who have been treated with estrogens. In these "glandular sweaters," the skin is normally dry and cool between flushes.

Certain *foods and medications* make people sweat. Coffee will do it. A shot of morphine given for pain not only controls discomfort but also results in perspiration at the height of its action.

Various diseases cause sweating even in the absence of fever:

- A cold, drenching sweat often precedes or accompanies the characteristic chest symptoms in an acute *heart attack.* But a similar sweat may also occur when you're seasick.
- Periodic sweating, the kind that comes and goes (in the absence of a hormonal change), is frequently caused by an *abscess*—a collection of pus somewhere in the body—and is accompanied by fever.
- *Diabetics* receiving insulin or oral medication may go into a cold sweat when their blood sugar drops

too low. At the same time, they experience profound weakness, nausea and a rapid pulse that feels "weaker" than normal.

The bottom line: Sweating is usually nothing to worry about. But excessive or unexplained sweating should be checked out with your doctor to determine the underlying cause.

Points to Remember

Symptom: Excessive sweating.

What It May Mean	What to Do About It
1. Normal response to heat or exercise.	Stay cool.
2. Emotional stress, anxiety.	Supportive care.
3. Fever.	No treatment unless it's very high. The fever attacks invading organisms, and the sweat cools the body.
4. Hyperthyroidism.	Treat with surgery, radiation or medication.
5. Menopause.	Estrogen replacement.
6. Treatment for prostate cancer.	Episodic. No therapy.
7. Reaction to certain foods and drugs (coffee, morphine).	Temporary. To be expected.
8. Earliest sign of a heart attack.	Get help if the sweating is accompanied or followed by chest pain or pressure.

9. Infection, abscess.	Treat the underlying cause.
10. Low blood sugar in diabetics.	Stabilize the sugar level.

WHAT YOUR FINGERNAILS AND TOENAILS CAN TELL YOU

For me, the world is divided into two kinds of patients—those who wait for symptoms to occur and those who keep looking for trouble! It's easy to recognize the latter, especially if you're living with one. The really committed among them go all the way. There they are, every morning, standing in front of the mirror, intently evaluating their protruded tongues. When they've finished that maneuver, they move on to the eyes. Are they bloodshot, bleary-looking? The women among them then hop into the shower to examine their breasts. The men check out their testicles.

Now, breast and testicular self-examination is very important, something everyone should do regularly. But forget the other two—you can't tell much of importance from a coated tongue or bloodshot eyes. There is, however, another part of the body, which these self-examiners often overlook, that *can* yield a great deal of information: the nails of the fingers and the toes. But you must first remove all the polish and, of course, any artificial extensions that some people find attractive.

I can think of almost forty different disorders which can be diagnosed just by looking at the nails—everything from compulsive nail-biting to anemia, lung disease, heart trouble, infection and brain malfunction. You can distinguish among them if you know what to look for. Note the color of your nails, their shape, their thickness, the presence of any markings on or under them and how firmly they are attached to the fingers. Here are some specifics:

- *Nail-biting* is difficult to conceal, unless you wear gloves. Fully one third of my patients are nail-biters, including one who is the top banana in a multibillion-dollar international corporation, a suave, debonair man with a stretch limo waiting for him —and with closely bitten nails. His chauffeur, on the other hand (also my patient), has nails that are properly cut and maintained! Nail-biting may be nothing more than a bad habit, but it may also reflect chronic tension and anxiety. If done to the point of bleeding, it is evidence of an uncontrollable compulsion.

- *Pale nails* signal anemia. It will not be apparent in your skin if you've spent time in the sun, but you can't camouflage your white nail beds unless you paint them. Whatever its cause, if anemia is severe enough and long-standing, your nails are not only pale, they're brittle. They also change their shape, becoming either flat or concave like a spoon, and develop ridges running up and down their length. If you notice any of these signs in your nails (the pallor always comes first), look at the creases in your palms and the color of the conjunctivae in the eyes. If they're pale, too, you can bet you're anemic. Your doctor will have to figure out why. It can be due to anything from a blood loss of which you are unaware (such as insidious oozing from hemorrhoids, or gastric irritation from too much aspirin) to a disease of the bone marrow (which isn't making the right kind of blood in the proper amounts), to a hidden tumor or to chronically heavy menstruation. Statistically, however, it's usually just a matter of diet—the iron you've *not* been eating.

- *Bluish nails* (*cyanosis*) mean there is not enough oxygen in the blood. Should you also be short of breath and develop a cough, see your doctor right away. You probably have some degree of heart failure or chronic lung trouble. On the other hand, if your nails are blue but you are neither short of breath nor coughing, you may have been exposed to a toxic chemical which has poisoned your red blood cells. In infants, cyanosis may be due to a congenital heart condition ("blue babies") which is surgically correctable.

- *Thick, distorted fingernails* may result from a number of diseases. A fungus infection will do it. If that's what your doctor suspects, he or she will get a little scraping from the nail and look at it under the microscope. Psoriasis, in which areas of the skin throughout the body are covered with silvery white scales, may also so distort the nails. If the problem is due neither to fungus nor to psoriasis, it may be caused by a vitamin deficiency, arteriosclerosis or a host of other diseases. See a dermatologist.

- *"Clubbed" fingernails.* If your fingernails are very rounded, like the back of a teaspoon, they may qualify for the term "clubbed." This happens in a variety of diseases, all of which are important—chronic infections, especially abscesses, cancer of the lung, chronic lung and heart disease, longstanding tuberculosis and several forms of congenital heart disease. Why these different conditions all cause the fingernails to become clubbed is a mystery. I suspect it's due either to some change in the oxygen content of the blood or to an alteration in the way blood flows to the fingers. If and when the underlying disorder is successfully treated, the clubbing may disappear.

But before you panic about the shape of your nails, remember that there is a difference between a healthy rounded nail and one that's clubbed. It's a matter of degree. You can tell them apart by looking at the nail from the side. It should normally form an angle of about 160 degrees where it meets the skin. A clubbed nail does not do so, and in effect it runs into the skin in a straight line.

- Everyone I know has, on occasion, seen little *white flecks* under the nails. They represent pockets of air. They're of no consequence and usually disappear on their own, although they may persist for years. Vitamin enthusiasts insist that they are caused by some deficiency or other. I doubt it.

- If you're a mystery buff, you probably know what the combination of *white lines* and horizontal *ridges* in fingernails means. It's a sure sign that someone is trying to do you in by slipping arsenic into your diet (without the old lace). But remember, these ridges run from side to side, not lengthwise as they do in anemia. I wish I could say that I foiled a murder attempt by spotting such ridges in an intended victim's fingernails, but I cannot tell a lie.

- Together, dry skin and nails that are *brittle* and separate easily from the nail bed constitute evidence of an underfunctioning thyroid. In that case, you'll also feel abnormally tired; your skin may have a lemon hue, and the pulse is slow; you're always cold and your coarse hair tends to fall out. Interestingly enough, *hyper*thyroidism, in which the gland is *overactive*, also leaves the nails brittle and loose; here, however, they are also characteristically concave, like a spoon.

- If when you look very closely at your nails you see

something that looks like a *splinter,* but you know isn't because it doesn't hurt, you may have stumbled across a very important piece of evidence pointing to subacute bacterial endocarditis (SBE). This is a condition in which heart valves already diseased (perhaps due to a congenital defect or to rheumatic fever) become infected. The infection makes its presence known with fever, weakness, lassitude and, very often, what looks like little splinters under the fingernails. These are actually small hemorrhages, and their presence is virtually 100 percent diagnostic of SBE. How do you get the infection in the first place? If you have a heart murmur, and allow the dentist to work in your mouth without your taking prophylactic antibiotics, the normal bacteria in your mouth enter the bloodstream and, bingo, end up on the heart valves.

There is one other totally unrelated cause of splinterlike hemorrhages under the nails: trichinosis, the infection you can get from eating raw or inadequately cooked pork. The other symptoms of trichinosis are diffuse muscle aches and pains and puffy, swollen eyes.

• Look at your nails. Notice that little white "half moon" at their base? That's, of course, normal. If your pituitary, the master gland of the brain, is diseased, those "moons" are lost. However, if your nails have a *whitish hue* at their base, you may have liver trouble, notably chronic hepatitis or cirrhosis (usually the end result of too much alcohol for too many years).

So, just like the skin, the fingernails are an excellent reflection of the state of your health. Many a life has been saved and medical reputations have been made by brilliant diagnoses based on a quick glance at a patient's fingernails.

Points to Remember

Symptom: Abnormalities of the finger- and toenails.

What It May Mean	What to Do About It
1. Bitten nails: anxiety, habit.	Psychological help.
2. Pale nails: anemia.	Determine the cause and treat.
3. Blue nails (cyanosis): heart or lung trouble, toxic chemical action on blood cells, congenital heart disease in infants.	Identify the cause and correct the abnormality.
4. Distorted nails: fungus, psoriasis, vitamin deficiency, arteriosclerosis.	Treat the underlying condition.
5. "Clubbed" fingernails: abscess, chronic infection, cancer of the lung, chronic heart disease.	Correct the underlying condition. Make sure it's not a normal variant.
6. White flecks: air pockets.	Does not require treatment.
7. White lines and horizontal ridges: arsenic poisoning.	Gastric washing if acute; bind the arsenic with chelation therapy if chronic.
8. Brittle nails: hyperthyroidism or hypothyroidism.	Extra thyroid if too low; surgery, radioactive iodine, medication if overactive.

9. "Splinters": subacute bacterial endocarditis, trichinosis.

See your doctor immediately.

10. White hue at the base of the nails: liver disease.

Treat the underlying disorder.

CHAPTER 12

PALPITATIONS, PULSES AND AN IRREGULAR HEARTBEAT

I'm always amazed at the number of patients who know how to examine their breasts or their testicles, who own sophisticated blood-pressure-monitoring machines, who even measure their own blood-sugar levels, but who do not know how to take their own pulse! It's by far the easiest self-evaluation test there is—and an important one.

HOW TO TAKE YOUR PULSE

With each heartbeat, blood is pumped into the circulation through every artery in the body. When you feel for this "wave" of the circulating blood with your fingers placed over a large artery close to the skin surface, you're "taking the pulse." The trick, however, is to find an artery that's large enough and that you can get at. There are lots of big blood vessels inside the body, but most are out of reach. The wrist is the traditional pulse-taking spot, but there are others: the sides of the neck, the groin, the top of the foot (in a line between the big toe and the one next to it, about one and a half inches up toward the ankle) and the inside of the ankle just by the bone. But you're probably not going to go to the trouble of feeling the neck, the foot or especially the groin if you're taking someone else's pulse—in public! So that leaves the wrist.

With the palm turned upward, the spot you're looking for lies on the wrist about a half inch from the base of the thumb. Sometimes you'll have to search around a bit with your fingers before you find it. The position of the artery isn't fixed; it varies from person to person. Sometimes it's a little over to the side, or closer to the midline, or higher up on the wrist. So don't just give up if you're having trouble— remember, *everyone* has a pulse somewhere or other.

Medical students are taught to use their middle finger and forefinger to feel a pulse—never the thumb. Why? Because the thumb is less sensitive and has a tiny pulse of its own, which can confuse things. However, if you are able to feel your own pulse or someone else's with your thumb, by all means do so.

WHAT YOUR PULSE TELLS YOU

Once you've found your pulse, what should you make of it? First of all, you want to know how fast it is. This tells you your heart rate. Count the pulse beats for a specific period of time—thirty seconds should be enough, but if you're not in a hurry, take as long as you like. If you're counting for thirty seconds, multiply the number of beats by two to obtain the heart rate per minute. So if you were to count thirty-five beats in those thirty seconds, two times thirty-five equals seventy—that's the rate your heart is beating per minute.

Although the normal rate at rest varies between sixty and one hundred per minute, most healthy people clock in between sixty-five and eighty-five. But it all depends on what you've been doing, what medication you're taking, whether or not you have a fever and how "physical" you are. For example, if you've just finished a game of tennis or chopped a cord of wood or made love, your pulse may go as high as 150 per minute. If, however, you've been resting quietly, it's more likely to be somewhere in the sixties or seventies.

If you're physically fit and do a great deal of exercise on a regular basis—running, swimming, tennis—your pulse rate at rest is likely to be *lower* than if your most strenuous exertion is getting up from the table or pushing an elevator button to go down one floor. I read somewhere that Björn Borg, the great Swedish tennis star, has a resting pulse rate in the thirties. In some three-martini-lunch businessmen I know, it's around eighty-five or ninety most of the time. But for the vast majority of us in between these extremes, the limits of the *resting* pulse rate are below one hundred (in the absence of fever) and above sixty.

IS IT NORMAL?

Like the frequency of bowel movements, we each have our own characteristic heart rate. The real question is, What's normal for *you*? First let's look at the possible causes of an *abnormally slow* heart rate:

- Are you taking digitalis to control an irregular heartbeat, or a beta blocker (Inderal, Tenormin, Corgard, Blocadren, Lopressor, Visken, Sectral) to treat high blood pressure, angina pectoris, a heart rhythm disorder, an anxiety state or migraine? These and several other medications, especially in combination, can slow the heart rate dramatically.
- If your pulse is consistently below sixty, and you're not an athlete and not taking any medication that could be responsible, you may have an *underactive thyroid*. This probability increases if, in addition to the slow pulse, you feel tired all the time, are cold when no one else is, are constipated, are losing your hair or finding that it has become

coarse, have periods that are heavier than you think they should be and have difficulty losing weight.

- Most of us think about the heart in terms of its arteries, valves and muscle. There is yet another critical component within the heart which helps determine the cardiac rate—namely, the electrical system. Specialized fibers conduct impulses to various regions of the heart. When these pathways are interrupted by disease or affected by medications of various kinds, *heart block* can ensue. When that happens, the cardiac rate may slow to dangerous levels.

More common than an excessively slow pulse is one that's *abnormally fast*. Here are some possible causes:

- If your pulse is consistently over one hundred at rest and you feel palpitations (a pounding in your chest) even while you're sitting quietly, look for these other symptoms: hair that has become silky thin, fine skin, a slight tremor of your fingers when your hands are extended (if you lay a sheet of tissue paper over them, does it shake?), weight loss for no apparent reason, nervousness and excessive perspiration. If this picture fits, you have an *overactive thyroid*.

Hyperthyroidism isn't the only condition that will race your pulse. A rapid heartbeat can reflect your body's attempt to compensate for some other problem. For example, a major function of blood is to carry the oxygen within its red cells to every nook and cranny, every organ, every bit of living tissue in the body. When you're anemic and blood is deficient in these red blood cells, or in iron (the mineral needed to carry the oxygen), the tissues are not adequately nourished. In order to compensate, the heart beats faster and faster to get more of the oxygen-poor blood to the target organs. In other words, it tries to make up in quantity what it lacks in quality. So, whatever the underlying cause of your anemia (remember, it's a symptom, not a disease unto itself), the heart rate tends to be higher. After the anemia is corrected, the rate slows down.

This cardiac compensatory mechanism—beating faster to make up for some deficiency—occurs in circumstances other than anemia. Thus, when the cardiac muscle is weak and not expelling enough blood every time it pumps, the heart rate accelerates to make up for the drop in output. In fact, cancer or any chronic kidney or liver disease can also trigger an abnormally rapid rate.

A very common cause of a surge in heart rate is too much medication, or the wrong kind. The greatest offenders are thyroid pills, caffeine and appetite suppressants. Doctors prescribe thyroid pills for true underfunction of the thyroid gland, and most people do not need more than two grains to replace what their own gland fails to produce. In that dosage, symptoms of thyroid underfunction clear up and the heart rate is normal. Unfortunately, some patients believe that if two grains are good for you, four grains must be even better. Application of this philosophy results in a rapid heart rate (and many other disquieting symptoms).

An underfunctioning thyroid gland isn't the only reason people take thyroid pills. Because this hormone increases the body's metabolism, thyroid supplements have for generations been abused by overweight individuals looking for a quick fix for their excess poundage. Big mistake. Unnecessary thyroid medication can cause not only heart rate irregularities, but blood-pressure elevation and worsened angina. If taken long enough, they will turn off your own gland from making enough hormone on its own.

Caffeine is addicting. For many people, there's nothing more satisfying or refreshing than a cup of hot coffee in the morning. Another at lunch can also add to your vitality in the afternoon, especially if you've had a cocktail which might otherwise sedate you. But really, that should be it. Persons addicted to caffeine drink lots more coffee (or carbonated soda pop that contains it) than they should. Some months ago I examined a woman who was consuming fifteen cups a day. When she reduced it to ten, she felt tired! Moreover, her resting pulse was—get this—120 beats per minute, for which there was no explanation other than the caffeine. When she was weaned from her addiction over a period of time, her heart rate dropped to eighty beats per minute. So if you're a caffeine addict, that's probably the reason for your elevated heart rate.

Some appetite-suppressant pills on the over-the-counter market also raise heart rate. The reason the Food and Drug Administration has allowed these substances to be purchased without a doctor's prescription is that they are safe when taken *exactly* as prescribed. But that's not always how people use them. Furthermore, even though the inserts in the packages do state that anyone with hypertension, heart problems or cardiac arrhythmias should check with his or her doctor before using these compounds, many individuals don't bother to read the inserts, and toss them out with the empty package. They assume that because a drug is sold over the counter, it's not really strong enough to do them any harm. So there are people who aren't aware of any underlying "contraindication" to the pills they're taking, and who develop untoward consequences from their use.

Most diet medications lose their effectiveness after a few weeks because one becomes "tolerant" to them. The tendency is to take more and more. The result is an overdosage and a further increase in heart rate.

The same active ingredient in diet pills (phenylpropanolamine—PPA) is also present in many cold remedies and in most nasal decongestants. If you've got the sniffles and are taking a medication to "open" your air passages, and you develop a rapid heart rate, the PPA may well be the cause.

Another group of drugs that can cause a fast pulse is the antiasthmatics. However, some preparations used in the treatment of asthma, namely Atrovent, cromolyn and the steroids, do not. Whether you take your spasm-breaking medicine by aerosol nebulizer or as one of the oral theophylline derivatives (Theo-Dur, Uniphyl, Quibron, Elixophyllin—there are a whole variety of them), you may notice a quickening of your heart rate. That's an expected pharmacological effect, but one we pay special attention to in individuals with heart disease.

Tobacco, particularly the nicotine in it, raises the heart rate, too. If there's any doubt in your mind about that and you're a smoker, just count your pulse before and after you deeply inhale a cigarette.

Generally speaking, *routine* pulse-taking is not necessary or desirable, but should be done when there's a reason. Some persons, when they feel "weak," check their pulse not for rate, but for strength or intensity. Patients have reported to me that their pulse is so feeble they can barely get it. They're certain that's why they feel so bad. In almost every case, that perception is false. The "poor quality" of the pulse in someone well enough to take it is simply due to the anatomy of the artery at the wrist: its distance from the skin, how much fat is covering it—factors which have no clinical relevance. But when "shock" has set in and the pulse really is weak, as might occur after a heart attack has severely damaged the cardiac muscle, or because there has been a significant loss of blood due to hemorrhage somewhere, there will be many other signs of "weakness." Under those circumstances, you're not likely to be checking your own pulse, anyway.

You may want to see how fast your heart is beating during exercise. I happen to think it's difficult if not well-nigh impossible to continue your exercise, count your pulse and look at your watch all at the same time. If you're trying to establish or maintain a target heart rate during physical activity, buy a pulse monitor, the kind that straps conveniently on your wrist like a watch or attaches to your earlobe.

People tend to check their pulse when they have become aware of their heartbeat. If you've just run a race, or been scared out of your wits by your neighbor's pit bull, your heart will pound. There are times when you may feel your heart beating irregularly. The most common cause is what patients call an *"extra beat,"* usually felt as a thump in the chest. If you take your pulse when you get this symptom, you'll find that your regular pulse is interrupted by a beat that comes earlier than anticipated and is followed by an unnervingly long pause before the heart resumes its normal rhythm.

Although frightening, this pause is not a sign of trouble; it *does not* mean your heart is going to stop. Nor is the extra beat really extra; it's just early. When that happens, the long pause is there to compensate for the premature beat, so that the heart can get back into step and resume its normal rhythm.

Most "extra beats" are harmless, but because they involve the heart, people worry about them. Remember that the heart is the toughest organ in the body. It works incessantly night and day, year in, year out.

A premature beat every now and then isn't going to do you or your heart any harm. These "extra" beats have a wide variety of triggers—stress, too much coffee or other stimulants, alcohol and other "recreational" drugs, fatigue, nervousness, tobacco or medications. They also occur for no apparent reason. They are best left alone. Medications that suppress them are often fraught with side effects. Unless they're really troubling you, do not insist on having them treated.

Despite the usually benign nature of most heart rhythm irregularities, some *are* of consequence. Any kind of heart disease, whether it's something as innocent as an uncomplicated mitral valve prolapse or as serious as congestive heart failure, is sometimes associated with important disturbances of rhythm, but not merely an occasional "extra" beat. *The significance of a disordered heart rhythm almost always depends on the other evidence and symptoms of heart disease that accompany it.*

When the heart beats so rapidly, or so slowly, *in a sustained manner* that it fails to deliver enough oxygenated blood to the tissues, the accompanying symptoms may include loss of consciousness, dizziness, lightheadedness, chest pain, perhaps even a stroke. In these situations, when the heartbeat is too rapid, we first try medication to slow it down. If that doesn't work, a brief electric shock may be necessary. When the heart rate is too slow, a pacemaker may be needed.

I believe that if we were all to become regular pulse-takers for no reason, we'd end up a rather frightened lot. There is no one whose heart rhythm and pulse are always completely regular. "Extra" beats are part of the normal heart action. But because heart disease is the number-one killer in our country, any perceived irregularity is viewed with alarm. So this piece of advice may surprise you: Unless you are monitoring your heart rate for a specific reason—you're taking some drug which can slow it, like digitalis or a beta blocker (where the next dosage is dependent on your pulse rate), or you have a target heart rate in your exercise program—don't bother taking your pulse. Examine your breasts, your testicles, your fingernails, your hair, your glands, and even stick your tongue out at yourself in the mirror —but stay away from your pulse.

Points to Remember

Symptom: Heartbeat irregularities.

What It May Mean	What to Do About It
1. Below 60 beats per minute: excellent physical training; medication; underactive thyroid; heart trouble.	If you're in good physical shape, keep up the good work. Otherwise, see your doctor.
2. Above 100 beats per minute at rest: fever, medication, any chronic disease, overactive thyroid, anxiety, anemia.	See your doctor.
3. "Extra" beats, usually benign if sporadic: due to caffeine, stress, fatigue, tobacco, alcohol, heart trouble.	Have your doctor check them out anyway, especially if you have other heart symptoms like shortness of breath, chest pain or pressure.

CHAPTER 13

HIGH BLOOD PRESSURE:
What the News Should Mean to You

This was not a good day for you. A routine checkup produced the definitely unexpected and unwelcome news that you have high blood pressure (hypertension). Suddenly all the bits and pieces of information you've heard about hypertension over the years—and ignored because your blood pressure was always normal—now come flooding into your consciousness. You remember phrases like "the silent killer," conversations with friends with hypertension who told you that the treatment is worse than the disease and they're now spending a lot less time with sex and a whole lot more in the bathroom emptying their bladders. You think, in particular, of your friend Joe, whose high blood pressure was diagnosed a few years back. Going out to dinner with him was a bore because poor Joe could order almost nothing on the menu. It seemed that everything he liked was loaded with salt. When you ate at his house, even while you nodded and smiled and said how good everything was, the food had the zest and flavor of paper pulp. Now *you* too will be leading Joe's kind of life.

Well, relax. Much of what you may have been led to believe is really not true. Hypertension *is* a silent killer, but *only* if left undiagnosed and untreated for a long time. Under those circumstances, the incessant pounding of the arteries under high pressure speeds up the process of arteriosclerosis everywhere. It may also cause them to balloon out and burst. So someone with *untreated* hypertension is a sitting duck for a stroke (the brain arteries clog or rupture), blindness (the eye arteries become diseased and blocked and they hemorrhage), heart attacks (the coronary arteries develop arteriosclerosis and are occluded), cardiac failure (the heart muscle is worn out pumping blood against the resistance of the elevated pressures in the body's arteries), kidney failure (its arteries also become arteriosclerotic and the kidneys stop working normally), aneurysms of the aorta (this major vessel distends and finally ruptures, a usually fatal event) and closure of the arteries in the legs (making it painful to walk any great distance).

Given the newer understanding of this disorder and the medications now available to control it, there's no reason for anyone to have high blood pressure these days. Diet, weight loss and exercise alone are sometimes enough to normalize elevated pressures. Occasionally, increases are only mild and temporary and they drop of their own accord. Doctors are also encountering more and more individuals with high blood pressure that is not salt-sensitive. In other words, such patients may safely consume reasonable amounts of salt without further elevating their pressure readings. Most persons can easily tolerate today's drug regimens—if one is needed. The intolerable side effects you've heard about are an exaggeration.

So, a diagnosis of high blood pressure isn't the end of the world. But in order to understand its implications both for your life and for your lifestyle, you should be familiar with the many faces of hypertension and know which specific variety you happen to have. Think for a moment about how the circulatory system works. In the very center, there is a pump—the heart. Every time it contracts, it empties its blood into a network of tubes—the arteries. Blood pressure refers to the pressure under which the blood flows through those arteries. Its level depends on three main factors.

The first is the *amount of blood* in the system. It's obvious that if the volume of blood circulating in this closed system is appreciably reduced, the pressure will drop. By the same token, if it is increased, the pressure often rises. The volume of blood in your circulation will *decrease* when you suffer a hemorrhage—that is, lose blood from either an injury, an operation or internally (as from a bleeding peptic ulcer). If the pressure drops too low, you go into shock —that is, a state of circulatory collapse.

What conditions result in an *increased blood volume*? One is too much salt in the blood, usually the result of kidney malfunction or, rarely, from tumors which cause the body to retain large amounts of salt. Some drugs, like the steroid hormones, can also induce salt retention, so that anyone taking this medication for any length of time may develop hypertension. So can heart failure, when the neck veins are distended, the feet are swollen and the lungs are filled with fluid. But in this latter case, the picture is dominated by a weak heart muscle, so that the pressure does not rise, but actually falls.

The second factor that determines blood-pressure levels is the *force* of the heart's pumping action. When the heart is weakened during or after a heart attack or by some other cardiac disease, it cannot pump its normal amount of blood. When that happens, the pressure may drop so low that the person goes into shock, very much like what happens after a severe hemorrhage.

But what can possibly give you *increased* cardiac output, and why on earth would that be bad? Well, just as one aspirin may be good for you but ten are not, by the same token a greater than normal output from the heart is undesirable because it strains the circulation. This can happen when the thyroid gland is overactive, when there is a leaky aortic valve in the heart and in several other less common conditions.

The third important factor governing your blood pressure level is the *"tone"* of the artery walls. There are tiny nerve endings in these walls which respond to messages from the brain and other organs, either dilating the arteries and reducing the pressure within them or constricting them and raising it. The arterial walls also react to a variety of hormonal signals. Whatever the mechanism, constriction of the artery wall raises blood pressure.

Here's how this tone mechanism works. You're coming home from the office late one night. You've parked your car, and just as you get out you feel a hand on your shoulder and are overcome by fear. At that moment, your adrenal glands secrete more adrenaline, causing the arteries to constrict. This is believed to be an evolutionary response to danger. Not only does the surge of adrenaline give you the ability either to run faster or to stand and fight harder, but should you be injured the constricted arteries help reduce the loss of blood. But fear isn't the only trigger that releases adrenaline. There's also a tumor called a *pheochromocytoma*. It causes high blood pressure by sending large amounts of adrenaline-like substances into the blood. It's not a common cause of hypertension, but if you have other symptoms of adrenaline surge without provocation —a racing, pounding heart or flushed skin, with lots of sweating for no good reason—it should be considered, especially if you're young. These adrenaline-like substances are also present in certain medications, which is why so many drugs carry the warning about their use if you have high blood pressure.

There are other causes of narrowed arteries, the

most important of which is *arteriosclerosis*. When the large vessels harden, they become less flexible, less compliant; they can't "roll with the punches" as they used to when a wave of blood ejected by the heart is propelled through them. This narrowing of arteries by arteriosclerosis and the resulting rigidity also elevate blood pressure.

So, then, the three main factors that contribute to an elevated blood pressure are (a) an increased volume of blood, (b) a greater than normal amount of blood pumped out by the heart with each beat and (c) increased tone in the arteries. In many cases, we can pinpoint the cause and treat it—sometimes even cure it.

CAUSES OF HYPERTENSION

Given this basic understanding of what high blood pressure is about, there are some clues and symptoms you can look for to see into which category you fall. Through your own knowledge and medical sleuthing, you may be able to tip your doctor off to the underlying cause in your case.

A good doctor is a biological detective, and every patient should be one, too. Not long ago I saw a woman of twenty-nine with an elevated blood pressure in the 180/100 range. Because she was so young, her arteries were going to take a terrible beating in the years ahead unless she was treated effectively. I ordered a full diagnostic work-up before starting therapy.

We came up with absolutely nothing abnormal. Her kidneys were fine; her hormone levels were normal; she wasn't on the Pill; she wasn't taking appetite suppressants or any other medication that could possibly be responsible for her hypertension. During one of her visits, however, we discussed her eating habits. I specifically wanted to know about her salt intake, and her appetite (since she was overweight). "Well, I love licorice," she said. "Unless I eat at least four long pieces a day, I become very constipated."

That casual statement solved the mystery of her hypertension! Licorice raises blood pressure when eaten regularly and in substantial amounts, as she was doing. I persuaded the young woman to abstain from licorice and to keep her bowels moving normally by increasing the amount of fiber in her diet. She followed my recommendations, and within ten days her blood pressure had returned to normal.

Now it's your turn to play medical Sherlock Holmes. If you have high blood pressure, ask yourself the following questions:

• Remember my first cardinal rule? Whenever you develop any symptoms, look first to your medicine cabinet. Many *appetite suppressants,* both over-the-counter and prescription (especially the amphetamine-based ones), can raise blood pressure. The Pill may do so, too, as can steroid hormones. One particular group of antidepressants called the monoamine oxidase inhibitors (marketed in the United States as Marplan, Nardil and Parnate) cause a dangerous blood-pressure elevation when taken along with aged cheese, red wine or chocolate.

• If your high blood pressure is first detected beyond the age of forty-five or fifty, chances are ten to one it is a case of *essential hypertension*—that is, of unknown cause. Even so, it can be treated.

• Are you pregnant beyond the sixth month? A condition called *toxemia of pregnancy* may occur at that time. Although not very common, it results in a level of blood pressure so high as to be life-threatening to the mother, and it often constitutes grounds for terminating the pregnancy.

- Was your blood pressure found to be elevated during a routine exam, or did you have symptoms? Hypertension is called the "silent killer" because it may be present for years without your knowing it. At some point, however, symptoms will occur. You may feel dizzy or short of breath, or have swollen feet, or experience pain in the calves of your legs when you walk, or have angina—all because the general circulation has finally become affected. It's much better to discover and treat hypertension before all that happens.

- Severe headaches accompanied by bouts of high blood pressure raise the possibility of the adrenaline-secreting tumor, *pheochromocytoma*. Women in their late forties and early fifties whose periods have become irregular will naturally attribute palpitations, nervousness, sweating and headaches to menopause; these symptoms, however, along with *unexplained weight loss,* should raise the suspicion of a pheochromocytoma.

- Does it hurt when you empty your bladder, and do you have blood in your urine? The origin of your high blood pressure is in the *kidneys*.

- Do you have to get up frequently at night to empty your bladder? In men this is often attributed to an enlarged prostate. But, male or female, if you need to urinate more than twice during the night without an obvious cause—you don't have diabetes, and haven't been drinking beer all evening or enjoyed a pot of tea before going to sleep—you may have high blood pressure.

- I mentioned earlier that taking steroids over a period of time raises blood pressure. In *Cushing's syndrome,* the body itself produces excessive amounts of these steroids due to a tumor in the adrenal glands, or in the pituitary of the brain. Patients with Cushing's have other easily identifiable characteristics. They often have a "buffalo hump" on the back; they may grow hair where it's not wanted—for example, on the face and the legs in women; they develop red blotches under the skin due to increased fragility of the small blood vessels located there; they bleed more easily. But the most telling clue is unexplained *weight gain*. If you haven't been gorging yourself, have had a steady weight all your life and have suddenly begun to gain weight, grow a mustache, develop a ruddy complexion and a hump in your back and have high blood pressure, you've got Cushing's.

A word about *low blood pressure*. Patients often complain to me that they tire easily, become dizzy when they stand up quickly, lack energy and have no get-up-and-go, because they've been "cursed" with low blood pressure. In most cases, low blood pressure is not abnormal unless, of course, you've been taking some medication which drops it (many heart drugs and high-blood-pressure pills can reduce your readings to an unacceptable level) or you have a very rare condition in which pressure is abnormally low. Its hallmark is recurrent spontaneous fainting, or loss of consciousness. So, if you're not taking such medication and you don't have that rare condition, your pressure really isn't low no matter what the numbers say. Do not take medication to raise it. Count your blessings. You'll live a lot longer if your pressure is low.

Points to Remember

Symptom: High blood pressure (hypertension).

What It May Mean	What to Do About It
1. Essential hypertension (the kind whose cause is not fully understood: 90–95 percent of cases).	Diet, weight loss, exercise, salt restriction in some cases (especially for blacks) and medication.
2. Adrenaline-secreting tumor (pheochromocytoma).	Surgical removal.
3. Arteriosclerosis.	Risk factor control.
4. Medication, appetite suppressants.	Change or avoid.
5. Toxemia of pregnancy.	Often grounds to terminate the pregnancy.
6. Kidney disease.	Medication or surgery.
7. Cushing's syndrome.	Surgery or medication.

CHAPTER 14

SLEEP:
Not Enough—or Too Much

I hear it so often from my patients. No matter what else ails them—a heart attack, high blood pressure, pneumonia, diabetes—they assure me that if they could only get a good night's sleep they'd be "fine." Although it's true that insomnia is the bane of millions, somnolence—or chronic sleepiness—troubles many people, too. They can't get going in the morning no matter how early they went to bed the night before or how soundly they slept. Not only that, but they nod off wherever they happen to be during the day—at a business meeting, the movies, a conference, or at the wheel of their car!

Let's look at the "sleep too much" contingent first, at their symptoms and the clues that can identify the cause of their problem.

WHEN IT'S ALL YOU CAN DO TO KEEP YOUR EYES OPEN

Drowsy all the time? Can't seem to keep your eyes open? Could it be the dreaded sleeping sickness? Certainly—if you live in the heart of Africa and have been nipped by one of those nasty, disease-carrying tsetse flies. Otherwise, forget it! As you will see, there are several "conditions" which can leave you with the energy of a zombie. But in the real world, in most persons chronic somnolence is psychological. Such persons are bored, depressed or taking some medication with soporific side effects. How can you tell whether *your* somnolence is all in your head?

All of us can, of course, remember a time when we slept more than usual just to avoid an unpleasant responsibility or one which we were unable to fulfill. I'm aware of it myself from time to time. For example, I worked for many months on this book, devoting to it every spare moment away from my office and my hospital rounds. That meant nights, weekends and "holiday." However, it's not always possible to write simply when you have the time to do so. One needs to "feel like it." When you don't, and are worried about meeting a deadline, a good way to deal with your anxiety is simply to doze off. There's no guilt in the Land of Nod. So, excessive sleep can be an escape mechanism.

Somnolence can also represent a flight from boredom or stress. Whenever my daughter takes my son-in-law shopping, he falls asleep in the store. The minute they leave, he's back to his vigorous self. As soon as they enter another establishment, he makes a beeline for the nearest comfortable chair and dozes off again. This arrangement seems to suit them both. She is not inhibited by his looking askance at her purchases, and he is spared the pain of witnessing the transaction!

The causes of somnolence are not, however, always so obvious. A patient of mine once posed a real diagnostic challenge. He was the head of a vast business empire and was known for his inexhaustible energy. He'd be up at four or five in the morning, work out, get to the office by seven and not return home until eight o'clock in the evening. He was *never* tired. But then one day something very unusual happened. He actually looked sleepy at his desk. He was even seen to yawn several times! It happened again a day or two later and then with frightening frequency.

Two or three weeks later he couldn't be counted on to stay awake during the most stimulating board meetings. The patient himself was, to say the least, embarrassed and puzzled. Maybe he wasn't getting enough sleep. He started going to bed earlier and earlier and awaking later and later. He stopped working out mornings and began to drink several cups of coffee with breakfast. That helped a little, but not enough. He still could barely keep his eyes open during the day. Mornings were his worst time. When all the home remedies had been tried and found wanting, Rip Van Winkle made an appointment to see me.

He arrived at 5 P.M., and I must say he looked rather good—and not at all sleepy. I questioned him in great detail, searching for some physical or psychological explanation for his sleepiness. Was he bored? Not at all. Was there some unpleasant aspect of his life he was trying to escape? Don't be absurd! Was he depressed? Only about his somnolence.

Then I ran through a list of his medications. Was he on any tranquilizers, antidepressants or sleeping pills? He admitted that he had in the past taken some very mild sleeping pills, but said he hadn't done so for weeks, not since this problem started. In fact, the only medication (if you could call it that) that he took regularly was two multivitamins with breakfast —and those never put anyone to sleep.

Still stymied, I went on to perform a careful and complete physical examination. I found him to be in excellent shape. Then I ran a battery of blood tests, looking for evidence of anemia, kidney disease, liver trouble, low thyroid function—all of which can cause sleepiness. They too were normal. I sent him to a neurologist, who in turn arranged a CAT scan of the brain. No problem whatsoever. What could it be? The next step was to get a psychiatric evaluation.

However, before I got around to making that sugges-
tion to the mogul, we figured it all out. You'll never
guess what it was that made this healthy man so
sleepy. I can tell you there were a couple of red faces,
mine among them, when the diagnosis was finally
established. Here's how it happened:

One day at breakfast with his wife, my patient
was finishing his orange juice and a couple of slices
of toast. He reached for his vitamins, which were in
one of those plastic containers dispensed by pharma-
cists. (The label on this one was missing.) He put two
capsules on the table while he poured another cup of
extra-strong coffee.

His wife looked at the vitamins. "What's that
you're taking, dear?" she asked.

"My vitamins. Without them I probably couldn't
survive."

She looked puzzled. "Honey," she said, "those vitamins look a lot like your sleeping pills."

Well, you can guess the rest. It seems that our
friend had inadvertently switched containers and for
these many weeks had been taking two sleeping pills
every morning with breakfast! They were almost
identical in size, shape and color to his vitamins!
Having had his morning fix, he went off to work—
and to sleep.

A whole slew of drugs, most of which are in the
tranquilizer family, can make you sleepy. Long-act-
ing sleeping pills will leave you with a hangover and
feeling drowsy the next day. So can the antihistamines present in many cough and cold remedies.
These antihistamines are, in fact, such potent sedatives that they are the main ingredient of many over-
the-counter sleeping aids. It's one thing to use them
to help you sleep at night, but if you're taking one
every four hours for some allergy, you're going to do
a lot of unexpected dozing during the day. Beta

blockers like Inderal and Tenormin (there are several more) can also slow you down very much.

Once you've eliminated boredom, depression and medication as the causes of your drowsiness, there are several diseases to be considered:

- The disorder most often associated with chronic sleepiness is an *underfunctioning thyroid gland*. If you're also constipated, overweight, losing your hair (which has become coarse) and are always cold and tired (no matter how much you sleep), your thyroid needs a boost.

- If you're a fan of Charles Dickens, you surely remember the fat boy in *The Pickwick Papers* who falls asleep at the drop of a hat—unpredictably, even standing up, and for long periods of time. In deference to Dickens, this affliction is known as the *Pickwickian syndrome*. Doctors also call it the *obesity-hypoventilation syndrome*. Normal breathing depends on enough carbon dioxide to stimulate the respiratory center in the brain. The sleepiness in this condition is due to too little carbon dioxide in the system. Since very fat people don't move the diaphragm very much, the flow of air in and out of the lungs is reduced. The resulting low level of carbon dioxide in the blood is almost anesthetic in its action on the sleep center in the brain.

- Obese persons may also suffer from *sleep apnea,* found mostly in men fifty years of age or older who are overweight and snore. Their breathing at night is irregular, with periods of ten seconds to a minute or longer during which they do not breathe at all. They wake up hundreds of times every night without knowing it, and so are very sleepy the next day. They're also impotent and have high blood pressure. (See pages 294–298, where I discuss this condition in detail.)

- If your teenage son falls into a deep sleep after eating, consider the *Klein-Levin syndrome,* a fairly rare hormonal disorder that affects adolescent males.

- If you've knocked your head "ever so slightly" *before* you became a sleep zombie, you may have done more damage than you think and caused a *subdural hematoma* (a collection of blood under the skull pressing on your brain). That's what happened to former President Reagan. This too can cause drowsiness.

- If along with your drowsiness you also have headaches, your eyesight isn't so good, there's weakness of an arm or leg, you've noted some difficulty speaking and you tend to be dizzy, you may have had a *stroke* or you may have a *brain tumor.* See your doctor.

- The need to doze off at any time can be part and parcel of any underlying disorder that is wearing you out—*liver disease, kidney trouble,* advanced *cancer,* any *infection,* even the common cold. Men with prostate trouble who have to get up every hour or two during the night to empty the bladder are often exhausted the next day. So are asthmatics or persons with heart failure who have difficulty breathing during the night. And let's not forget the roommates of melodious snorers.

- There is a sleeping disorder called *narcolepsy* in which there are uncontrollable attacks of sleepiness occurring unpredictably and which have nothing to do with feeling tired. Typically people with narcolepsy will suddenly fall asleep for a few minutes, almost without warning. They then wake up abruptly as if nothing had happened, and they either remain free of attacks for days or weeks or have another one a few minutes later. There's nothing abnormal about the sleep itself, which, for all intents and purposes, looks like a natural nap and from which they can be awakened as easily as anyone who has simply dozed off.

It all sounds rather benign, doesn't it? After all, what's wrong with a refreshing little sleep during the day? Winston Churchill did it every afternoon during the war when he was Prime Minister. The difference is, Churchill and other normal persons plan their nap, prepare for it and settle down into it. The narcoleptic has no warning. He or she falls asleep anywhere at any time—driving a car, operating a chain saw, walking down the stairs, even making love.

Narcolepsy can be recognized and distinguished from normal sleep by the accompanying symptoms. For a brief period, seconds or minutes, either when they're about to fall asleep or just after they've awakened, the affected individuals experience paralysis of the legs or hands, so that they will drop what they have been carrying or suddenly fall to the ground. This loss of power is only temporary, and muscle strength is soon completely regained. Some persons with narcolepsy also see, hear and smell things that aren't there before or after the attack.

The cause of narcolepsy is unknown. Between spells, these persons are perfectly healthy and every test performed on them is normal. Happily, a drug called Ritalin effectively controls the symptoms of this bizarre disorder.

So if you have trouble keeping awake while those about you are bouncing around full of energy, ask yourself whether you're depressed. Then check your medications, every single one of them. Beyond that, the cause may lie in any disease ranging from anemia to low thyroid to narcolepsy. But don't just "live with it" simply because there's no pain involved. See your doctor. He or she may well be able to give you a new lease on life.

Points to Remember

Symptom: Excessive drowsiness.

What It May Mean	What to Do About It
1. Depression, anxiety, boredom, stress.	Try to solve your problems with or without help.
2. Medications (tranquilizers, sleeping pills, antihistamines, heart pills, beta blockers).	Switch or stop them.
3. Hypothyroidism.	Thyroid supplements.
4. Obesity-hypoventilation syndrome (Pickwickian syndrome).	Weight loss.
5. Sleep apnea.	Mechanical breathing aids during the night.
6. Klein-Levin syndrome.	Hormones.
7. Brain injury (subdural hematoma) or disease.	Identify cause and treat.
8. Kidney and liver disease, cancer, infection.	Requires appropriate treatment.
9. Narcolepsy.	Stimulants (Ritalin).

INSOMNIA: REAL OR IMAGINED?

"I just can't sleep" is one of the three most common complaints with which doctors have to deal. (The other two are the size of the fee and the amount of time patients sit around in the waiting room.)

Everyone has sleepless nights now and then—because of jet lag, grief, worry, anxiety, exhilaration or excitement. That's different from the chronic situation in which night after night you toss and turn, unable to get the rest that your body needs.

Let's look at some obvious causes of insomnia first. There are several environmental and behavioral situations which can interfere with a good night's sleep. Your *bedroom* may be poorly ventilated—too stuffy, too hot, too dry or overly air-conditioned. The bed may be too hard, too soft or too short. You may have gotten into the habit of working at bedtime when you should have been preparing for sleep, so that your thoughts are racing long after you've turned off the lights. Sex can be relaxing, but some people are so *stimulated* by it they have trouble falling asleep afterward. You'd think that working out with a late-night run or twenty minutes on a rowing machine would tucker you out, but it often has the reverse effect.

What you eat and drink, and when, can also interfere with sleep. *Alcohol* at bedtime may help you get to sleep, but will frequently awaken you in a few hours. *Nicotine* from cigarette smoking late at night and *sugar* from a snack munched shortly before bedtime can both keep you up, as will *caffeine,* whether in coffee, tea or a cola drink. (Oddly enough, caffeine doesn't affect everyone the same way. There are those who can handle two cups of black coffee after a late dinner and still enjoy a good night's sleep, while if I, for example, have just half a cup after five in the afternoon, I'll toss and turn all night.)

Aging is another cause of sleeplessness. The older you get, the less sleep you need. For example, at one month an infant will snooze away a whopping twenty or twenty-one hours a day. This drops down to about eighteen hours at six months and fifteen hours at a year. At puberty the daily average is ten or twelve hours. Most adults do best with about eight hours of sleep a night until age sixty, after which six hours suffices.

There are also quirks of perception that contribute to the problem of sleep deprivation. I'd bet that if we were secretly to observe a large number of persons who complained of not having slept a wink, we'd find that a substantial number of them in fact enjoy a good many winks. But they're not lying. It's just that the time awake, staring into space or tossing and turning, seems much longer than it really is. By comparison, the time asleep is, at least for them, nonexistent. One is rarely aware of slipping in and out of the sleep state.

Of course, your perception about your insomnia may be correct and you may in fact have slept neither very well nor for very long. If so, here are some possible causes for you to consider:

- Many older people have a "polyphasic" sleep rhythm—that is, they *nap* so frequently during the day that they are unable to sleep very deeply or for long periods at night. This is especially true of those with lots of time on their hands who just sit around, read or watch TV.
- At the other end of the spectrum, your infant's sleeping problems are usually due to some physical discomfort—*colic, indigestion, hunger,* a foul diaper, or you may have bundled the child up either

too heavily or not warmly enough. Children may have trouble with their *teeth* or have *worms.* Some kids experience nightmares that keep them awake, or they suffer from leg cramps. It's important to discuss all these possibilities with the pediatrician, who may want to look for more serious and subtle neurological conditions of which a parent is not necessarily aware.

- An *overactive thyroid* gland interferes with sleep, leaves you jumpy, irritable, chronically wet from perspiration, with a rapid pulse and with weight loss despite a ravenous appetite. Persons with *low* thyroid may have the same symptoms when they take too much replacement hormone.

- Can't get to sleep? Have you started a *new drug,* whether prescription, over-the-counter or illicit? The ones most often associated with sleeplessness are those taken to lose weight (amphetamines or phenylpropanolamine—PPA), nasal decongestants, diuretics (because they have you voiding so often at night), high-potency vitamins, antidepressants and other mood-altering drugs.

- *Abruptly stopping a medication* to which you've become accustomed can keep you up at night. You made a New Year's resolution to stop taking sleeping pills—and you've kept it. Now you're not getting any sleep at all. Your body has become dependent on the drugs, and for the time being you can't do without them. Persevere. You will, sooner or later.

- Several diseases whose symptoms come on or worsen at night interfere with sleep. Classic examples are an *enlarged prostate* in men and *cystitis* (inflammation of the bladder) in women, both of which make you "go" every little while. Getting up frequently throughout the night is enough to disrupt anyone's sleep pattern. Duodenal ulcers often act up during the night. Heart failure and lung disease can disturb you after you've gone to bed, by making you short of breath. In severe cases, angina pectoris can arouse you, too. Anything that causes *physical discomfort* (arthritis is notorious) will keep you from having a good night's sleep.

My advice at this point may surprise you somewhat. Throughout this book, I've emphasized when to see your doctor about a given problem and why it's important to do so. But as far as insomnia is concerned, unless you can identify a real physical cause like an overactive thyroid or some other disease, it's better to try to solve the matter yourself. Given the current trends in medicine, in which physicians find themselves increasingly hard-pressed for time, when the one-on-one relationship between patient and doctor is being replaced by the allegedly more "cost-efficient" group practice, there is a tendency for many health professionals to deal with insomnia by prescribing sleeping pills because they simply haven't the time to listen to your story and discover why you cannot sleep. Except in unusual and temporary circumstances, that's no answer; it will only leave you hooked eventually. Here's one situation you'll most often need to deal with yourself—with support from family and friends.

Points to Remember

Symptom: Insomnia.

What It May Mean	What to Do About It
1. Depression, grief, anxiety.	Try to deal with it without drugs.
2. Bed or bedroom not conducive to sleep.	Correct the problem.
3. Excessive physical or intellectual stimulation at bedtime.	Avoid it.
4. Caffeine, food, alcohol or stimulants at bedtime.	Avoid them.
5. Excessive sleep during the day.	Keep busy and awake.
6. In children, colic, hunger, indigestion, teething, worms.	Consult your pediatrician.
7. Hyperthyroidism.	Treat it appropriately.
8. Medication (excessive thyroid replacement hormone, amphetamines).	Adjust the dose or eliminate the medication.
9. Abrupt withdrawal from sleeping pills.	Persevere.
10. Interference with sleep by various diseases— enlarged prostate, pain of arthritis, heart or lung problems.	Treat the underlying cause.

WHY ARE YOU SO TIRED?

Fatigue, a feeling of exhaustion, is not the same as drowsiness. *Any* disease, acute or chronic, physical or psychological, can deprive you of energy. So never ignore the onset of utter fatigue that is not immediately explainable. This symptom deserves a thorough investigation, which may, in the end, reveal anemia (due to any number of causes ranging from a nutritional deficiency to a malignancy), implicate some medication you're taking or identify a chronic infection or a hormonal disorder.

Feeling tired, then, is a "nonspecific" symptom which challenges the diagnostic ingenuity of the doctor, and yours as well. Unfortunately, it is such a common complaint and so often due to psychological causes that its potential seriousness is too often ignored, even by good doctors. Patients too are at fault. Instead of getting the problem checked out, they're apt to drink more coffee or get hold of some pep pills to increase their energy. That's dangerous, because the stimulants briefly eliminate the fatigue and so mask an important indicator of disease (apart from the fact that they may be habit-forming). They're also risky, especially for the elderly and those at any age with heart disease, high blood pressure or heart rhythm disorder.

Let's assume you're tired and really don't know why. You don't work too hard, you keep sensible hours, you're not sleep-deprived, you don't drink too much, you're not traveling back and forth across time zones and suffering from jet lag, you're not taking sleeping pills regularly, you're not on any medication like beta blockers (fatigue is one of their principal side effects), you also don't have any apparent illness and you're not depressed. So why the fatigue? Here are some possibilities to consider:

- If you've felt this way for months and are convinced that you were "born tired," you probably have *psychogenic fatigue*. There's no disease, with the exception of low thyroid function, that will keep you exhausted for months and years without making its presence obvious in other ways.

- If you wake up tired even after a restful night, you're probably depressed without knowing it. In most diseases, a good night's sleep results in some improvement, but the energy level drops as the day wears on. By the same token, if you're fatigued without any relation to effort, that is, you feel just as exhausted sitting around doing nothing as you do after a workout, chances are the cause is emotional.

- Are you having sexual problems? For men, impotence can trigger fatigue either as an excuse ("I'm too tired"—a headache is the equivalent symptom in women) or as a symptom of depression.

- If you are on some unusual or crash diet, your fatigue may be *nutritional* in origin.

- Have you recently recovered from *the flu* or *infectious mononucleosis*? Both can leave you fatigued for a long time. Mono is caused by the Epstein-Barr virus (EBV), and some doctors believe that this infection may become chronic, leaving the patient tired and depressed for months or years. I don't happen to agree. Most such cases are, in my opinion, due to psychological or emotional factors, provided all other physical causes have been ruled out. However, some virus other than EBV, as yet unidentified, may be the culprit, especially if in addition to your fatigue you have a sore throat, tender glands and a low-grade fever.

- Are you taking *diuretics*? Not only do they make you lose water and potassium (most people now know that), they can also drain you of magnesium, low levels of which can leave you exhausted.

- If you're tired, have noted a new onset of constipation and diarrhea and there's blood in your stool, you may have a *bowel tumor*.

- Have you developed a persistent cough along with the fatigue? Cancer of the lung is a possibility, especially if you're a smoker. But even in this day and age you must also consider the possibility of tuberculosis, whose incidence is on the increase, especially among older people in nursing homes.

- Whenever patients complain to me of fatigue and loss of interest in food, I think of depression, *drug toxicity* or chronic infection. In short, I take them seriously.

- When the fatigue is accompanied by fever, there's obviously something physical going on, like a hidden infection somewhere.

- It's sometimes difficult to distinguish between simple tiredness and *muscle fatigue*. There are several diseases which selectively strike the muscles, leaving them (and you) weak. So think for a moment. Do you have double vision that comes and goes, or difficulty in speaking from time to time, do you have trouble swallowing, or are you tired out just chewing a steak? *Myasthenia gravis,* a condition in which the muscles and the nerves don't interact normally because of a chemical imbalance between them, may be the culprit. Double vision never accompanies fatigue of emotional origin.

- If you're tired and gaining weight, *low thyroid function* and emotional depression are both possibilities. You can recognize the former by the constellation of typical symptoms which accompany it: constipation, dry skin, profuse menstrual flow, cold intolerance and so on.

Fatigue is a treacherous symptom, and its root cause may be difficult to determine. Until such time as it is, you may be dismissed as neurotic by family, friends and even your doctor. Don't buy it! That diagnosis made capriciously and without the appropriate evaluation can be disastrous. Consider all the possibilities I've mentioned above. Keep track of your temperature several times a day. If it's elevated on a daily basis, show the sheet to your doctor. Look for telltale symptoms. Record your weight and let your doctor know whether it goes up or down and how much. Your fatigue may be psychogenic, but always give yourself the benefit of the doubt by thinking of the other possibilities.

Points to Remember

Symptom: Fatigue.

What It May Mean	What to Do About It
1. Any disease whatsoever.	If it persists, undergo a thorough medical evaluation.
2. Psychogenic fatigue.	Determine the nature of the problem, and try to solve it —with or without help. Avoid masking matters with pep pills.
3. Poor nutrition.	Dietary counseling.
4. Recent flu, mononucleosis or other viral infection.	Plenty of rest and patience.
5. Diuretics.	Replace lost potassium and magnesium.
6. Bowel tumor.	Surgery.

7. Cancer of the lung.	Medical treatment or surgery.
8. Medications.	Review with your doctor.
9. Muscle disorder.	Medical management.
10. Low thyroid function.	Thyroid hormone replacement.

CHAPTER 15

YOUR URINE:
You Don't Have to Taste It to Test It

You wake up one morning feeling a bit out of sorts. It may have been a bad dream, or something you ate or drank the night before. In any event, as is your wont, you check your tongue in the mirror; nothing remarkable there except for the coating you normally see from time to time. You then continue your morning ablutions, one of which is emptying your bladder. Yikes! Your urine is bright red! "My God," you say, "what terrible disease do I have?" It doesn't look like blood, because it's too light and too bright. What could it be?

We'll get to that in a moment, but first let me emphasize that *normal* urine has a variety of scents and colors. As you will see from the following anecdote, however, you need only two of your senses, smell and vision, to appreciate them.

This is a story well known among medical students and doctors the world over. It's said to have taken place on the very first day of classes at a medical school in the Northeast. All 110 entrants, full of enthusiasm, aspirations and noble ideals, were being welcomed by their dean. He spoke at length of the rigors of their profession, of the demands that would be made of them as doctors and the standards their school expected them to meet. In addition to selflessness and devotion to the sick, he emphasized the need to develop a keen sense of observation. This, he told them, was a fundamental requirement for the practice of good medicine.

The dean hammered home the point that there was no aspect of the body's function that should be permitted to elude their most critical scrutiny and evaluation. "You must utilize every one of your five senses to the fullest," he asserted. He then dismissed the class for a few minutes, arming each student with a small plastic cup in which to deposit his or her own urine specimen. When they had all returned, cups full, the dean placed his own container on the table in front of him. "Urine," he said, "is a vitally important by-product of our metabolism. It should be examined in every way possible, because it can reveal a great deal of information about how the body is functioning. Now I want you to do exactly as I do." With this, he dipped a finger into the urine—and then he put his finger into his mouth and licked it! The entire class as one, without so much as a cleared throat, did the same—after all, there was no sacrifice too great to make on this, the first day of their medical careers. When they had finished (many of them disgusted—one student was overheard to say, "Tasting my own pee is bad enough. I'll never do it with anyone else's"), the dean smiled. "Now you have all learned your first lesson about observation," he said. "*I* put my little finger in the urine and licked my forefinger."

Well, he was right about one thing. The characteristics of your urine are important in the diagnosis of disease. Fortunately, neither patient nor doctor need taste it these days, because there is a grand array of laboratory equipment available to analyze what you excrete. Years ago, however, urine was taste-tested to identify the sweetness characteristic of diabetes mellitus.

Examining your own urine can help you solve many otherwise perplexing symptoms—pain in the back or the lower abdomen, fever whose origin is not clear, headache, sudden onset of high blood pressure, swelling of the fingers and face, to name but a few. But in order to understand what certain changes in the urine may reflect, you need to know how it is made.

Urine is formed by the kidneys, whose function it is to maintain the chemical equilibrium of the body. The kidneys, one on each side, filter the blood that circulates through them, retaining those substances which the body needs and excreting the rest. Two thousand liters of blood are recirculated through both kidneys every twenty-four hours, yet only one and a half to two end up as urine! Healthy kidneys do not permit the loss of any substance required by the body, so they reabsorb the sugar, certain minerals, proteins, red and white blood cells and other vital elements in the blood that passes through them. One tests the urine by looking for things in it that shouldn't be there.

TESTING YOUR URINE

The first and simplest test of urine is to *look* at it. Don't worry if it appears murky or cloudy. That may merely reflect the phosphates in the meat or other foods you've been eating. In women, normal vaginal secretions often confer a cloudy appearance to the urine. If the weather has been hot and you've been sweating without having adequately replenished your liquids, your urine will be concentrated and hence darker in color. Indeed, most changes in urine color have to do with how much water you've been drinking. The more dilute the urine, the paler yellow it's apt to be. When you're *dehydrated*, it's deep gold in color.

If your urine has the hue of tea or mahogany, it contains *bile*. To confirm its presence, pour some out into a container (one that has a cap!). Close the container and then shake it vigorously. If the urine foams, bile is present. Now take a look in the mirror. You may not have noticed that you're jaundiced. Both these symptoms signal a *liver disorder*.

Red urine usually means *blood,* and that's a major danger signal of *cancer, infection* or *stones* in the urinary tract. It's almost never a normal variant, and it demands an immediate visit to the doctor. But red urine can also be due to the beets or borscht (beet soup) you had last night! Laxatives which contain phenolphthalein will also turn the urine red (Ex-Lax is the best-known example).

Dyes present in some candies, foods and drugs can alter the color of urine. I remember one patient who was alarmed when she noticed her urine was green! She had been taking Urised, for spasm of the urinary tract. This medication contains a harmless dye that turns the urine green. Some bacteria which can cause urinary infections produce a blue pigment, which, when mixed with the yellow urine, also give it a green color.

Tranquilizers like Thorazine and Compazine may turn the urine red or brown. Vitamin pills, especially those containing B complex, give it an orange hue, as well as a characteristic odor. Pyridium, for the relief of the pain of bladder irritation, makes the urine bright orange. *Pus* from an infection somewhere in the urinary tract will leave it looking milky yellow.

Now here's something really bizarre. Aldomet, a medication for treating high blood pressure, can turn urine black. It starts out yellow, but the moment it hits the water in the toilet bowl it becomes black—a shocking sight if you're not prepared for it. The color change is due to a chemical called hypochlorite.

Then there's the *odor* of urine. When you eat asparagus a unique powerful scent is imparted to the urine shortly thereafter. Other foods confer their own characteristic aromas. So remember, when your urine smells different, is cloudy or has a peculiar color, your first thought should be, What have I been eating or drinking recently? Have I been taking enough water, and what about that vitamin supplement? Don't worry about some dreadful disease you're not likely to have, *except if the urine is bloody*.

Points to Remember

Symptom: Abnormal urine.

What It May Mean	What to Do About It
1. Wide range of normal colors and odors, reflecting food, medication, vitamins.	Nothing.
2. Dark yellow: dehydration.	Replace fluids.
3. Mahogany- or tea-colored: bile present, liver disease.	Diagnose and treat.
4. Red: blood—a major danger signal of cancer, infection, stone.	Requires complete evaluation.
5. Milky yellow: pus, infection.	Identify the source and treat it with antibiotics.

CHAPTER 16

WHEN YOU'RE THIRSTY ALL THE TIME

When you're thirsty, you usually know why. It's a warm summer day, you've just finished a grueling three-set match of tennis and you've been sweating to beat the band. Any wonder, then, that the first thing you do is head straight for the water fountain at the side of the court and drink deep? Or maybe you haven't been so active. Instead, you had a fabulous Sunday brunch and you were "lax," threw caution (and your diet) to the winds and ate bagels with cream cheese and smoked salmon, together with some delicious matjes herring, all washed down with a couple of spicy Bloody Marys. You're thirsty the rest of the day, but that doesn't surprise you, considering all the salt and spices you consumed.

But suppose it's cool outside, you haven't been exercising, you haven't eaten anything salty, but still you're thirsty. In fact, looking back, you realize that you've been "dying of thirst" for the past few days, even weeks, and it's the kind of thirst that you just can't seem to quench. That's abnormal.

Being thirsty and drinking abnormally large amounts of water are not the same thing. People who drink great quantities of water aren't necessarily thirsty. They do it because they like to, or are trying to lose weight, or have had kidney stones and want to prevent another attack. There's also a rare *psychological* disorder in which large amounts of water are drunk compulsively. (Frankly, I have never seen a case and know very little about the disorder or why

402

it occurs.) Real abnormal thirst, however, is different. It's not something you choose. You drink because you must.

When considering excessive thirst and its consequences, remember that what goes in must come out. Because you're constantly trying to quench your thirst, you're also continuously emptying your bladder. I was in China some years ago, attending seminars at several hospitals. Before each session, the participants would sit around drinking endless quantities of delicious jasmine or Beijing tea. The subsequent proceedings were frequently interrupted by calls of nature for both the Chinese and the American doctors. It was then that I conceived the now universally used formula, $T = P$!

INTAKE AND OUTPUT

Doctors commonly write the order to "measure intake and output" in a seriously ill patient. They want to know the patient's fluid balance, and whether he or she is consuming and eliminating fluids in appropriate amounts. A normal balance is the result of the interaction of several hormones, an excess or deficit of any of which can cause thirst and/or water retention. In other words, if you're losing lots more fluid than you're drinking, you're going to be thirsty. If you're consuming a much greater volume than you're eliminating, you'll have different problems, the most important of which is congestion of the lungs if you have any underlying heart disease.

The major hormone involved in the regulation of fluid intake and output is called vasopressin, or *antidiuretic hormone* (ADH). You know what a diuretic is—it makes you "go." The antidiuretic hormone has the opposite effect. It causes your body to retain fluid. In normal persons, how much of this hormone is produced at any given moment depends on the fluid intake. So, when you drink large amounts of water, less vasopressin is made, thus permitting your body to excrete what it doesn't need. The sensation of thirst is also terminated, so you stop drinking until the fluid balance is restored. On the other hand, if you're lost in the desert without water, your brain will send more vasopressin (ADH) to the rescue. This allows you to retain whatever precious little water there is left in your system. So, normally, the more/less you drink, the more/less you excrete— all meant to keep the body's water supply constant. That is the theoretical basis for my famous $T = P$ equation!

There is a specific disease called *diabetes insipidus* (not to be confused with diabetes mellitus, the sugar disorder) which causes a deficiency of ADH by affecting an area in the brain that controls the hormone's production. Since there is no longer enough antidiuretic action, there is little or no control over how much urine you pass. Put another way, it's as if you were always on a diuretic. So you're constantly thirsty, drinking to replace the huge amounts of urine excreted. But be sure to distinguish between large amounts of urine and frequent visits to the john in which only small quantities are passed. The latter is what happens in the presence of cystitis (inflammation of the bladder), a urinary tract infection or an enlarged prostate.

Some types of *kidney disease* interfere with the kidneys' ability to respond to ADH even though the levels of that hormone are normal. The net result, however, is the same—increased thirst and a tremendous volume of urine.

Diabetes insipidus is relatively rare. There are no more than fifteen cases among every hundred thousand hospitalized patients. A much more common cause of chronic thirst and increased urine output is the other kind of diabetes, the one associated with too much sugar—*diabetes mellitus,* or sugar diabetes. (*Mellitus* is the Latin word for "sweet.") Although this is a treatable disorder, there are millions of diabetics in the United States who are either undiagnosed or inadequately treated.

The reason high blood sugar leads to abnormal thirst is that the body gets rid of the excess sugar via the urine. But since the kidneys can't pass sugar cubes, the body must provide extra water to dissolve the abnormal sugar load presented to the kidneys. When the diabetes is out of control, with high blood- and urine-sugar content, the body runs short of water, triggering the thirst response.

FINDING THE CAUSE

Now that we've looked at the main possible causes of increased thirst, how can *you* tell what's causing you to chug all that water?

- Do you have an increased appetite along with your unquenchable thirst, and have you lost weight to boot? That suggests diabetes mellitus. So does a vaginal itch, which diabetic women develop because of an overgrowth of yeast that thrives in the sugar-rich environment. If you've been breaking out, especially with boils, suspect diabetes, too.
- Was the onset of your thirst and enormous urine output sudden or gradual? A sudden onset suggests a psychogenic origin, while a gradual one is more likely to be diabetes insipidus (providing, of course, you don't have the symptoms of diabetes mellitus).
- If you're passing more than five liters of urine a day, you have diabetes insipidus, kidney disease or

a psychogenic problem. If it's less than that, diabetes mellitus is more likely. But rather than hang around measuring liters and liters of urine, it's much simpler to buy some strips of diagnostic tape at a drugstore and see whether it tests positive for sugar. It won't in diabetes insipidus or kidney disease or if the cause is psychogenic.

- Do you have to get up frequently at night to empty your bladder? If your abnormal thirst is psychogenic in origin, you'll usually be able to sleep through the night or at most get up just once or twice.

- What fluid best quenches your thirst? People with diabetes insipidus are fussy. They almost always prefer ice water to soda pop or tea. But if the problem is psychogenic, anything that's wet will do. Again, if the thirst is intermittent, the cause is probably psychogenic in origin.

- If water is not available or is withheld, do you still void large amounts of urine? If so, you have true diabetes insipidus. But if the urine volume decreases as consumption goes down, then it's probably psychogenic.

If your excessive thirst and urination are due to diabetes insipidus, you'll want to look for other neurological symptoms which may tell you why the production of ADH has been reduced. So:

- If you had a stroke recently, the area of the *brain* that regulates the formation of that hormone may have been damaged.

- Are you female with a history of breast cancer? The malignancy may have spread to involve the source of ADH production in the brain.

- Have you developed headaches recently, or changes in vision? These symptoms also raise the possibility of some disease process in your brain.

The bottom line: Thirst is usually the reaction to exercise or salty foods, or just a habit. Drinking lots of water is usually good for you. However, beyond a certain limit your desire to do so excessively may reflect an underlying disease, either physical or emotional. Examining the characteristics of your thirst as described above will almost always tell you why you have it. You can then hand the diagnosis to your doctor in a silver goblet!

Points to Remember

Symptom: Abnormal thirst.

What It May Mean	What to Do About It
1. A recent salty, spicy meal.	Satisfy your thirst.
2. Compulsive thirst.	Psychological help.
3. Diabetes insipidus.	Neurological consultation to determine why the brain has stopped making the antidiuretic hormone (ADH). Kidney work-up too.
4. Diabetes mellitus.	Proper control of blood-sugar levels.
5. Kidney disease.	Evaluation and treatment.
6. Brain disorder.	Thorough medical evaluation.

CHAPTER 17

YOUR GENETICS AND LIFESTYLE:
Their Impact on Your Symptoms

A symptom is a distress signal—the effect that some disease or disorder has on your body. The meaning of that signal depends to a great extent on your biological profile—the mix of your genetics and your lifestyle, the stuff with which you were born and what you have made of it. You're either more vulnerable to certain diseases or more resistant to them, depending on your family health record, your sex and your sexual preference, such personal habits as smoking, drinking and the use of "recreational" drugs, your age, your occupation and even your marital status. For example, why has the cough that started with a "cold" hung on so long? In most cases, it's nothing to worry about—it just does sometimes. But if you're a heavy smoker, there's always the possibility of lung cancer. If you're gay and promiscuous, or an IV drug user, then AIDS must also be considered.

Here is how some of these personal characteristics can influence the interpretation of many of the symptoms described throughout this book.

THE EFFECTS OF AGE

Your age is a personal matter. Telling a casual acquaintance how old you *feel* is one thing, confiding how old you *are* is quite another. Sure, there is the occasional lapse in a hallmark year—like a fiftieth or sixtieth birthday—when a well-meaning, loving spouse spills the beans by throwing a big surprise party for you. But after it's over, privacy is again the rule—unless, of course, someone is keeping track.

People misrepresent their age for all kinds of reasons, even to their doctors. Some do it because they're vain; others fear for their careers. But perhaps a more frequent reason older patients lie about their age is their belief that doctors don't take "senior citizens" seriously, dismissing their complaints with "You know, you're not as young as you used to be" or "What do you expect at your age?"

For whatever reason you choose to do it, is telling your doctor that you're two or three years younger than you really are all that important? Probably not, provided that all the insurance forms are correctly filled out—and that you yourself appreciate the fact that there are specific diseases to which everyone becomes more vulnerable as the years go by. For example, all of the following disorders occur with increasing frequency after middle age, something to be borne in mind whenever you're evaluating a new symptom:

- *Cancer*—anywhere from head to toe.
- *Arteriosclerosis*—hardening of the arteries. Its major complications are heart attacks and strokes (but there are others).
- *Osteoporosis*—fragility and easy fracture of bones (especially in women after menopause) due to loss of bone calcium.
- *Diabetes*—the kind that runs in families, is often associated with excess weight and does not usually require insulin.
- *Alzheimer's disease.* Your chances of getting it after age sixty-five are about 15 percent.
- *Cataracts.* They begin to show up after age forty.
- *Glaucoma*—increased eye pressure, which un-

treated leads to blindness (so get yourself tested for it annually after age thirty-five).

- *Nerve deafness*—when you miss all the clever repartee at the theater and prefer loud musicals or pantomimes to dialogue.
- *Constipation*—when the daily movements you had when you were younger are now a memory, and each one is an event.
- *Osteoarthritis*—in which weight-bearing joints such as the knees and those in the back become painful.
- *Peptic ulcers*. Men are more vulnerable early in life to these ulcers of the stomach and the small intestine, but women catch up after menopause.
- *Gout*. The likelihood of your getting a hot, red, swollen and very painful big toe increases with age (but this disease does occur in younger people too, especially men).
- *Parkinson's disease*—a neurological disorder caused by a deficiency in the brain of a chemical called dopamine. Most patients are males over the age of sixty-five.
- *High blood pressure*. Although everyone's blood pressure increases somewhat as the years go by, if it gets too high you are at increased risk for stroke, heart disease, kidney trouble, blindness and blocked arteries anywhere in the body.
- *Hernias*. Internal organs of the body are kept where they're supposed to be by intact muscles. When these muscles weaken, tissues push out or slip through them—here, there and everywhere. After age sixty, two kinds of hernias in particular are prone to develop—*hiatus hernia* and *inguinal hernia*. The former occurs when the stomach slides up into the chest through a weakened diaphragm muscle, causing an array of symptoms which mimic those of heart disease. Inguinal hernia, on

the other hand, is a bulging in the groin which becomes apparent on standing, coughing or straining. Older men with enlarged prostate glands that obstruct the outflow of urine are subject to this type of hernia because they have to strain to empty the bladder. (If surgery becomes necessary, such individuals are usually advised to have the prostate fixed, too, for otherwise the hernia will simply recur.)

• These are the disorders most likely to explain the majority of your symptoms as you grow older. But remember, not everyone develops high blood pressure or glaucoma or Parkinson's disease in the golden years. In fact, as of the most recent count, 82 percent of "elderly" Americans are actually in reasonably good health and well able to take care of themselves. And if you're worried about Alzheimer's disease, only 5 percent of Americans end up in nursing homes because of impaired mental status.

• Finally, although the aging process is unavoidable, many of the symptoms associated with it can be treated—a good reason to see your doctor periodically as you grow older.

THE "STRONGER" SEX

Women live longer than men. Much of this biological "strength" is probably due to their hormones, which seem to protect them from the ravages of heart attacks, the number one killer of males. Recent studies, however, suggest that the differential in life span between the sexes may also reflect the fact that men have always smoked more than women and thus suffered from all the diseases to which tobacco makes one vulnerable. But that's changing. While men are kicking the habit in ever greater numbers these days, more and more women are embracing it. If this trend continues, the difference in life expectancy may well be narrowed or even disappear.

Although most major diseases can and do affect both men and women (except, of course, for those that involve their sex organs), certain ones occur more frequently in one sex than in the other. Bear this predilection in mind whenever you attempt to interpret any symptom. For example, if you develop back pain, and you're a female in your sixties, it's most probably due to osteoporosis (unless, of course, you've had breast cancer which now involves your bones). But a similar complaint in a man the same age should first suggest arthritis, and then cancer of the prostate that has spread to the bones.

Following are some of the conditions in which there is a significant statistical predilection for one sex or the other:

- *Acute bacterial pyelonephritis*—an infection of the urinary tract which begins in the bladder and then spreads up to involve the kidneys. It's much more common in women, because they are more prone to bladder infections (cystitis). So if you're female, look to the bladder for the origin of your chills, fever, back pain and nausea. In males, such kidney infections usually start in a diseased prostate.
- *Arteriosclerosis.* This disease, in which arteries in various parts of the body become narrowed and blocked, is the number-one killer of both sexes in the Western world. (Cancer is second.) Women are generally spared before menopause, unless they are diabetic, have high blood pressure or any clotting disorder, or are taking the contraceptive pill and smoke cigarettes. Thereafter the incidence is the same as in men. So, if you're under age fifty, still menstruating, and having chest pain, coronary ar-

tery disease should *not* be high on your list of possible explanations. Also, a woman's vulnerability to the ravages of arteriosclerosis is the same as a man's if she's had a hysterectomy in which both ovaries were removed, and has not had adequate hormonal replacement.

• Despite the fact that hundreds of thousands of hysterectomies are performed every year—often unnecessarily—I'm always surprised at how few women really fully understand this operation. The term "hysterectomy" is very loosely used. When the uterus is removed but the ovaries are spared, menopause does not occur even though the monthly periods end. Menstruation requires the uterus, because that's where the blood comes from. But menopause occurs only when the ovaries, which make estrogen (the female hormone), either are taken out or are no longer working. So if you've had a hysterectomy in which even only a small portion of one ovary has been left behind, you will neither become menopausal nor vulnerable to arteriosclerosis.

• *Autoimmune disorders.* These develop when the immune system gets all mixed up and, instead of protecting you, makes you sick. That happens when its so-called "troops" end up attacking normal body tissues as if they were bacteria, viruses or cancer cells. These autoimmune diseases, more and more of which are being recognized, *strike women much more commonly than they do men.* The most important ones so far identified are:

• *Graves disease*—overfunction of the thyroid gland, a condition which usually causes the eyes to bulge or "pop" and makes you nervous and irritable.

- *Rheumatoid arthritis*—the deforming type of joint disease.
- *Systemic lupus erythematosus (SLE)*—in which arteries to virtually every part of the body become inflamed. Symptoms depend on which blood vessels are affected. In the heart, the result may be angina; in the brain, a stroke; in the kidneys, pain and blood in the urine; and so on. If you're a young woman with several seemingly unrelated symptoms in different regions of the body, think of SLE, the great mimic. Even doctors don't consider this disease as often as they should, and patients sometimes go undiagnosed for years.
- *Carpal tunnel syndrome*—probably an autoimmune disorder in which a nerve at the wrist is compressed by locally inflamed and swollen tissues. The result is pain and weakness in the hand. Surgery is usually required to release the trapped nerve. However, when the problem develops during pregnancy, which it sometimes does, it often clears up spontaneously after delivery.
- *Colitis,* a form of inflammatory bowel disease causing chronic pain, cramps, diarrhea and/or constipation, may be due to some autoimmune malfunction.
- *Raynaud's disease (or syndrome)* produces spasm of the small blood vessels in parts of the body exposed to cold. When the temperature drops, the tips of the fingers, toes and nose blanch and become painful. This is an autoimmune disorder to which women are more susceptible than men. If your bride complains that her fingers hurt when she rinses the dishes in cold water, buy her a dishwasher—or do the dishes yourself. She's probably not malingering.
- *Myasthenia gravis*—the autoimmune disorder from which Aristotle Onassis suffered in the last

years of his life. It causes weakness of muscles, mainly those controlling eye movement, swallowing and breathing. Women are stricken more often than men. It's interesting that myasthenia gravis often seems to develop after a serious illness or emotional shock. Onassis was my patient, and I'm convinced that in his case the untimely death of his only son in a tragic plane crash contributed to the onset of the myasthenia gravis.

- *Cancer.* Most malignancies affect both sexes equally, but some have a greater predilection for one than for the other. For example, males are more prone than females to the following cancers: esophagus (food pipe), three to one; kidneys, two to one; larynx, four to one; the lips, two to one; pharynx (throat), three to one; stomach, almost two to one; tongue, seven to one.
- I suspect that the higher incidence of these particular tumors in men (with the possible exception of stomach cancer) reflects their greater use of tobacco—not just cigarettes but also pipes, snuff and chewing tobacco. Despite the statistics, two of my last three patients with cancer of the tongue were women—and both were heavy cigarette smokers.
- The following conditions are *more frequent in women than in men:*
- *Breast cancer.* Despite a female/male ratio of 150 to one, breast cancer is not exclusively a disorder of women. I have found it in several men in my own practice. I'm not suggesting that males should routinely examine their breasts or have mammograms, but, man or woman, never ignore any lump anywhere, including the breast.
- *Thyroid cancer*—three to one. These malignancies are often curable, so report at once any irregular

lump in the midline of your neck, especially if it *doesn't* hurt.

- *Gallbladder disease.* Gallbladder cancer, stones and infection occur much more frequently in women, probably because the female hormone (estrogen) interacts in some way with bile in the gallbladder. Taking the Pill (which contains estrogen) also makes a female more susceptible to gallbladder disease. So bear this predilection in mind when trying to interpret a pain in the right upper portion of the abdomen, especially if you're female and using an oral contraceptive.

- *Headache (migraine).* As with gallbladder disease, the reason migraine predominates in women is probably hormonal. These headaches often clear up after menopause.

- *Lactose intolerance*—due to the deficiency of an enzyme, lactase, which digests lactose, a dietary sugar. In the absence of this enzyme, the lactose remains in the gut, causing distention, bloating, gas and often diarrhea, whenever milk or a milk product is consumed. It is one of the most common intestinal disorders in this country. No one knows why it affects women more than men, and blacks more than whites. My own family is plagued by it, but curiously only the males. Our women feast with impunity on luscious cheese cake and creamy pastries for dessert, while the men must make do with fruit salad.

- *Lung embolism.* This occurs when a piece of a blood clot in a vein breaks away (embolizes) and ends up blocking a blood vessel in the lung. This causes chest pain, cough, bloody sputum, a little fever and, if the traveling clot is big enough, death. Women are more vulnerable to pulmonary embolism because such clots usually form in the veins of the legs and the pelvis. Childbearing predisposes women to varicose veins in the legs, and chronic pelvic inflammatory disease leads to trouble in the pelvic veins. So whereas a young man with chest pain should always be checked out for heart disease, sudden discomfort in the same area in a young woman should always raise the suspicion of pulmonary embolism.

• *Mitral valve prolapse.* This was unknown both to doctors and to patients until twenty-five years ago. Today the "floppy valve," as it is sometimes called, is a very commonly diagnosed disorder occurring much more frequently in women than in men. It is due to abnormal structure and function of the mitral valve, one of four within the heart. The symptoms with which mitral valve prolapse is associated may include unprovoked chest pain, shortness of breath, palpitations, migrainelike headaches and panic attacks. So, if you are a young woman with any or all of these complaints, don't allow yourself to be written off as neurotic just because your electrocardiogram is normal. If your doctor hasn't thought about it, ask him or her to look for mitral valve prolapse. It is easily diagnosed with the stethoscope and confirmed by an echocardiogram.

• *Multiple sclerosis (MS)*—a neurological disorder in which women have a slight numerical edge over men. It appears early in adult life, follows a chronic, insidious and ever-worsening course, and causes a variety of neurological symptoms. If you're a young woman and develop visual problems which come and go, intermittent weakness of a limb or unexplained numbness and tingling, multiple sclerosis is to be considered. But if you have headaches too, migraine is a better bet.

• *Osteoporosis*—overwhelmingly a disorder of older women who lose calcium from the bones, which become deformed, brittle and easily fractured. Interestingly enough, male alcoholics, especially those who consume large amounts of antacids because their stomach has been irritated by the booze, also have a high incidence of osteoporosis. So if you're beyond menopause and suddenly have back pain or break a hip when you cough vigorously, or seem to be developing a humpback, and are shorter than you used to be, you've probably got osteoporosis.

- *Peptic ulcers,* which have the same predilection for men as arteriosclerosis; in other words, pre-menopausal women don't get them very often. So if you're still having your periods and you suffer attacks of pain and discomfort in your upper abdomen, gallbladder disease, which strikes women so much more often than men, is a better bet than peptic ulcer. But regardless of your sex and age, remember that prolonged use of or large doses of aspirin or related painkillers—or steroid hormones —can cause ulceration of the upper intestinal tract.

- *Sexually transmitted diseases.* These do not usually discriminate between men and women, but there is some variation in vulnerability. For example, there are two chances in ten that a man will "catch" gonorrhea after having sex with an infected woman; in the reverse circumstance, the female's risk doubles to four in ten. The incidence of AIDS is higher in men, not because of any greater biological susceptibility to this disease, but simply because more men than women engage in anal intercourse and use intravenous drugs.

- You can now appreciate the importance of your sex when trying to make a "differential diagnosis" of any particular symptom. Remember, however, that your biological wheel has many different spokes, of which sex is only one.

EQUAL BUT NOT THE SAME

Your genes, your heritage, your cultural and ethnic background and your economic circumstances all help determine which diseases are most likely to affect you and with what severity. Appreciating this vulnerability, together with other personal factors, can help you sort out the more likely diagnostic possibilities when you develop a certain set of symptoms. But be very careful not to generalize about racial predispositions and characteristics. This is sometimes done to tout biological "superiority" or "inferiority" where none really exists. Also, in a world where substantial numbers of people intermarry or migrate—for political, religious or economic reasons—the profile of a given race or people may change from generation to generation. For example, racially "pure" Japanese who have left their homeland to live in Hawaii have a higher incidence of heart disease than do their relatives who stayed behind. And those who have gone on to mainland America are at greater risk than those who settled in Hawaii. That's mostly because of the change in their diet, but I'm certain that climate, stress level, the hardness or softness of the drinking water, also play some role.

What is true for migrating Japanese also pertains to other populations on the move. For example, when Jews who had been living in Yemen for generations migrated to Israel, their disease statistics began to approach those of native-born Israelis. Specifically, the low incidence of arteriosclerosis they enjoyed in Yemen disappeared. So, defining the susceptibility of Asiatics, Hispanics, Jews and blacks to any disorder can be a tricky business. Given that caveat, there are a few observations which are, nevertheless, valid.

THE HEALTH PROFILE OF BLACKS

The conditions to which blacks are *genetically* more vulnerable include:

• *Sickle cell anemia (SCA).* Its symptoms usually start in the first year of life, and the disease claims the bulk of its victims long before maturity. Affected children are chronically anemic, sickly and jaundiced and are periodically racked with pain. One of every four hundred blacks in this country, and a smaller but still significant percentage of Hispanics (one in 1,500) have SCA. If you're black or Hispanic, you should know all about this disease, since it is not only terrible but preventable.

Sickle cell anemia is due to an abnormal hereditary variation in the structure of hemoglobin, a protein found inside the red blood cell. Hemoglobin is important because the oxygen molecule carried by the red blood cell is attached to it. Red cells with normal hemoglobin are round, flexible and pliable. When they come up to a blood vessel that's smaller than they are, they can change their shape, squeeze into it and discharge their cargo of oxygen. By contrast, in patients with sickle cell anemia the red blood cells have a curved or "sickled" shape because of their abnormal hemoglobin. They are rigid, without the normal flexibility. And because they are now unable to change their configuration they cannot get into the tiny blood vessels, and end up obstructing them. It's very much like what happens when a heavy flow of traffic approaches a major conduit like a bridge or a tunnel whose four lanes have suddenly been reduced to one because of construction or an accident. That's the kind of traffic jam that occurs at the entrance to those vessels too small for the sickled cells to enter. The tissue in which this blockage occurs, and it can be anywhere—brain, heart, lungs, joints or bones—is thus deprived of oxygen. The symptoms of the disease depend on which organs are affected in any given attack. A crisis or flare-up occurs when the percentage of sickled red cells suddenly increases, usually because of a decrease in available oxygen in the environment.

In addition to their altered shape, sickled cells also have a shortened life span. While a normal red blood cell survives 120 days, sickled cells break up after only thirty to fifty days. A yellow pigment (bilirubin) present in hemoglobin is then released into the bloodstream, and stains the skin, the whites of the eyes and other body tissues yellow, the condition known as jaundice. This premature destruction of red cells also leaves the patient anemic.

In order for a black baby to have full-blown sickle cell disease, he or she must inherit one gene for the disease *from each parent*. Persons with only a single sickle cell gene have the sickle cell *trait*— that is, they do not suffer from the disease, but can transmit it. So if only one parent has this gene, the offspring can acquire the trait but will never develop the disease. If *both* parents carry the gene, their children have a 25 percent chance of inheriting sickle cell disease. Ten percent of all blacks have the sickle cell *trait;* one in four hundred suffers from the disease. If every black or Hispanic man or woman contemplating parenthood were to have his or her blood tested and then make an appropriate decision about whether or not to have children, sickle cell anemia would virtually disappear.

There is an interesting theory as to why the black race, specifically, was genetically endowed with sickled cells. The kind of hemoglobin responsible for these cells is resistant to the most deadly form of malaria, a disease that has long been, and remains, a major cause of death in Africa. Since that's where blacks have their roots, they may have been so genetically programmed in order to protect them from the ravages of malaria.

• G6PD *(glucose 6 phosphate dehydrogenase) disease*—another kind of hemoglobin abnormality, this one due to the lack of a certain enzyme. Here the blood cells retain a normal shape, but, as in sickle cell anemia, they break up prematurely. G6PD affects only black *males* and is passed along to them by their mothers. Even though it gets relatively little attention (perhaps because the name is such a jawbreaker), many blacks are affected by the disease.

Unlike sickle cell anemia, G6PD disease does not shorten life. Its symptoms, severe anemia, jaundice and general illness, can occur at any age. An attack is often provoked by infection, or by any of several drugs including the sulfas, chloramphenicol (an antibiotic), quinine (present in tonic water and often used to control night leg cramps) and quinidine (a cardiac medication prescribed in the treatment of heart rhythm disorders). In most cases, however, a black person will suffer an acute attack after eating fava beans. So if you're a black male and you intermittently develop anemia, jaundice and generalized malaise, have your hemoglobin analyzed, especially if you can correlate any of these symptoms with drinking a gin and tonic, or eating your favorite dish made with fava beans.

• *Prostate cancer.* For some unknown reason, this is eight times more common in blacks than in whites. So every black man should be on the lookout for this particular malignancy in order to have it detected before symptoms appear. Prostate cancer, when early enough to be cured, is usually totally "silent." By the time it produces symptoms, it is usually too late to cure. *The best way to detect early prostate cancer is to have a routine rectal examination every year after age forty.* All it takes is the doctor's finger—no fancy or expensive tests.

• *Hypertension.* High blood pressure is the most important condition for which blacks should be on the lookout *throughout their lives.* In the United States, one in four blacks has hypertension. Their readings are generally higher than they are in whites, and complications are more frequent and often more severe.

   No one really knows why high blood pressure hits blacks so often and so badly. It may have something to do with their ancestors having come from hotter climes; as a result, a black body is genetically programmed to retain salt, normally lost in sweat. That may be desirable in the tropics, but in New York, say, where excessive heat is not a problem, it may cause hypertension. If you're black, it's a good idea to reduce your salt intake even if your blood pressure is normal, and to have your pressure checked at least twice a year. Remember, hypertension is a "silent killer"; you have to *look* for it. When it does cause symptoms, they usually consist of a throbbing headache, nosebleeds from time to time and the feeling of fullness in the head.

• *Lactose intolerance*—another condition found more often in blacks (as well as Jews and Asians). Although rarely serious, it can make life pretty miserable. Persons with lactose intolerance are deficient in lactase, the enzyme that digests the lactose in your diet (lactose is a sugar present in milk and all its derivative foods). Undigested lactose makes for gas, bloating, cramping and diarrhea one to two hours after you eat it. *Seventy percent of blacks in the United States are lactose-intolerant.*

Whatever your ethnic background (but especially if you're black, Jewish or of Asian descent), if you can relate your gas and cramping to milk or any food containing it, try a lactose-free diet before spending your money on a work-up for gallbladder or gastrointestinal disease. If you are lactase-deficient, chances are your symptoms will disappear.

There are a host of other diseases from which blacks have a higher death rate than whites—diabetes, lupus erythematosus, glaucoma, circulatory problems and cancer. I believe that poverty and its consequences (primarily failure of early diagnosis and inadequate treatment) contribute greatly to those statistics.

WHAT GREEKS, ITALIANS, ARABS—AND SOME JEWS— HAVE IN COMMON

Imagine this. In the course of a routine checkup, your doctor finds that you're anemic. The possible causes range from poor nutrition to excessive bleeding. You're asked about your eating habits and it's determined that you're not a food faddist. There's plenty of fish and meat in your diet, as well as lots of leafy green vegetables. Despite the anemia, you don't feel tired. You assure the doctor that your menstrual flow is not excessively heavy, that you're not regularly taking aspirin (which might erode the lining of your stomach and cause chronic insidious blood loss), and you don't have hemorrhoids. Your stool is then checked for the presence of blood and none is found.

At this point, your doctor may pursue the work-up with more sophisticated and expensive procedures to solve the problem. However, if your ancestral roots are in any country bordering the Mediterranean Sea, the thing to do is to analyze your hemoglobin for thalassemia (Mediterranean anemia). Thalassemia is a hereditary disorder in which an abnormality of hemoglobin results in anemia. It may be mild or severe. If you're thalassemic, don't waste your time taking extra iron, B_{12} shots or other vitamins. They don't help.

Interestingly, thalassemia is found in virtually every population living in the Mediterranean area. That means you're susceptible if your roots are Arabic, Jewish, Greek, Italian or in any other country near that sea—no matter where you're living now.

"Funny, You Don't Look Jewish!"

It's very difficult, in most cases, to generalize about the genetic vulnerability of Jews, largely because they're a people and not a race. Although their geographic roots are in the Middle East, over the past centuries only a small number of Jews remained in the Arab world or in what is now known as Israel.

Despite the present diversity of the Jewish people, there are ten uncommon genetic diseases to which they are almost exclusively susceptible. These include such rarities as Tay-Sachs disease and spongy degeneration of the nervous system. In virtually all these disorders, symptoms appear early in life, and death folows soon thereafter.

I have already referred to some of the more benign disorders that occur more frequently in Jews, like lactose intolerance. Jews, especially those whose family tree is rooted in Central or Eastern Europe

(Ashkenazi), are also more vulnerable to diabetes mellitus, coronary artery disease, Buerger's disease (blockage of the arteries in the legs) and inflammatory bowel disease—but no one really knows why. It's probably a combination of genetics and environment.

To sum up, certain diseases are more common among specific ethnic groups and races than others, but this is often due more to environmental conditions such as poverty, diet and availability of medical care than to genetic factors. Inherited diseases, however, do play a role in determining your susceptibility to a particular disorder. Persons who are potential carriers of *fatal* hereditary diseases *must* seek genetic counseling before having children.

MARITAL STATUS AND ITS IMPACT

Neither doctors nor patients pay enough attention to marital status when evaluating certain symptoms. An unhappy marriage and whether you are divorced, single or widowed all have important health consequences. In fact, if your spouse has just died or you are recently divorced, be very careful for the next twelve months of your life, because during that time you're especially vulnerable. For example, among the elderly in this group there are six times more deaths from pneumonia than among those whose marriages have remained intact.

If your marriage breaks up, the chances of your developing some acute illness within a year increases by about 30 percent. *Divorced persons* are particularly susceptible to headaches, genitourinary disorders and diseases of the skin. They also have an increased incidence of syphilis—probably because of greater exposure to risky sex when they're alone.

Separation also results in a sixfold increase in the number of visits to the psychiatrist.

Widowers between fifty-five and sixty-five have a 60 percent higher death rate from all causes than do married men the same age. They suffer more from new-onset coronary artery disease, elevated blood pressure, diabetes, rheumatoid arthritis, osteoarthritis and respiratory problems. But if they remarry within a year, they not only escape all these consequences, they apparently live healthier and longer lives than their counterparts who did not lose their wives!

Single men don't do as well as those who are happily married, but they have a much rosier outlook than those whose marriage is on the rocks, has broken up or has been terminated by death of the wife.

Some doctors believe that the explanation for these statistics lies in the critical interaction among the *brain* (the seat of all emotions), the *nervous system*(which transmits information from the brain to the rest of the body via nerves, and which also controls the production of hormones) and the *immune system*, which determines the level of resistance. When we are under stress, angered, depressed or frustrated—by divorce, separation or bereavement—the number of immune cells that protect against cancer and infection is reduced for as long as fourteen months. In one study that compared thrity-eight apparently happily married men with the same number whose marriages had broken up in the preceding twelve months, there was a 30 percent decrease in the number of immune cells in the divorced and separated groups. The greater the attachment to, preoccupation with and longing for their ex-mates, the sharper the drop.

There's an important message in all of this. First, marriage may be about the best thing that can happen to you—but only if it is a happy one. Singles are better off in every way than those in a troubled union; so don't enter into marriage casually. Finally: If you're lonely and develop any unusual symptoms, don't assume they're psychological. They may, in fact, have a very real physical component that requires treatment.

IF IT RUNS IN YOUR FAMILY

All of us enter the world with forty-six chromosomes in every one of our cells, the result of a combined contribution by both parents. Each chromosome contains thousands of genes which determine most of our characteristics—eye color, hair hue, height, intelligence and so on. However, genes are much more than just a blueprint for looks and brains. They also determine your health status. Knowing your family's medical history will help you appreciate your own risks and, therefore, what a given symptom may mean.

But be careful! I have so often heard patients with a family history of some particular disease say, "What's the use? It's going to get me no matter what I do. It's all in my genes, so I may as well eat, drink and be merry—while I can." Such nihilism is occasionally justified, as, for example, in Huntington's chorea, an inherited brain disorder that causes no symptoms whatsoever until middle age; then there is a devastating downhill course that ends in death. If one of your parents had Huntington's disease, you have a 50 percent chance of having inherited it yourself, and at the moment there's nothing you can do to avoid it. The same is true for sickle cell disease, if you happen to have inherited its genes from both parents.

But relatively few family-related diseases are that

serious or so purely genetic. Environment usually plays at least an equally important role in their development. Despite an apparent familial tendency, a disease may be not "in the blood" but in the air. For example, I look after a family, many of whose members had cancer of the lung. Genetic? Maybe, but the fact that they were all heavy smokers surely contributed to their disease. I wonder how many of them would have developed cancer if they had never smoked. By the same token, when several members in a black family have high blood pressure, a low-salt diet and proper medication can effectively control the disease and prevent its complications, whatever the genetics involved. So in most cases, there is no reason to adopt a nihilistic attitude because of an adverse family history.

Here are some of the more common and important conditions that seem to run in families. Remember, however, that in each one the environment also plays an important role.

- *Alcoholism* (yes, it's a disease). Whether or not you're an alcoholic is in part determined by your family tree. A genetic factor has been identified in some 35 to 40 percent of alcoholics and "alcohol abusers" (the dividing line between the two is very, very thin). If one or both parents have a drinking "problem," you are at four times the risk of becoming alcoholic yourself as compared to children of parents who don't drink at all. So, if you think you may be an alcoholic or are well on the way to becoming one, look into your family history. Regardless of what you find, if you have any anxiety about your drinking habits, consult a trained counselor.

- *Alzheimer's disease.* There is no other disease, with the possible exception of cancer, which generates as much anxiety in the blood relatives of those who have it—and not entirely without reason, for your risk of getting Alzheimer's is increased by about 10 to 15 percent if the disease affected a close relative early in life. But before you attribute to Alzheimer's any change in behavior or memory loss, make sure that other more common causes like chronic alcoholism, poor nutrition, brain injury and multiple untreated strokes have been accounted for. *Almost half the cases diagnosed as Alzheimer's turn out to be due to some other, often treatable or preventable condition.*

- *Arteriosclerosis.* Arteries can become clogged anywhere in the body—the legs, heart, brain, kidneys, even the eyes. Although this condition sometimes runs in families, there are almost always accompanying risk factors which you can control and thus reduce your own vulnerability. For example, your high blood pressure can be treated; you can lose weight; you can lower your cholesterol by diet and/or drugs; you can exercise, stop smoking and develop a better outlook on life. You should take all these steps, regardless of whether or not arteriosclerosis is especially prevalent among your relatives. Don't count on a good family history to protect you if you're a two-pack-a-day cigarette smoker who is overweight and has high blood pressure and an elevated cholesterol level. But if you're over forty years old, have noticed some chest pressure when you exert yourself and are wondering whether or not it's angina, you should take the symptom very seriously and have it evaluated without delay, especially if your father or other male relatives had coronary disease when they were young.
- *Breast cancer.* If your mother and a sister both had breast cancer, your *lifetime* risk for developing it is

about 30 percent even if your mammogram is normal and you can't feel any lump in your breast. If your mother was fine but two of your sisters had it, your risk is 15 percent. The probability of a breast lump being malignant doubles if your mother *or* your sister had breast cancer before menopause. That risk increases *sixfold* if your mother and a sister both had the disease.

But these are only statistics. Here's what really counts. If you find a lump in your breast, no matter whether you're young or old, male or female, with a good family history or a bad one, have it immediately and thoroughly evaluated.

Every woman should have a screening mammogram at age thirty-five, every two years after age forty and annually after fifty. But don't depend entirely on the mammogram. Examine your breasts every month and make sure your doctor does, too, at every visit.

• *Colon and rectal cancer.* There are strong familial determinants for this disease. When President Reagan developed cancer of the bowel, we learned that his brother too had had it some years earlier. If an immediate blood relative has colon cancer, your own risk for it is increased some two to five times. So, always be on the lookout for and immediately report to your doctor the cardinal symptoms of colon and rectal cancer: *any* change in bowel habits (sudden onset of constipation or diarrhea, or alternating diarrhea and constipation), blood in the stool, narrowing of its diameter (so that it resembles a ribbon) and unexplained new abdominal symptoms like pain, cramping or spasm. I also recommend that you test for blood in the stool at least twice a year with a kit you can buy at any drugstore at very little cost. It's one of the best investments you can make.

- *Diabetes.* The classic symptoms of this disease are increased thirst and urination (what comes in must go out), weight loss and, in women, vaginal itching due to yeast in the sugar-rich urine. No other condition I know gives you all three symptoms.

   There are actually two kinds of diabetes: adult-onset and juvenile, or insulin-dependent. The former accounts for 90 percent of all cases and, as its name suggests, occurs later in life, usually in overweight persons. Statistically, your risk of developing it doubles with each decade and every twenty pounds of excess weight. Most adult-onset diabetes can be controlled by diet and weight loss, or by oral medications. However, if you continue to lose weight beyond the goal set for you, and become very thirsty, you'll know you're not succeeding and probably need insulin.

   The 10 percent of diabetics who are insulin-dependent usually develop their symptom in childhood or early adult life. When insulin is needed to control sugar levels in the adult-onset form of the disease, its use does not mean that these patients have the same complications as do those whose diabetes started when they were children.

   Although both forms of diabetes have a high blood sugar in common, they are not the same disease. Their familial risk factors are also quite different. For example, if both parents have adult-onset diabetes, 60 percent of their children will develop the condition before age sixty. However, when one child has insulin-dependent diabetes, the likelihood that a brother or sister will also become diabetic is much less than that.
- *Emphysema.* Patients with this lung disease lose the tiny sacs (alveoli) through which the lungs exchange the oxygen inhaled for the carbon monoxide exhaled. In some cases, the cause is an

inherited enzyme deficiency. The main symptoms of emphysema are shortness of breath, wheezing and recurrent episodes of bronchitis. Because of the large amount of air retained in the lungs in this disease, the rib cage is expanded and the chest becomes barrel-shaped. Your chance of getting emphysema is increased if any immediate family member suffers from it. If you have this disease at any stage and are a smoker, quit immediately. Smoking makes things worse. Better still, never start, especially if you are genetically vulnerable.

- *Hypertension.* Whether or not you develop high blood pressure is probably determined 60 percent by your genes and 40 percent by your environment. But, as I indicated earlier, regardless of the genetics involved, everyone with high blood pressure can and should be treated by a combination of weight loss, diet (especially salt restriction, where it's indicated) and drugs.

- *Migraine headaches.* This condition afflicts about 5 to 10 percent of the population, and those who suffer it are often clustered in families. For example, if both your parents have it, chances are seven out of ten that you do (or will), too. If only one parent has migraine, that figure drops to 4 percent —still pretty high. So, if you've grown up in a "migraine" family, and you develop recurrent sickening one-sided headaches, preceded by a variety of warning signals (flashing lights, strange noises), you probably have migraine.

- *Obesity.* If you're excessively fat, you may, of course, have a glandular disorder (statistically unlikely); you may be eating too much and exercising too little (very likely); or it may be your unavoidable genetic destiny (much more likely than we used to think). The responsible gene is now being hunted, but it may take years to find. In the meantime, your best bet is to assume that the poundage is due to your lifestyle and not to your genetics, and act accordingly.

• *Prostate cancer.* This disease is especially common in blacks and may also run in families. The sons and brothers of men with prostate cancer appear to be at three times the average risk of dying from this malignancy. So, if there's a strong incidence in your family, be sure to have your prostate checked by simple digital (finger) rectal examination each year after age fifty. Remember, this is one cancer which, when detected early, can often be cured.

• *Psoriasis.* This condition, whose causes are unknown but which may be related to an autoimmune disorder, is the bane of 1 to 2 percent of Americans. It causes large areas of the skin, especially the scalp, to become scaly and quite unattractive. Mercifully, it does not often involve the face. If either of your parents or any siblings has psoriasis, your risk of developing it is about one in ten, which is roughly ten times greater than that of the general population.

These are just a few of the common conditions that appear to have familial ties. There are many others—duodenal ulcers, bronchial asthma, uterine and stomach cancers, schizophrenia and even osteoarthritis. So when you're trying to decide what disease a certain symptom reflects, look into the kinds of disorders that have cropped up among your blood relatives over the years. Your family tree should be of more than social significance to you. Remember, however, that although many diseases tend to run in families, most can be modified by eliminating specific, personal risk factors in your own environment. An adverse family history should lead to activism, not nihilism.

IS YOUR JOB KILLING YOU?

Your occupation determines to some extent how likely you are to develop certain diseases, and it should influence how you interpret any given symptoms. If exercise is supposed to be good for you, why are men in very physical jobs more likely to die from heart disease than are high-pressure executives? Why do they also have more cancer? No one knows for sure, but the physical activity *is* protective, and almost certainly not responsible for these unexpected findings. The answer may lie in dietary differences; or perhaps blue-collar workers do not have access to high-quality medical care; or they delay the necessary treatment because they may not recognize early signs of disease.

Regardless of the nature of your work, here are the kinds of situations that render you more likely to have job-related symptoms:

- Your supervisor is "nonsupportive," or, to put it bluntly, he or she is giving you a hard time.
- Your chances for promotion, for more authority and for a greater salary in the future are small. In other words, you're trapped and you know it.
- Your work load seems too much for you to handle.
- You don't feel you've been given responsibility commensurate with your ability.
- You'd rather be doing a different job.
- You're a female clerical worker (that puts you at twice the risk for heart disease as compared to a housewife).
- You're either a blue-collar worker or frustrated at your job, but your wife, on the other hand, is a successful executive.

Now let's take a look at some common symptoms and their possible *physical* relationship to the work you do:

- You have headaches and your eyes burn, ache or sting. If your job involves close work, and you spend all day concentrating on visual detail (reading fine print, drawing, making small, accurate measurements), it's probably all due to eye strain. The same symptoms can result from sitting at a video display terminal for hours at a time without enough breaks.
- Does your job require a lot of photocopying? The bright flash of light from some machines can cause temporary blurring of vision and "after images." So keep the cover down on the machine and close your eyes or look away when the light goes on.
- Do your stuffy nose and heavy breathing clear up on weekends, only to return every Monday morning? You may have the "tight-building syndrome," first recognized in the 1970s. At that time, we were preoccupied with saving energy and minimizing the loss of heated or cooled air from the work site. So new buildings had either no windows or ones that couldn't be opened. In many older buildings, windows were nailed shut and caulked and their sashes weatherproofed. Sounds okay on paper, but the trouble is, in addition to trapping air, such buildings seal in all kinds of indoor pollutants, especially fumes—from the rug shampoo and formaldehyde disinfectant the cleaning crew uses, from the old wet-process copier that hasn't been traded in for a new model, from your typewriter correction fluid, marking pens, glue and room air deodorizers. These all accumulate in an airtight room, causing not only a stuffy nose and labored breathing, but chronic headaches, nausea, dizziness, sore throats, eye and skin irritations, dry cough, allergies and even sleep disorders. What's

more, the humidifiers and air conditioners necessary to control the humidity and temperature in
these sealed buildings provide an ideal environment in which bacteria or fungi can breed. The
best-known consequence of that is Legionnaire's
disease, from which so many people died before
the cause was determined. So if you work in one of
these airtight buildings and have developed repeated chest colds or allergies, don't blame your
coughing coworkers or the receptionist's perfume!

• If you type all day long and have developed numbness, tingling and perhaps weakness in your fingers, don't assume that you have arthritis. The
constant movement of your fingers and wrists can
sometimes inflame their tendons. If you perform
any repetitive motion all day long, you may end up
with pain in your shoulder, elbow, wrist or fingers,
depending on which joint you're abusing.

• If you've suddenly discovered you have high blood
pressure, reflect on the kind of work you do and
how you're handling it. For example, an air-traffic
controller's job is associated with a higher incidence of hypertension than are most other occupa-
tions. A noisy work environment can also raise
blood pressure (and your cholesterol level too).

• If you've developed a chronic cough but don't
smoke and have never had bronchitis, think about
your occupation. If you are a ceramist or a potter,
or if you work in a dusty environment with fiber
art, jewelry or metal sculpture, you may be inhaling silica and other dusts. These can cause a
chronic cough and varying types of lung disease—
including silicosis (often a forerunner of lung cancer).

There are specific risks accompanying other occu-
pations—cancer of the kidney in coke-oven workers,

malignant tumors of the bladder in rubber and dye workers, leukemia among radiologists and X-ray technicians as well as among workers in the rubber industry. In almost every case, these risks can either be minimized or eliminated by proper public-health measures. If you suspect that an illness is related to the machines you use or the materials you are exposed to in your work, take the steps necessary to protect yourself and improve your work environment.

ESPECIALLY IF YOU ARE GAY (AND PROMISCUOUS)

Homosexual men are especially vulnerable to several diseases, one of which is invariably fatal (AIDS), others potentially so (hepatitis B) and all very unpleasant (virtually every sexually transmitted disease from herpes to syphilis). But if you are male or female, straight or gay, and are sexually active, you should be aware of the early symptoms of the so-called "venereal," or sexually transmitted, diseases.

AIDS, the New Plague

It's no longer an "epidemic," which is defined as the spread of a disease within a community. Since AIDS (acquired immune deficiency syndrome) now involves the entire planet, it has, in fact, become "pandemic"—geographically widespread.

At first, AIDS was confined largely to homosexuals, among whom it was transmitted sexually, and to intravenous drug abusers, who spread it by sharing contaminated needles. They remain at high risk for the disease, but it now also threatens anyone who received a blood transfusion between 1979 and 1985 (before we learned how to screen blood for the virus that causes the disease), the partners of bisexuals, children born of infected mothers, and health-care professionals. To what extent it will ultimately spread to the larger population remains to be seen. Certainly, the incidence among heterosexuals is increasing and, as of early 1988, amounted to 4 percent of cases. So no one is immune.

AIDS is caused by the HIV virus, which destroys the body's immune system, leaving it vulnerable to a variety of "opportunistic" infections, so called because they take advantage of the body's inability to fight back. There is presently no cure, nor is one in sight in the immediate future. Prevention remains the key to control of the disease.

The Symptoms of AIDS

Someone with AIDS falls sick with a variety of symptoms—those either directly caused by the virus itself or stemming from secondary, opportunistic infections. The first evidence of the viral infection may consist of a generalized swelling of the lymph glands —in the neck, the groin and the armpits. In contrast to other causes of glandular enlargement, these don't go away. Thus far, one person in five who has developed these glandular swellings has gone on to develop the full-blown disease. (How many more will do so as the years go by remains to be seen.) In the rest, the glands simply remain swollen in what appears to be an arrested phase of the disease, called ARC (AIDS-related complex).

Instead of causing glandular swelling, the virus may make its presence known in much the same way as infectious mononucleosis: fever, night sweats, utter fatigue, aching muscles, joint pains, headaches, sore throat, diarrhea, swollen glands and a faint body rash. If you are in a high-risk category and develop any combination of these symptoms that continues for two weeks or more, AIDS is a real possibility.

Instead of affecting the whole body in this way, the AIDS virus may attack a particular organ system right off the bat. One of my patients, an older man, homosexual and promiscuous, was admitted to the hospital for removal of an enlarged prostate gland. The operation was successfully completed without complications. Then, just as we were making plans to discharge him, he suddenly became totally confused and irrational. He didn't know who or where he was and was puzzled by all the strangers in white milling about him. I thought initially that he had had a stroke. He was in fact suffering from an acute case of AIDS. The virus had made its way to the brain, causing his dementia. He died one month later.

The AIDS virus can strike anywhere in that way: the bowels, producing diarrhea; the kidneys, paralyzing their function; the skin, with an uncommon form of cancer called Kaposi's sarcoma; and the lungs (where 50 percent of all patients first become affected), with a form of pneumonia called *Pneumocystis carinii*. Kaposi's sarcoma causes a rash, enlarges the lymph glands, invades the intestinal tract (giving abdominal pain, fever and diarrhea) and can also strike the lungs, leaving you short of breath and coughing. Symptoms of *Pneumocystis carinii* pneumonia, which is caused by a fungus, consist of a dry cough and shortness of breath. If you are a high-risk individual, and you develop such a cough for no apparent reason (you don't smoke or work in a dusty environment or have any allergies), see your doctor. The diagnosis of AIDS pneumonia is confirmed by a chest X ray, analysis of the sputum and, at some point, a positive antibody test for the virus.

If you are at high risk and have recurrent fungal or other unusual infections in the mouth and haven't been taking antibiotics or other medication, you may have AIDS. The disease shows up in this way because the body's weakened immune system can't rid your mouth of the fungus.

The diagnosis of AIDS, even when strongly suspected, cannot always be immediately confirmed, because the usual antibody blood test may not become "positive" for months or years after exposure. That's one of the problems with receiving a blood transfusion, even today. Blood from an infected donor who was in this "silent phase" before the body had produced antibodies to the virus will screen "negative." So, although the risk of contracting AIDS from a blood transfusion is much less than it used to be, it still exists, and is estimated to be one in forty thousand.

Other Diseases Which Affect Homosexuals

Although AIDS has completely overshadowed the other sexually transmitted diseases, every sexually active individual, but especially promiscuous homosexual men, should also be on the lookout for the symptoms of other infections. For example:

• The tipoff to the diagnosis of *syphilis,* which is caused by an infectious microorganism, is the appearance of a painless "cold sore" on the genitals, the mouth, in the anal area—wherever sexual contact has occurred—which disappears without leaving a trace. You should have no trouble distinguishing it from herpes sores, which keep cropping up in the same location, are preceded by itching, burning or pain for several days and crust over before clearing up.

Even though the syphilitic chancre, as the sore is called, vanishes without treatment, the disease itself does not. It enters the so-called secondary stage in a matter of weeks and causes a variety of characteristic symptoms: fever, enlarged lymph glands, headache and skin rash. Untreated, the infecting organism then passes into the tertiary stage, retreating into the interior of the body, where it silently continues to wreak havoc over the years. Although the disease is not contagious at this point, as it is in the primary and secondary stages, it can cause devastating symptoms in the heart, the liver, the eyes, the brain and many other organs.

No one is immune to syphilis, but 50 percent of all cases occur in the gay community. A congenital form of the disease can also be passed on by an infected expectant mother to her unborn child. A course of penicillin or other antibiotics is all it takes to cure the infection in its primary or secondary stages. It is much more difficult to treat in the tertiary stage, after organ damage has occurred.

• A discharge from the penis can reflect either a nonvenereal irritation or the sexually transmitted diseases *gonorrhea* or *chlamydia,* both of which are caused by infectious organisms. You can distinguish between the latter two by the nature of the discharge: yellowish green pus in gonorrhea; thin, watery and colorless in chlamydia. Should you develop a painful, swollen joint (knee, ankle or elbow) weeks after the appearance of the discharge from the penis, that's further evidence of gonorrhea. What have the joints got to do with this sexually transmitted infection? The "gonococcus" bug responsible for all the trouble gets into the bloodstream and, unless treated, may settle down in a joint and infect it too. Like syphilis, both gonorrhea and chlamydia are curable with the appropriate antibiotic.

• There's a high incidence of *hepatitis B* among

homosexuals. Unlike hepatitis A, which almost always clears up completely, hepatitis B can progress to chronic liver disease, cirrhosis, liver cancer and even death. Hepatitis-B vaccine provides virtually complete protection against the virus that causes the disease. So, if you are gay and haven't had your shot, go to your doctor immediately and get one. The original vaccine was made from human blood products, and many people were afraid to take it for fear of getting AIDS—even though there was no basis for that fear. The newest vaccine is produced by a recombinant-DNA technique which does not require human blood in its manufacture. So now there is no excuse whatsoever not to have it.

The symptoms of hepatitis B are appetite loss, apathy and sluggishness, a low-grade fever and perhaps pain in several joints. Then comes the jaundice—the yellowish tinting of the skin and the whites of the eyes. The diagnosis is confirmed by specific blood tests. The course of treatment includes bed rest, the proper diet, appropriate medications, complete abstinence from alcohol, steroids and interferon.

- *Hemorrhoids* are dilated veins of the rectum or the anus, and homosexuals who practice anal intercourse are particularly prone to this disorder. Hemorrhoids are usually due to poor bowel habits, multiple pregnancies, nervous stress or chronic constipation. But gay or straight, man or woman, never assume that blood on the toilet tissue is due to hemorrhoids alone—even if you are certain you have them. Sometimes the blood you see is the signal of a cancer lurking higher up in the bowel. Check out the colon just to make sure you do not have two concurrent conditions.
- If you are gay and develop diarrhea for no appar-

ent reason, suspect the "gay bowel syndrome," an infection and irritation of the lower bowel induced by anal intercourse.

Every homosexual should be familiar with the characteristic symptoms of the diseases to which he is particularly vulnerable and, when they appear, seek treatment immediately. But *all* sexually active individuals, male and female, straight or gay, are vulnerable to a wide variety of venereal infections. The greater the number of sex partners, the higher the risk. Abstinence is the only certain means of prevention, but there are other ways you can reduce your risk considerably. Choose your sex partners with care. Use a condom. Do not engage in unsafe sexual practices. Many of these sexually transmitted diseases can be prevented, treated or cured.

ALCOHOL: "HOW MUCH IS TOO MUCH?"

Doctors define "excessive" intake of alcohol as fourteen or more drinks per week. Is drinking less than this amount necessarily safe? Probably not. It now seems that "light" consumption also can be hazardous. This news makes me sad because I love good wine and enjoy some with every evening meal. So how much is too much? To answer that question, you need to know what happens to the alcohol you consume.

When you drink on an empty stomach, the alcohol is absorbed quickly and completely and enters the bloodstream in short order. The presence of food, especially fat, decreases the rate at which the alcohol gets into the circulation. You may think you're diluting the impact of your cocktail by adding a carbonated beverage. In fact you're doing just the opposite; mixing the booze with some fizzy concoction actually speeds up its absorption.

Once the alcohol is in the bloodstream, it goes directly to the liver, where fully 95 percent of it is "broken down" (the remaining 5 percent is excreted through your breath, urine and sweat). That's pretty efficient performance by the liver. The trouble is, it can process no more than an ounce of whiskey per hour (that's less than a single can of beer or one glass of wine). If you drink more than that, the excess hangs around in your body, doing all kinds of things, usually bad, to virtually every organ. For example, booze dilates blood vessels everywhere, including the skin. (The reason chronic alcoholics have a "Rudolph the Red-nosed Reindeer" nose is because its small capillaries have been dilated for so long.) When the widened blood vessels in the brain, the liver and elsewhere snap back to their original diameter after some alcohol-free sleep, you experience the familiar morning-after hangover.

A hangover is the least of the health hazards you face. Here are some others:

- If you're a drinker, you are prone to heartburn, gastritis, nausea and stomach ulcers, because of the irritation and erosion of your stomach lining by excessive amounts of alcohol over the years.
- Alcohol increases your risk for several different cancers, notably of the mouth, the esophagus and the stomach—especially if you're also a smoker. So a sore in the mouth that doesn't go away, trouble swallowing, or pain in the belly worsened by eating should all prompt a thorough search for such a tumor.
- If, a few days after a drinking binge that ended in vomiting, you develop a fever, a cough and pain in the chest, it's probably not the flu, but "aspiration

pneumonia"—some of the vomit got into your lungs during a retching spell.

- Over the long term, the liver is the organ hardest hit by heavy drinking. Initially, it is enlarged by fat deposits laid down in its cells, a condition known as "fatty liver." This does not usually give any symptoms, but your doctor may detect an increase in the size of the liver when he examines you. If at this point you go on the wagon, nature forgives the insult and your liver will usually return to normal.

However, if you continue to drink, you go on to the next phase, "alcoholic hepatitis," whose symptoms are jaundice, nausea, discomfort in the right upper portion of your abdomen and maybe a little fever, very much like the way you feel when you have the garden variety of infectious hepatitis. If you're a heavy drinker, alcohol is the more likely culprit than the suspect shellfish you ate recently. Hepatitis A from rank shellfish has a mortality rate near zero, while 10 to 30 percent of those with alcoholic hepatitis who continue to drink will die.

The final, irreversible and often fatal stage of alcoholic liver disease is *cirrhosis*. When you consume alcohol heavily over the years, scar tissue gradually replaces the normal liver cells. Cirrhosis compromises all the vital and myriad functions of the liver, which can no longer release its stored sugar on demand, so you become hypoglycemic if you miss a meal or two; it doesn't make the proteins needed to clot blood, so you bleed and bruise easily; it doesn't detoxify many of the medications you require, and you become intolerant of them; it doesn't produce the necessary antibodies and other proteins in the required amounts, so you fall prey to all kinds of infections. The final, frightening episode in the life of the patient with advanced liver cirrhosis is often a massive hemorrhage from ruptured varicose veins in the throat which resulted from the backup of blood from the scarred liver. Statistically, women drinkers, especially blacks, are most likely to develop liver disease, even if they consume smaller amounts of alcohol than men. They also have a higher risk of dying once the liver has been damaged. But any heavy drinker is vulnerable to the scenario portrayed above.

Habitual excessive drinking also wipes out brain cells, so that a chronic alcoholic may become demented. In fact, alcohol is second only to Alzheimer's disease as a cause of mental deterioration in adults. If someone you love who has imbibed generously over the years develops poor short-term memory, disorientation, hallucinations, emotional disturbances, double vision and loss of muscle control, the cause may be booze, not Alzheimer's. The big difference between alcoholic dementia and Alzheimer's disease is that abstention from alcohol can prevent further deterioration and sometimes even result in improvement, while with Alzheimer's the path is inexorably downhill.

Although a glass or two of wine eases tension, stimulates the appetite and triggers a sense of well-being, for most people alcohol is a depressant. Even in "moderation" it can induce mood swings and impair sexual performance in males. Men who drink heavily have a 40 percent drop in their level of testosterone, the male hormones that give you the urge—and the capacity to do something about it.

Alcohol hurts the heart too. Heavy drinkers have more heart attacks, probably because testosterone deficiency promotes clot formation in the coronary arteries. Alcohol can also poison the heart muscle and weaken its pumping action. If you're a heavy drinker and have become short of breath, need two or three pillows at night to prop you up and notice that your feet are swollen, the alcohol has pummeled the cardiac-muscle fibers into docility and failure. This damage is further compounded by nutritional deficiencies when alcoholics forgo food for booze, which, although high in calories, is nutritionally void.

Alcohol, in addition to damaging the heart, can also irritate it, even in small amounts. A few drinks can make it beat very fast or irregularly, giving you palpitations, dizziness, chest pain and occasionally loss of consciousness. Because this is more apt to happen when you're partying over a long weekend, this sequence of events has come to be known as the "holiday heart." You're especially vulnerable to it if you have a preexisting cardiac-rhythm disorder.

The only good news about alcohol's impact on the heart is that it is often reversible. I've seen patients literally at death's door from congestive heart failure who, with the appropriate medication, nutrition and *complete abstinence from alcohol* have lost many of their symptoms.

The very disturbing recent news about alcohol is that women who drink lightly—only three or four cocktails a week—may be more vulnerable to breast cancer. If this observation is substantiated by future research, then stop drinking, period. For the time being, if you've got a strong family history of breast malignancy, you should at least reduce your alcohol intake.

Most bars now post warnings that drinking alcohol during pregnancy can cause birth defects. The most serious is the *fetal alcohol syndrome,* which occurs when the mother is alcoholic and results in mental retardation of the child as well as in various physical deformities. However, even just a drink now and then can be dangerous to the unborn, especially during the first three months of pregnancy. The children of drinking mothers tend to weigh less at birth; they have smaller heads; their limbs, fingers and face may be deformed, and the heart may contain defects. Occasionally, the infant appears to be perfectly normal at birth, and it's only in adolescence that learning, perceptual and behavior problems become apparent.

If a drink relaxes you after a hard day, it must also lower your blood pressure. Right? Wrong! It *raises* your blood pressure. And that's not a good thing if you have hypertension to begin with. I've seen many patients whose blood pressure has been difficult to control because of the alcohol they consume. Booze is hard on the brain too. Drinkers are more susceptible to hemorrhagic strokes (a blood vessel in the brain ruptures). Nerves too can be damaged by alcohol (alcoholic neuropathy), with resultant weakness and sharp, lancing, shooting pain in the limbs.

A year or two ago I might have been able to end this depressing discussion with some good news. At that time there was some indication that one or two drinks a day raises the level of HDL cholesterol (the "good" fraction which helps protect against heart disease). Unfortunately that theory has lately been challenged by some cardiologists, but not diehard wine enthusiasts like myself.

What's the bottom line? Should we go back to Prohibition? Are we to stop drinking completely, or can we still safely enjoy a nightcap? If you go by the statistics alone, you're probably better off cutting it out. But in the real world I recommend abstinence for people who have the following conditions:

A family history of alcoholism.
Pregnancy.

Liver disease of any kind.

Active ulcers.

Cardiac-rhythm disturbance or heart failure.

High blood pressure that's not well controlled.

A family history of breast cancer.

Heavy smoking. The combination of tobacco and alcohol is especially hazardous for several forms of cancer.

Older persons taking other medications, especially tranquilizers.

That should do it. Almost everyone else may continue to enjoy an occasional "cheers."

CIGARETTES: THE NAILS IN THE COFFIN

There is no greater single *avoidable* health hazard in America than tobacco. Beyond the halitosis, the stained fingers and teeth, the foul-smelling clothes, the "smoker's cough," tobacco means 300,000 deaths every year, mainly from cancer (not just in the lungs, but anywhere in the body) and heart disease— not only deaths, but oh so much pain and suffering!

Cigarette use puts you into a totally different health category from that of the nonsmoking population. Since you have two strikes against you right off the bat, you are forced to treat *any* suspicious symptom very seriously. So if you're a smoker:

• You dare not assume that the chronic tickle in your throat that persists at the tail end of a cold is "nothing." It may be the first symptom of a lung cancer.

• If you were formerly able to climb two flights of stairs without any trouble and now find yourself huffing, puffing and very uncomfortable, you must consider emphysema, chronic bronchitis or some other lung disease.

- You're urinating with greater frequency; it may be painful and on occasion you've even seen blood in the urine. If you're a nonsmoker, think of simple enlargement of the prostate. A smoker, however, must also consider cancer of the bladder, to which cigarettes leave one more vulnerable.

Here are some of the mechanisms by which tobacco makes you sick:

Consider the lungs first. The respiratory tract is lined with tiny hairs called "cilia" whose job it is to sweep mucus and any foreign matter in your bronchial tree up to your throat, from which you can spit it out. When you inhale tobacco, these little hairs are paralyzed. While you're asleep and not smoking, the cilia begin to recover, and they start pushing accumulated gunk upward during the night. In the morning, when you awake, that's what you cough up with the familiar "smoker's hack." After years of smoking, the cilia are eventually destroyed and don't bounce back during the night. So now the mucus in the respiratory tract that has trapped the pollutants and other foreign matter you've inhaled just sits there instead of being swept up and out. It's a perfect breeding ground for bacteria, and it explains why smokers have so many colds, respiratory infections and chronic bronchitis.

Tobacco smoke also aggravates *emphysema,* a disease in which the lung is less elastic and its alveoli—the air sacs that permit the exchange of oxygen for carbon dioxide—are destroyed. With fewer of these alveoli around, there is a smaller surface area available for this vital gas transfer. As a result, someone with emphysema may expend 80 percent of his or her energy getting enough oxygen just to breathe; the average nonsmoking adult uses only 5 percent for that purpose.

Then, of course, there's lung cancer. Eighty-five percent of lung cancers in men and 75 percent in women are linked to smoking. Maybe you've decided to play it "safe" and have stopped inhaling or have switched to a pipe or cigars, or only take snuff or chew tobacco. You're just kidding yourself. All you're doing is exchanging lung cancer for cancer of the lip, the mouth, the tongue and the throat. But you name the organ—pancreas, kidneys, stomach, even the cervix: all are more vulnerable to cancer in smokers. That's why cigarette smoking is *the* major cause of cancer deaths in the United States.

Smoking causes problems to the yet unborn. Pregnant women who light up have a much greater risk of ending up with a stillbirth or a *miscarriage*. Pregnant smokers also suffer from premature rupture of the membranes and from hemorrhage, and their babies weigh less at birth. In a recent study of three-year-olds, children who were shorter or had learning disabilities and were not as sharp as their peers in mathematical ability could blame it all on a mother who had smoked while pregnant.

Patients often ask me, "How can cigarettes be bad for me when they give me such a lift?" Let me tell you why they get that "lift" and what it actually does to them. When a smoker inhales, he or she drags into the lungs a mixture of tar, nicotine and as many as four thousand other poisonous gases and compounds, including cyanide, volatile aromatic hydrocarbons and carbon monoxide. These poisons enter the bloodstream and go right to the heart. Within seven seconds, the nicotine is pumped from the heart to the brain, where it is absorbed, triggering the release of substances called "catecholamines." These catecholamines produce an adrenaline-like effect, increasing heart rate and blood pressure. That's what gives the "lift." So lighting up one cigarette after another throughout the day maintains this "great feeling" at the expense of the vascular system. If you're a smoker, check it out yourself. Count your pulse and, if you can, record your blood pressure before your first cigarette of the day. Then take a puff and see what happens. Chances are, your pulse rate will increase by twenty beats per minute, your pressure will rise by ten to twenty points, and, I hope, you'll never smoke again. That's what made *me* stop thirty years ago!

A more serious consequence of this "wonderful feeling" is a release of free fatty acids into the bloodstream. These ultimately settle in the arteries and block them. That's why smoking doubles your risk of having a heart attack and increases the danger of sudden cardiac death some two- to fourfold. What's more, when a smoker suffers a heart attack, he or she is more likely to die than is a nonsmoker—and suddenly, within the hour. In addition to releasing these artery-blocking fatty acids, the inhaled smoke throws the blood vessels into spasm and narrows them. When that happens, you feel a constriction in your throat and chest which is the hallmark of angina pectoris.

Secondary or passive smoking—just being in the same room with someone who smokes—is harmful, too. I wish the airlines would ban smoking entirely, instead of only on flights of less than two hours' duration as they now do. Why don't you ask them to? I did!

Longtime cigarette smokers often have this attitude: "What's the difference? I've been smoking for so many years that stopping now won't do any good." That's simply not true. No matter how long you've smoked, if you quit right now your risk for *all* diseases will rapidly be reduced. After ten smoke-free years, the likelihood of your developing heart disease will be no greater than that of a person who has never smoked, even if you were a one-pack-a-day smoker! After ten to fifteen years, an ex-smoker's life expectancy, as well as the odds of getting lung cancer and cancer of the larynx, are the same as they are in those who never smoked at all!

If you're a smoker and have thus far been unable to quit, a good first step is to switch to a low-tar, low-nicotine brand. Although there's no such thing as a "safe cigarette," the American Cancer Society has found that those who smoke low-tar and -nicotine brands have a 16 percent lower death rate than high-tar and -nicotine smokers—and a 26 percent lower risk of cancer.

Smoking is more than a bad habit; it is an addiction, which means that it usually is very difficult to quit. But the hazards to your health are so enormous that you owe it to yourself, and to those who care about you, to try.

DRUGS (LEGAL AND ILLEGAL): PASSPORT TO A PERMANENT "VACATION"

Who knows why they do it? Some say that among the affluent it's to help them cope with stress, deal with frustrations, minimize depression or allay anxiety. Among the poor and disadvantaged, it may be to escape from reality and enter a world of pleasure and fantasy to which they otherwise have no access. Whatever the reason, millions of Americans use, depend on or are addicted to mood- and mind-altering drugs. It's legal when your doctor prescribes them; it's criminal when you do it on your own. In my view, the dividing line between the two is a thin one, and the end result, at least medically, is often quite similar.

When you take any of these drugs, the first experience may be wonderful, but the second time around it's not quite as thrilling. And as you go on you need more and more of the drug to achieve the desired effect. The inevitable consequences are dependence, tolerance and addiction. As the dosage increases and the intervals shorten, the craving becomes more intense. Nor can you ever be certain of your supply. If you have become dependent on a prescription drug, your doctor may not let you have as much as you need because the Drug Enforcement Agency is looking over his shoulder. If, on the other hand, you obtained your supply from a pusher, you may no longer be able to afford the habit. And when, for whatever reason, the supply can't keep up with your body's demand, withdrawal symptoms become unbearable.

When It's Legal

Americans spend more money on "happy pills" than they do on prescribed contraceptives and cold remedies. That's the size of the market! Although Valium is the prototype, doctors are constantly being bombarded with advertising material from pharmaceutical houses pitching "new," "safer," "less addicting," "more effective" and "less toxic" mood-altering drugs. Many psychiatrists have even stopped listening to the patient's problems—which take too long to solve. "Just swallow this pill three times a day before meals and you'll feel better." Of course, these medications can be a godsend for patients with real psychiatric disorders—manic depressives, phobics, schizophrenics. My criticism is that they are too often dispensed in lieu of advice to people with everyday problems.

Here are some of the consequences I have seen among those who regularly use or are dependent on

456   *YOUR GENETICS AND LIFESTYLE*

these so-called tranquilizers or "psychotropic" agents:

- *Irregular heartbeat.* Many of the antianxiety and antidepressant drugs can give you extra heartbeats and palpitations. Although these sometimes make you uncomfortable, they're usually not dangerous. But they can be, if you've got a heart rhythm problem to begin with or suffer from some underlying heart disease.

- *Effect on blood pressure*—up or down. If you're on an antihypertensive agent, adding tranquilizers will usually lower your reading and leave you dizzy and/or lightheaded. On the other hand, a group of agents called "monoamine oxidase inhibitors," which usually reduce blood pressure, can shoot it sky high if you happen to drink red wine, eat chocolate or enjoy some aged cheese with them. This combination has caused strokes and even death.

- *Alcohol intolerance.* Remember the Karen Quinlan case? She is said to have gone into a coma from the combination of too much Valium and alcohol. Don't for one moment think that Valium is the only drug with which that can happen.

- *Impotence.* Tranquilizers can "relax" you right out of the desire and the ability to perform sexually.

- In addition to these representative specific adverse effects, the "psychotropics" can also cause the usual drug reactions, allergic responses, fevers and unpleasant interactions with other drugs.

When It's Illegal

Whether you puff a joint of marijuana, sniff cocaine or self-administer drugs intravenously, in addition to the potential consequences of the chemical itself, you're opening a legal Pandora's box. One man was compelled to withdraw from his nomination to a seat on the Supreme Court; countless others have been arrested and imprisoned for sharing, using or simply being in possession of illegal drugs. So consider these consequences when toying with the temptation to enjoy a "thrill."

Everything I've said about prescription drugs obviously applies to illegal substances as well. In this latter group, however, there is the additional danger of never knowing for sure exactly what you're getting. Despite the dangers of regularly using prescribed tranquilizers, you can at least depend on the purity of the product you're buying at the pharmacy; but there's no telling how much of what contaminant you're going to inhale, inject or swallow when you make a street purchase.

Here, then, are some of the problems, aside from addiction and withdrawal, inherent in the more widely used so-called "recreational" drugs. This is not a complete list, only the highlights of what I myself have observed among some users.

• *"Speed" (amphetamines)*. These drugs used to be the mainstay of the psychiatrist's armamentarium against depression. They were also the most widely prescribed appetite depressants. Currently, not many doctors recommend them as a mood elevator, and their use as "diet" pills is forbidden in most states. So they have been taken to the streets, where they are called "uppers" or "bennies" and they are sold to induce a "high." The reasons to keep away from them are:

1. Possible dependence.
2. They raise blood pressure.
3. They speed the heart rate.

4. They can cause abnormal heart rhythm.
5. "Speed" is particularly dangerous when taken intravenously.
6. An inadvertent overdose can lead to death.

• *Marijuana.* Pot, grass or whatever else you want to call it can alter your behavior and impair memory, judgment and other brain functions. It is not addictive, but can result in:

1. Atrial fibrillation (a rapid, irregular heart action that has serious consequences).
2. Decreased fertility in males. (I'm not sure exactly how accurate that observation is, but some doctors are sure it's so.)
3. Diminished sexual performance in men after prolonged use.
4. Worsened respiratory disease. If you suffer from chronic bronchitis, the irritant action of the deeply inhaled smoke can aggravate your symptoms.

• *Cocaine.* Remember when you were assured that whatever adverse effects cocaine induced, it wasn't addicting? Forget it. Along with heroin, coke is one of the most potent addicting substances there is. In its powder form it is sniffed up the nose; in liquid form, it is injected intravenously at the risk of a fatal overdose or contracting AIDS.

Cocaine causes a wide range of serious cardiac and neurological disorders. When a patient is brought unconscious to the emergency room, doctors usually think first of such common disorders as insulin shock (too little sugar reaching the brain), diabetic coma (the consequence of too high blood sugar), heart attack, stroke, poisoning or some form of brain disease. But these days, what with the rampaging cocaine epidemic—especially in its purified form, "crack"—there are more and more neurological emergencies, coma and paralysis all due to cocaine.

Cocaine also irritates the heart muscle, throwing its contractions out of synch. Several of my own patients have suddenly developed atrial fibrillation, which is quite uncomfortable and potentially dangerous. Much more frightening, however, was a recent case involving a previously healthy woman of forty. She was on a cocaine romp with some of her friends when, suddenly, in the midst of all the "fun," she felt a terrible pressure between her breasts. It became so bad she had to be taken to the hospital, where the emergency room doctors diagnosed an acute heart attack.

Why should this happen in a pre-menopausal woman without risk factors for coronary artery disease? She had normal blood pressure, was not diabetic, her family history was good, and, as it turned out, so was her cholesterol level. What do you think her coronary angiogram showed? Her coronary arteries were "clean," completely free of obstructing arteriosclerosis plaques. The cocaine had thrown them into a severe and prolonged spasm which so narrowed the arteries that the flow of blood to the heart muscle was cut off (a consequence as serious as if the vessels had actually been diseased).

• *Crack.* This form of cocaine is now the greatest menace on the American drug scene, because:

1. A dose is much cheaper than a dose of any other form.
2. It is perhaps the most addicting agent now being sold on the street. The period of "satisfaction" is intense, but very short-lived, so that "crashes" oc-

cur frequently unless aborted with more of the drug.
3. It can lead to stroke, heart attack, lung failure and sudden death.

The symptoms associated with smoking crack are due either to the direct toxic action of the drug itself or from its withdrawal. Here's why crack is lethal: Cocaine is a white powder made up of the active drug in combination with other substances and contaminants. When this powder is inhaled in the nose, it takes several minutes to be absorbed from the nasal lining to the bloodstream and into the brain. During the process of converting powdered cocaine into crack, the "buffers" and contaminants are burned off, leaving pure, very highly concentrated cocaine in crystal or rock form. When this is puffed (usually in a glass pipe), the inhaled smoke reaches the lungs instantly. That's where it does the most damage. But then, from the lungs, the cocaine is absorbed almost immediately into the bloodstream, and only seconds later it hits the brain. So the "high" from crack comes on much more quickly than when the cocaine is snorted. It is also of much shorter duration and leaves the user with an intense craving. The result is repeated dosing, often in the same night. No small wonder that death occurs so often with this drug, or that crack is so violently and quickly addicting.

- *Heroin*, which is derived from the opium poppy, is highly addicting. Today it constitutes an entirely new risk for those who use it. Since heroin is "mainlined," that is, injected intravenously, often with shared and contaminated needles, many such addicts have developed AIDS. Less dramatic, but still very important, is the risk of endocarditis, a serious and sometimes fatal infection of the heart valves, stemming, again, from the introduction of infected needles into the bloodstream. Hepatitis B, the worst kind of hepatitis there is, is also a high-risk complication of intravenous heroin use.

• Heroin is extremely addicting because of the way it works on the brain. As you know, the body produces its own opiates, usually in response to exercise, sex, water (curiously enough) and other pleasant stimuli. Our own natural opiates are what make us feel so good. When you're taking heroin for any length of time (the interval differs from person to person), the brain stops making its own opiates. After all, why bother when so much is coming in via the needle? So now, no matter what usually pleasurable stimulus you happen to encounter, it will do nothing for you, because your brain isn't responding with its own opiates anymore. The only thing that will make you happy is a heroin fix.

The consequences of addiction to any of the so-called "recreational" drugs are very grave, including behavioral and personality changes, respiratory and cardiac problems, severe neurological disorders and death. Are any of them worth it? You be the judge.

You may not be able to change many of the major factors that contribute to your risk profile, such as your age, sex or race, but you can, and should, make every effort to avoid or conquer any personal habits, such as the use of tobacco, alcohol and addictive drugs, that pose a serious threat to your health and your life.

A FINAL WORD

If you feel sick, you now have at your disposal some guidelines to help you decide whether or not your symptoms are serious enough for you to call your doctor—and when to do so. If you believe *or even suspect* that time is of the essence, don't dally—even if it's in the middle of the night. There's nothing that upsets a conscientious and caring doctor (the kind you should have) more than a patient who has waited until morning to call with an urgent problem. A stroke or a heart attack, a perforated or obstructed bowel, an internal hemorrhage or a ruptured ectopic pregnancy, a high fever with a stiff neck, an unexpected seizure, a temporary weakness of an arm or a leg—these are just some of the cases in which the few hours lost because you hesitated to disturb your doctor's sleep can make a difference between life and death. If you've got the kind of relationship with your doctor that leaves you uncomfortable about calling him or her at such an "awkward" time, then either redefine that relationship or change doctors.

Some physicians give their home phone numbers to their patients. Many do not—and for good reason. They may be out of town, so there may not be an answer at their home when you ring. Or a housekeeper can't be relied upon either to take a proper message or to find the doctor; or, as happens so often in group practices, the physician you usually see is "off call" and away. So, generally speaking, you're better off dialing the office number and asking the answering service to find whoever is working that night. But make sure now, *before you get sick,* that there's a *person* at the other end, and not an answering machine. I for one would never stay with a doctor who has an instrument and not a live human being taking calls at night.

All of the above notwithstanding, more and more patients find it more convenient in a crisis situation to go directly to an emergency room rather than lose time trying to locate their doctor. That's a good idea. In most cases, your own physician will have you do that anyway—especially during the night. By the time he or she has gotten dressed and traveled to your home, precious minutes will have been wasted. What's more, the wherewithal to evaluate your problem properly, the X rays, electrocardiogram, blood tests and consultants required, are not available at your place. Wherever possible, the emergency room you go to should be in the hospital where your own physician is on staff, so that he can direct your care once he gets there. If you've called an ambulance, ask the driver to take you to that particular emergency room if it doesn't happen to be the nearest one to your home. Unless it's hours away, which it shouldn't be, most ambulance services will oblige. The important thing is to know all this *before* you take sick.

Finally, my last cardinal rule: *When in doubt, call for help.* Don't take any chances with your health and your life. It's better to be safe than sorry. Never hesitate to cry wolf!

ACKNOWLEDGMENTS

I am very grateful to the following colleagues, who reviewed those portions of the manuscript in which they have special interest and expertise. Their suggestions were invaluable, their knowledge vast:

Stanley J. Birnbaum, M.D., Professor of Obstetrics and Gynecology, Associate Director of OB/GYN, The New York Hospital-Cornell Medical Center

Harry L. Bush, M.D., Associate Professor of Surgery (Vascular), The New York Hospital-Cornell Medical Center

Robert Coles, M.D., Clinical Associate Professor of Ophthalmology, Mount Sinai School of Medicine, New York

Howard Goldin, M.D., Clinical Professor of Medicine (Gastroenterology), The New York Hospital-Cornell Medical Center

Antonio M. Gotto, Jr., M.D., D. Phil., Chairman, Department of Medicine, Baylor College of Medicine, and Chief, Internal Medicine Service, The Methodist Hospital, Houston, Texas

Wilbur James Gould, M.D., Attending Physician (Otolaryngology), Lenox Hill Hospital, New York; Director of Vocal Dynamic Laboratory, Lenox Hill Hospital

Robert Greenberg, M.D., Associate Clinical Professor of Dermatology, The New York University Medical Center

Catherine C. Hart, M.D., Assistant Professor of Medicine (Infectious Disease), The New York Hospital-Cornell Medical Center

Daniel Libby, M.D., Clinical Associate Professor of Medicine (Pulmonary), The New York Hospital-Cornell Medical Center

Steven K. Magid, M.D., Assistant Professor of Medicine (Rheumatology), The New York Hospital-Cornell Medical Center, Hospital for Special Surgery

James McCarron, M.D., Clinical Associate Professor of Urology, The New York Hospital-Cornell Medical Center

Samuel Rapoport, M.D., Clinical Assistant Professor of Neurology, The New York Hospital-Cornell Medical Center

George Reader, M.D., Professor of Medicine, The New York Hospital-Cornell Medical Center; Livingston Farrand Professor and Chairman, Department of Public Health

Leon Root, M.D., Chief, Children's Orthopedic Service, The Hospital for Special Surgery, New York; Professor of Clinical Surgery, Cornell University Medical College, New York

Stephen Scheidt, M.D., Professor of Clinical Medicine and Assistant Dean for Continuing Medical Education at The New York Hospital-Cornell Medical Center

G. Tom Shires, M.D., Professor and Chairman, Department of Surgery, The New York Hospital-Cornell Medical Center; Dean, Cornell University Medical College, New York

My thanks to Fred Hills, Burton Beals and Toni Burbank for their valuable editorial advice. I am especially grateful to Graham Yost, who helped me edit the mass of data I collected in order to write this book. Elaine Glasner did a superb job typing and retyping successive drafts, long before I finally provided her with a word processor.

INDEX

abdominal pain, *65–82*,
    170, 266, 418, 431,
    440, 445, 446
abortion, 169, 173
abscesses, *108*, 112, 182–
    183, 184, 189, 351,
    353, 355, 358
  in gums, 114
  in lungs, 284, 287
  in rectum, 132
  in throat, 260, 263
ACE (angiotension-
    converting enzyme)
    inhibitors, *282–283*,
    285, 287, 313
acetaminophen, 67, *180*
acid reflux, 26, 27, *63–64*,
    261, 302, 303, 305
Acyclovir, *92*
Adalat, 137
Addison's disease, *345*, 347
adrenal glands, 176, 337,
    345, 373
  tumors of, *174–175*, 177,
    338
age, *408–411*
AIDS (acquired immune
    deficiency syndrome),
    92, 184, 185, 284,
    286, 287, 312, 316,
    408, 418, *438–441*,
    460
AIDS-related complex
    (ARC), 439
air-swallowing, *124*, 128
alcohol, 12, 13, 14, 74, 77,
    78, 121, 229, 257,
    259, 368, 369, 417–
    418, 429, 444–450
  belly distention and, *125*
  DTs and, 194, *223*
  elderly and, 228, 229
  flushing and, 339–340,
    341–342, 343
  hypertension and, *447–
    449*
  impotence and, 309–310,
    313, *315*
  liver and, 67, 68, 96, 97,
    151, 171, 315, 357,
    445–447, 450
  nerves and, 38, 44, 449
  numbness and, 211, 212
  sensitivity to, 339–340,
    343, 456
  sleep and, 295, 297, 387,
    391
  stool and, 162, 272, 278
  throat and, 286, 293,
    298, 302, 303

alcohol (cont.)
  tremors and, 206, 208–
    209, 210
Aldactone, 96, 123
Aldomet, 96, 123, 137, 182,
    266, 313, 321, 400
allergies, 113, 116, 119,
    129, 130, 140, 143,
    145, 188, 190, 238,
    240, 243, 274, 279,
    283, 286, 288, 326,
    327, 331
alopecia areata, 333–334,
    335
Alzheimer's disease, 215,
    220, 221–222, 227,
    228, 230, 409, 411,
    429–430, 447
amebiasis, 183
amiodarone, 346
amitriptyline, 194
amphetamines, 223, 375,
    389, 457–458
ampicillin, 25
amyloidosis, 113, 114
amyotrophic lateral sclerosis
    (ALS; Lou Gehrig's
    disease), 262
anemia, 22, 24, 46, 162,
    188, 211, 212, 266,
    289–290, 294, 348,
    354–355, 356, 358,
    363–364, 369, 392,
    422
  hemolytic, 265, 266, 268
  Mediterranean, 424–425
  pernicious, 344, 346, 348
  sickle cell, 420–422
aneurysms, 79–80, 83, 300,
    302, 303, 371

angina, 8, 22, 35, 37, 55–
    56, 63, 64, 202, 291,
    365, 390, 414
  mesenteric, 79
  see also chest pain
anorexia nervosa, 248
antacids, 73, 271, 418
antibiotics, 21, 24, 25, 142–
    143, 181, 243, 248,
    251, 266, 277, 329,
    346, 347
antidiuretic hormone
    (ADH), 403–404,
    406
antihistamines, 181, 382,
    386
anus, pain in, 85–87
aorta, 79
appendicitis, 75–76, 81, 86,
    87
appendix, 75
appetite, loss of, 247–249,
    443
appetite suppressants, 364,
    365–366, 375, 378
Apresoline, 137, 181–182
Arabs, 424–246
ARC (AIDS-related
    complex), 439
armpit, lumps in, 118–120
arsenic poisoning, 345, 356,
    358
arteries, 43, 45, 112, 140,
    141, 371, 372, 373
  carotid, 28, 30
arteriosclerosis, 38–39, 79,
    83, 164, 235, 242,
    243, 244, 245, 311,
    314, 315, 355, 358,

370–371, *374*, 378,
409, 412–413, 430
arthritis, 19, 20, 29, 30, 31,
34, 35, 37, 38, 39,
40, 42, 46, 51, 52,
54, 83, 84, 186, 188,
255, 390, 412, 437
osteo-, 46, 49, 50, 410,
427, 434
rheumatoid, 42, 46, 48–
49, 50, 186, 242–
243, 245, 414, 427
see also gout
aspirin, 113, 142, 162, 180,
243, 248, 272, 354,
418
asthma, 283, *286*, 287, 291,
292
astigmatism, 17
Atabrine, 346
atropine, 223
Atrovent, 366
autoimmune disorders, 49,
143, 159, 160, *186*,
190, 259, 413–415

back pain, *30–34*, 187, 219,
399, 412, 418
bacterial infections, *25*, 47
balanitis, 93, 94
baldness, 332–336
barbiturates, 48, 181, 208,
223
bedwetting, 214–221
Bell's palsy, 204, 205
bellyaches, *see* abdominal
pain
beta blockers, 96, 123, 200,

271, 313, 362, 369,
382–383, 386, 392
beta carotene, 264, 346,
347
birth control pills, 47, *54*,
58–59, 68, 96, 99,
100, 137, 168, 169,
171, 173, 187, 233,
235, 251, 256, 258,
266, 323, 345, 346,
347, 375, 416
blacks, health profile of,
420–424
bladder, 78, 103–105, 110,
157, 159, 160, 161,
216, 217, 389, 404
cancer of, 451
infections of, 82, 157,
412
polyps in, 157
tumors in, 157, 438
blastomycosis, 183
blindness, 204, 205, 371
blind spots, 232, 234
Blocadren, 362
blood, bleeding, 15, 47, 50,
107–108, 140–177,
188, 285, 341, 354,
355, 372, 377
in brain, 15, 16
cancer of (leukemia), 29,
113, 114, 127, *143*,
329, 331
medications and, 140,
142–143, 148, 149
in stools, 162–167, 272,
276, 394, 431
in urine, 157–161, 376,
400, 401, 414

blood, bleeding *(cont.)*
  vaginal, abnormal, 168–
    173
blood clots, *see* embolisms;
    phlebitis
blood pressure:
  high, *see* high blood
    pressure
  low, 197–198, 377–378
blood sugar, 405; *see also*
    diabetes mellitus
blushing, 339–343
boils, 109, 131, 405
bones, 354, 412
  cancer of, 32–33, 34,
    187, 188
bony spurs, 42, 45
bowel, 65, 66, 72–73, 75,
    76, 78, 79, 270, 345
  cancer of, 75, 81, 86,
    271, 272, 280, *431*
  infections of, 185
  inflammatory disease of,
    50, 51, 77, 275, 276,
    279, *414*
  irritable, 77, 81, 82, 83,
    129, 271, 272, 274,
    275, 276, 279
  polyps in, 330, 345
  tumors in, 77, 271, 272,
    274, 330, 394, 395
bowel movements, 165,
    166, 269–270, 431
  see also constipation;
    diarrhea
brain, 234, 239, 240, 427
  bleeding in, 15, 16
  infections of, 228, 229,
    297
  injury to, 384, 386

seizures and, 191–195
  tumors in, 175, 177, 192,
    194, 195, 204, 205,
    213, 214, 221, 228,
    229, 231, 233, 236,
    239, 240, 252, 256,
    258, 297, 304, 306,
    313, 384
breasts:
  bleeding from, 157
  cancer of, 61, 95, 97,
    118–119, 120, *120–
    123*, 406, 412, 415,
    430–431, 448, 450
  cysts in, 95, 121, 122,
    123
  infections of, 122
  injuries to, 97, 122, 124
  lumps in, 118–119, 120–
    124
  medication and, 96, 97,
    122–123, 124
  pain in, 95–97
  tumors in, 157
breathing problems, 281–
    306, 415; *see also*
    shortness of breath
bronchiectasis, *155*, 284,
    287
bronchitis, 24, 155, 282,
    284, 285, 286, 287,
    433
brucellosis, 183–184
bruises, 142, 143
bursitis, *35*, 37

caffeine, 77, 364, 365, 369,
    387–388, 391
  see also coffee

calcium, 271, 417
cancer, 29, 30, 47, 50, 52, 61, 73, 74, 75, *107*, 108–109, 111, 126, 129, 140–141, 168, 174–175, 180, 252, 255, 276, 285, 290, 344, 346, 347, 348, 364, 384, 386, 400, 409, 412, 415, 434, 440, 445, 450, 452
  of bladder, 451
  of blood (leukemia), 29, 113, 114, 127, *143*, 329, 331
  blood in stool and, 163, 165
  of bones, 32–33, 34, *187*, 188
  of bowel, 75, 81, 86, 271, 272, 280, *431*
  of breasts, 61, 95, 97, 118–119, *120–123*, 406, 412, 415, 430–431, 448, 450
  of cervix, *170*, 171, 173, 321
  of esophagus, 262, 263, *415*
  of kidneys, 61, *415*, 437
  of larynx, 415
  of liver, 61, 268
  of lungs, 61, 142, *153–154*, 155, 156, 282, 285–286, 287, 292, 346, 355, 358, 394, 396, 408, 450, 452
  of ovaries, 82, *126*, 129, 173
  of pancreas, 74, 80, 81,

109–110, 166, 268, 329
  of penis, *93*, 94
  of pharynx, 415
  of prostate, 32–33, 61, 309, 351, 352, 412, 422–423, *434*
  of rectum, 431
  of stomach, 61, 77, 81, 150, 151, *415*
  of testicles, 91, 92, *130–131*, 132
  of thyroid, 415
  of tongue, 22, 24, 415
  of uterus, *170*, 171, 173
  of vocal cords, 301
  see also tumors
canker sores, 21, 23
Capoten, 282, 313
captopril, 282, 313
cardiac arrhythmias, *see* heartbeat, irregular
cardiac failure, 283, *371*
carotene, 264, 346, 347
carotid arteries, 28, 30
carotid sinus, 198, 203, 305
carpal tunnel syndrome, 414
cataracts, *231*, 236, 409
catecholamines, 452
CAT scans, 172, 188, 225, 227
celiac disease, 275
cervix, 98–99, 169, 321, 325
  cancer of, *170*, 171, 173, 321
  infections of, 173, 321
  polyps on, 169
  tumors of, 169

chemotherapy, 249, 251, 252

chest pain, 62, 187, 368, 416–417, 448
  from heart, 53–56
  from lungs, 56–61
  see also angina

chicken pox, 119, 180, 327–328

children:
  bedwetting in, 215, 216, 220
  earache in, 19–20, 149–150
  hair loss in, 335
  insomnia in, 388–389, 391
  shortness of breath in, 291
  sore throats in, 25, 26–27

chills, 185, 266, 412

chlamydia, 321, 329, 442

chloramphenicol, 422

chlorpromazine, 96, 123, 305

chlorpropamide, 266

cholesterol, 430, 449

cirrhosis, 125, 129, 150, 151, 266, 268, 357, 446–447

Clindomycin, 164

cocaine, 145, 208, 458–460

coccidioidomycosis, 183

codeine, 10, 248, 251, 270, 271, 274

coffee, 206, 351, 352, 368
  see also caffeine

Colace, 273

colchicine, 277

colds, 15, 284, 287, 366, 408

colitis, 33, 70, 76, 81, 86, 87, 414
  ulcerative, 50, 164, 185, 274, 276

colon, 86, 164, 274
  polyps in, 271, 274
  see also bowel

Compazine, 206, 208, 400

congestive heart failure, 368

conjunctivitis (pink eye), 17, 18

constipation, 133, 165, 256, 269–274, 275, 330, 362, 383, 394, 410, 414, 431

contact dermatitis, 327, 331

contraceptives, oral, *see* birth control pills

Corgard, 362

coronary artery disease, 8, 427

coronary-bypass surgery, 136

cortisone, 223, 233, 342, 345

cough, 155–156, *281–288*, 299, 300, 355, 394, 408, 416, 437, 440

CPR, 196–197, 202

Crohn's disease, 50, 76, 81, 164, 185, 274, 276

cromolyn, 366

Cushing's syndrome, 144, 145, 176, 177, 255, 258, 337, 342, 343, 377, 378

cyanosis, 355, 358

cystic fibrosis, 277, 280

cystic mastitis, chronic, *95–96*, 97, 121, 123
cystitis, 101, 104, 105, 142, 157, 389, 404, *412*
cysts:
  in armpits, 119, 120
  in belly, 127
  in breasts, *95*, 121, 122, 123
  in ovaries, 76, 82, *86*, 87, 99, 100, 169, 337, 338
  in scrotum, 131

deafness, *241–246*, 410
decongestants, 213, 214, 248, 366, 389
dehydration, 274, 399, 401
Demerol, 10, 248
depression, 392, 393
dermatitis, 327, 331
Diabenase, 340
diabetes insipidus, *404–405*, 406, 407
diabetes mellitus (sugar diabetes), 24, 194, 195, 201, 209, 210, 219, 220, 221, 255, 313–314, 329, 331, 351–352, 353, 398, 404–405, 406, 407, 409, 427, *432*
  digestive system and, 271, 274, 275, 276, 280
  ears and, 243, 244, 245
  eyes and, 234, 235, 237
  nerves and, 38, 39, 44, 211, 212

  skin and, 326, 340, 341, 343
diaphragm, *35*, 36, 66
diarrhea, 49–50, 76, 81, 86, 133, 162, 163, 165, 178, 185, 271, *274–280*, 342, 394, 414, 416, 424, 431, 439–440
digestive system, 247–280
  see also specific organs
digitalis, 96, 123, 200, 223, 247–248, 250, 252, 277, 313, 362, 369
Dilantin, 114, 206, 208
dilatation and curettage (D&C), 175, 177
diphtheria, 26, 27
discs, spinal, 31–32, 35, 36, 82, 84, 219, 221
diuretics, 38, 41, 74, 142, 182, 243, 313, 389, 393–394, 395, 403–404
diverticulitis, 33, 70, 73, 77, 80, 81, 86, 87, *164–165*
diverticulosis, 164
diverticulum, 262, 263
double vision (diplopia), 232, 233, 239, 240, 394
drugs, recreational, 184, 194, 208, 223, 267, 368, 408, 418, *454–461*
  see also medication
DTs (delirium tremens), 194, 223
duodenum, 77, 162

Dyazide, 182
dysmenorrhea, 98
dyspareunia, 100–103
dyspepsia, 73

ears, 19–20, 149–150, 241–
    246, 250
  diabetes and, 243, 244,
    245
  infections of, 19–20, 149,
    150, 250
ectopic pregnancy, 76, 82,
    169, 173
eczema, 149
ejaculate, 161–162, 320–
    321, 324
Elavil, 194
elbow pain, 51–52
elderly, 411
  alcohol and, 228, 229
  bleeding into skin in, 144,
    145
  hypothermia in, 229
  itching in, 330
  medication and, 221–223,
    229
  nutritional deficiencies in,
    221–222, 229
  sore throats in, 26
  stimulants and, 392
Elixophyllin, 366
embolism, 43, 140, 235,
    255, 284
  in kidneys, 83, 85, 157
  in lungs, 54, 57–59, 64,
    153, 154, 156, 187,
    190, 287, 289, 292,
    294, 416–417
  in rectum, 111

  in testicles, 110–111
emphysema, 289, 292–293,
    432–433, 451
enalapril, 282, 313
endocarditis, 47
endometriosis, 32, 34, 76,
    78, 82, 99, 100, 101
epididymitis, 89, 91, 130,
    132
epilepsy, 192–193, 195
Epstein-Barr virus (EBV),
    393
erthromycin, 164, 266
Esidrix, 182
Esimil, 137
esophagus, 54, 63–64, 65,
    162, 262, 263, 270
  cancer of, 262, 263, 415
  infections of, 260, 263
  tumors in, 260, 263
estrogen, 96, 137, 413, 416
ethacrynic acid, 243
exercise, 175, 177, 178,
    258, 273, 274, 291,
    325, 361–362, 367,
    369, 371, 407
exhaustion, 392–396
Ex-Lax, 400
exostoses, 106, 111
eyelids, drooping of, 237–
    240
eyes, 14, 16–18, 231–240,
    353, 354, 357, 371,
    384, 415
  aging and, 231–232
  Bell's palsy and, 204, 205
  bloodshot, 147
  bulging, 115–116
  diabetes and, 234, 235,
    237

infections of, 147, 234, 236
injuries to, 16–17, 18, 234, 236
objects in, 16–17, 18, 147
pain in, 16–18
spots before, 233, 234
sty in, 16–17, 18

facial paralysis, 204–205
fainting, 196–203
fallopian tubes, 319–320, 321, 325
familial Mediterranean fever, 186
familial polyposis, 345, 347
farsightedness, 17, 231
fatigue, 15, 392–396, 439
fever, 13, 14, 16, 17, 18, 171, 172, *178–190*, 266, 278, 290, 333, 335, 339, 343, 350, 352, 369, 393, 394, 399, 412, 416, 439, 440, 443, 445
fiber, 271, 273, 274
fibroids, uterine, 169, *170*, 171, 173, 217
    see also tumors, in uterus
fibromas, 106–107, 111
fingernails, 353–359
flank pain, 83–85
floppy valve, 417
flu, 17, 46, 47, 50, 180, 393, 395, 445
flushing, 339–343, 373
food poisoning, 249, 252, 277, 280
foot pain, 41–45

fractured skull, 146, 147, 149, 150
fungal infections, 259, 260, 286, 287, 334, 335, 355, 358, 440–441

gallbladder, 65, 66, 68–69, 108, 109–110, 112, 251
    belly distension and, 125, 129
    disease of, 54, *251*, 253, 416, 418
    stones in, 68, 69, 266, 268
gas, *124–125*, 271, 275, 416, 424
gastritis, *73*, 81, 82, 162, 445
gastroenteritis, 278
genetics, 408–461
genital herpes, 92, 94, 169
genital warts, 132
genitourinary tract, infections of, *104*, 105, 168
Gentamicin, 164, 243
German measles, 29, 30, 116, 119
giardia, 278
glands, 393
    adrenal, see adrenal glands
    lymph, see lymph glands
    parathyroid, 32
    pituitary, see pituitary gland
    swollen, 24, 25, 28–29, 116–117, 118, 185–

glands *(cont.)*
186, 238, 329, 341, 439, 440
thyroid, *see* thyroid gland
glandular disorders, generalized, 174–176, 177
glaucoma, 14, 16, 18, 147, 233, 234, 235, 236, *410*
globus hystericus, *261*, 263
glomerulonephritis, 159, 160
goiter, 117, 118
gonorrhea, 26, 27, 48, 51, 93, 321, 442
gout, 38, 40, *41–42*, 44, 45, 47, 48, 50, 410
Graves disease, 413
Greeks, 424–426
groin, 87–89, 129–130
G6PD (glucose 6 phosphate dehydrogenase) disease, 422
gums, 24, 114–115, 148–149, 345, 347

hair, 356, 362–363, 383
excess, 336–338, 377
loss of, 332–336, 362, 383
Haldol, 233
halo effect, 232, 233, 234
hand, pain in, 414
hay fever, 286
head, injuries to, 14, 16, 22, 146, 147, 150, 192, 195, 224–225, 227, 229, 244, 384, 386

headaches, *11–16*, 17, 18, 204, 205, 323, 376, 384, 399, 406, 423, 426, 439
migraine, 11, *12*, 15, 18, 234, 236, 237, 239, 240, 244, 251–252, 416, 417, 433
hearing problems, 241–246
see also ears
heart, 255, 300, 326, 357, 369, 371, 372, 373, 392
chest pain from, 53–56
tumors in, 202
heart attack, 35, 37, *54–56*, 61, 64, 192, 195, 201, 203, 289, 291, 304, 315–316, 351, 352, 371, 372–373, 411, 447–448
heartbeat:
irregular, 365, 373, 456
palpitations, 348, *360–369*, 376, 417, 448
heart block, 200, 328, 363
heartburn, 63–64, 65, 445
heart disease, 8, 22, 24, 355, 358, *368–369*, 449
legs and, 134–135
stimulants and, 392
swollen abdomen and, 126, 129
heart failure, 390
congestive, 368
heart murmur, 24
heart rate, *see* pulse
heat exhaustion, 180

heatstroke, *180*, 189, 195
hematoma, subdural, 14, 16, *225*, 227, 229, 384, 386
hemophilia, 143
hemorrhage, 15, 16, 112, 116, 140, 141, 142–145, 147, 172, 202, 203, 371, 372
hemorrhoids, *85*, 86, 101, 103, 111, 132, 133, 141, 163, 165, 272, 330, 331, 354, 443
hepatitis, *66–68*, 80, 151, 249, 252, 304, 346, 357
  A, 66, 446
  alcoholic, 446
  B, 47, 67, 68, 151, 438, 442–443, 460–461
  viral, 125, 167
hernia, 73–74, 87–88, 89–90, 92, 128, 129, 130, *410–411*
  hiatus, 26, *54*, 63, 65, 74, 81, 252, 261, 263, 410–411
heroin, *458*, 460–461
herpes:
  genital, *92*, 94, 169
  zoster (shingles), 17, 18, 62, 64, 70–71, 76, 81, 83, 84, 96, 327–328
herpetic sores, 22, 23, 441
hiccups, 303–306
high blood pressure (hypertension), 15, 16, 141, 234, 244, 255, 291, 300, 314, 342, 364, 365, *370–378*, 383–384, 392, 399, 400, 410, 423, 427, 433, 437
  alcohol and, 449
  medication for, 181–182, 203, 266, 271, 277, 313, 321, 338, 362
  medications and, 372, 375, 378
  nose bleeds and, 146
hirsutism, 336–338, 342
Hispanics, 419
histoplasmosis, 183
hives, 327
hoarseness, 262, 286, *298–303*
Hodgkin's disease, 119, 129, 340, *341*, 343
homosexuals, 67, 408
  sexually transmitted diseases and, 438–444
hormonal imbalance, 309–310, 318, 324, 325, 337–338, *351*
hormones, 338, 340, 411
Horner's syndrome, *238*, 240
hot flushes, 339, 343
Huntington's chorea, *228*, 230
Hydralazine, 181–182
Hydrodiuril, 182
hymen, 168, 174, 176
hyperparathyroidism, 32
hypertension, *see* high blood pressure
hyperthermia, 180
hypertrichosis, 336

hyperventilation, 201, 203, *288–289*, 291, 293
hypoglycemia, 201, 203, *256*, 258
hypothermia, *225*, 229
hysterectomy, 170, 217, 413

ibuprofen, 151
imipramine, 194
immune system, 427
Imodium, 278–279
impotence, 93, 297, *307–319*, 383, 393, 456
incontinence, urinary, 214–221
Inderal, 96, 200, 362, 383
Indocin, 151
infections, 15, 47, 50, 51, 52, *111*, 116, 118, 129, 130, 171, 188, 213, 214, 215, 265, 277, 278, 279, 355–356, 358, 384, 386, 393, 394
  bacterial, *25*, 47
  of bladder, 82, 157, *412*
  of bowel, 185
  of brain, 228, 229, 297
  of breasts, 122
  of cervix, 173, 321
  diarrhea and, 280
  of ear, *19*, 20, 149, 150, 250
  of esophagus, *260*, 263
  of eyes, 147, *234*, 236
  of female reproductive system, *101*, 103
  fungal, 259, 260, 286,

287, *334, 335, 355*, 358, 440–441
  of genitourinary tract, *104*, 105, 168
  of gums, *114*, 115, 148, 149
  of kidneys, *83–84*, 85, 157, 159
  of liver, 268
  of lungs, 70, *155*, 286
  of lymph glands, *119*, 120
  in mouth, *113*, 114
  in pelvis, *88*, 325
  of penis, 94, 95, 102, 103
  of pericardium, *126*, 129
  of respiratory tract, 153, 287
  of sinuses, 16, *17–18*, 20
  of teeth, *19*, 20
  of testicles, *130*, 131, 132
  of throat, *260*, 263
  of urethra, 93, *157–158*, 159, 161
  of urinary tract, 160, *218–219*, 220, 400, 401, 412
  viral, *17*, 18, 24, 25, 27, 47
  yeast, 113, 114, *329*, 405
  see also specific infections and organisms
infertility, 308, *319–325*
inflammatory bowel disease, *50*, 51, 77, 275, 276, 279, 414
injuries, 111
  to arteries, 140
  to back, 31, 34
  to brain, 384, 386

to breasts, 97, 122, 124
to eardrum, 149, 150
to eyes, 16–17, 18, 234, 236
to head, 14, 16, 22, 146, 147, 150, 192, 195, 224–225, 227, 229, 244, 384, 386
to joints, 50
to legs, 58
to neck, 30
numbness and, 210–211, 212
to rib cage, 54, 64
to shoulders, 35, 37
to spinal cord, 211, 212, 217, 310
to testicles, 89, 91
to tongue, 22, 23
to vagina, 172, 173
to veins, 140
insect bites, 327, 328, 331
insomnia, 379, 387–391
interstitial cystitis, *104*, 105
intestines, *see* bowel
iron supplements, 162, 163
irritable bowel syndrome, 77, 81, 82, 83, 129, 271, 272, 274, 275, 276, 279
isoniazide, 194
isosorbide dinitrate (Isordil), 14–15
Italians, 424–426
itching, 326–331
  rectal, 330, 331
  vaginal, *329–330*, 331, 432
IUD (intrauterine device), 99, 100, 169, 323

jaundice, 21, 23, 68, 69, 252, *263–268*, 329, 331, 346, 347, 400, 420, 422, 443, 446
Jews, 424–426
jobs, 435–438
joint pain, 38, *45–51*, 439, 443
  see also arthritis

kanamycin, 243
Kaopectate, 278–279
Kaposi's sarcoma, 440
kidneys, 24, 71, 81, 82, 83–85, 103, 105, 109, 192, 195, 207, 227, 243, 245, 252, 256, 326, 329, 331, 364, 371, 372, 376, 384, 399, 412, 414
  cancer of, 61, 415, 437
  disease of, 378, 386, *404–405*, 407
  legs and, 135, 138, 139
  embolism in, 83, 85, 157
  infections of, 83–84, 85, 157, *159*
  tumors in, 157
kidney stones, 76, 82, *83–84*, 88, 89, 91, 92, 105, 157, 159, 161, 400, 401
Klein-Levin syndrome, *384*, 386

labetalol, 321
labyrinthitis, *250*, 253
lactase deficiency, *275*, 280

lactose intolerance, 77, *416*, 423–424, 425
laryngitis, 285, 287, *298– 303*
larynx, cancer of, 415
laxatives, 158, 277, 400
lead poisoning, 211, 212, *225–226*
legs:
  pain in, *37–40*, 58, 133– 139, 143
  phlebitis in, 134, *135*, 138, 139
leukemia, 29, 113, 114, 127, *143*, 329, 331
levator dehiscence, 239
life expectancy, 411–412
lifestyle, 408–461
lincomycin, 164
lipoma, *106*, 111, 119, 120
lisinopril, 282, 313
lithium, 223
liver, liver disease, *66–68*, 80, 108, 143–144, 192, 195, 207, 227, 265, 309–310, 318, 326, 329, 345, 359, 364, 384, 386, 400, 401
  alcohol and, 67, 68, 96, 97, 151, 171, 315, 357, 445–447, 450
  cancer of, 61, *268*
  cirrhosis of, 125, 129, 150, 151, 266, 268, 357, *446–447*
  infections of, 268
  legs and, 135–136, 137, 138, 139
  tumors in, 268

  see also hepatitis
Lomotil, 278–279
Lopressor, 362
loss of appetite, 247–249
Lou Gehrig's disease (amyotrophic lateral sclerosis; ALS), 262
lump in the throat, 261
lumps, 106–139, 187, 341
  in armpit, 118–120
  bleeding and, 107–108
  in breasts, 118–119, *120– 124*
  in groin, 130–132
  in neck, 116–118
  in rectum, 132–133
  rule of sevens for, 111
  in testicles, 130–132
lungs, 54, 108, 214, 277, 281, 390, 403, 437, 450, 451
  abscesses in, *284*, 287
  cancer of, 61, 142, *153– 154*, 155, 156, 282, 285–286, 287, 292, 346, 355, 358, 394, 396, 408, 450, 452
  collapsed (pneumothorax), *59– 61*, 64
  embolism in, 54, *57–59*, 64, 153, 154, 156, 187, 190, 287, 289, 292, 294, 416–417
  infections of, 70, *155*, 286
  tumors in, 238
lupus erythematosus, 49
Lyme disease, 49, 51, 183, 186, 187, *328*

lymph glands, 24, 28–29, 88, 108, 112, 118, 119–120, 129, 130, 440
  infections of, *119*, 120
lymphoma, *29*, 128

macular degeneration, *236*, 237
magnesium, 394
malaria, 183, *265*, 422
malignant melanoma, *344*, 347
malnutrition, *see* nutritional deficiencies
mammograms, 121, 122, 123, 431
marijuana, *456–458*
marital status, *426–428*
Marplan, 375
mask of pregnancy, *345–346*, 347
mastitis, chronic cystic, *95–96*, 97, 121, 123
Maxzide, 182
measles, 327
  German, 29, 30, 116, *119*
medication, 229, 271, 361
  appetite loss and, 247–248
  bleeding and, 140, 142–143, 148, 149
  blood pressure and, 372, 375, 377, 378
  bowel movements and, 270
  breasts and, 96, 97, 122–123, 124

digestive system and, 271, 274, 277, 280
  elderly and, 221–223
  fainting and, 199–200, 203
  fatigue and, 396
  fever and, 181–182, 189
  flushing and, 343
  hair loss and, 334, 335
  headache and, 14–15, 16
  hearing loss and, 243, 245
  heart rate and, 362, 364, 368, 369
  high blood pressure and, 372, 375, 378
  hirsutism and, 337–338
  impotence and, 312–313, 316, 318
  infertility and, 320
  insomnia and, 389, 391
  itching and, 328
  jaundice and, 266
  nausea and, 250–251, 252
  seizures and, 194, 195
  shortness of breath and, 290, 294
  skin color and, 346, 347
  somnolence and, 382, 385, 386
  sweating and, 351, 352
  swelling of limbs and, 47–48, 50, 136–137
  tremors and, 206, 209
  vision and, 236
  vomiting of blood and, 151, 152
  see also specific medications
memory loss, 221–223

men, life expectancy of, 411–412

Ménière's disease, 244, 246

meningitis, 16

menopause, 101–102, 169, 173, 176, 177, 337, 338, 339, 341, 343, 351, 352

menstrual periods, 95–96, 256, 321–323, 325, 354, 363, 394, 412–413
  absence of, 173–177
  excessive flow in, 171
  painful, 98–100
  PID and, 99, 100
  water retention and, 133
  weight loss and, 174

mesenteric angina, 79

methyldopa, 182

migraine headaches, 11, 12, 15, 18, 234, 236, 237, 239, 240, 244, 251–252, 416, 417, 433

milk, 256, 258, 275, 416, 423–424

minoxidil, 332–333, 338

miscarriage, 98, 452

mitral valve prolapse, 368, 417

Moduretic, 182

moles, 344, 347

monilia, 114

monoamine oxidase inhibitors, 375, 456

mononucleosis, 25, 27, 29, 30, 72, 116, 118, 119, 127, 393, 395

morphine, 10, 248, 271, 351, 352

motion sickness, 249, 253

mucus, 281

multiple sclerosis (MS), 21, 207, 210, 219, 237, 417

mumps, 90, 92, 109, 130, 131

muscles, 396
  aches in, 357
  spasm in, 29, 30, 33, 34, 37, 40, 54, 60, 62, 64, 83, 84
  sprains of, 51
  strains of, 51, 52
  weakness in, 394, 415, 417

myasthenia gravis, 233, 238, 240, 259, 262, 263, 302, 303, 394, 414–415

nails, 353–359

Naprosyn, 151

narcolepsy, 384–385, 386

narcotics, 10

Nardil, 137, 375

nasal decongestants, 213, 214, 248, 366, 389

nausea, 12, 13, 249–253, 267, 412, 445, 446

nearsightedness, 17, 233

neck:
  hump in, 342
  injuries to, 30
  lumps in, 116–118
  pain in, 27–30

Nembutal, 181

nerve deafness, *241, 245,* 410
nerve irritation, 54
nerves, 39, 44, 414, 425, 427
  alcohol and, 38, 44, 449
  diabetes and, 38, 39, 44, 211, 212
nervous stomach, *124–125,* 129
neuralgia, 22, 24
neuroma, *44, 45, 244, 246*
neuropathy, 38, *44*
niacin (nicotinic acid), 341, 343
nifedipine, 137
nipples:
  bleeding from, 157
  see also breasts
nitroglycerin, 14–15, 55, 63, 199–200, 202, 203
noise damage, 244–245, 246
noises in ear, 241–246
nose:
  bleeding from, *145–147,* 149, 151, 153, 423
  polyps in, 145, 146, *213,* 214
  tumors in, *145,* 146
numbness, 39, 40, *210–212,* 417, 437
  injury and, 210–211, 212
nutritional deficiencies, 21, 23, 114, 148, 149, 325, 345, 348, 349, 392, 393, 395
  in elderly, 222, 229
  obesity, 41, 45, *253, 257,* 259, 294, 297, 433–434

obesity-hypoventilation, 383, 386
obstructive sleep apnea, *295–297,* 298, 383–384, 386
oral contraceptives, *see* birth control pills
osteoporosis, 32, 34, 409, 412, *417–418*
ovaries, 169, 319, 321, 413
  cancer of, 82, *126,* 129, 173
  cysts in, 76, 82, 86, 87, 99, 100, 169, 337, 338
  tumors in, *76, 82,* 338

pain, 7–105
  referred, 19, 24, 31–32, 35–36
  see also specific pains
painkillers, 248, 251, 418
paleness, 348–349
palpitations, heart, 348, *360–369,* 376, 417, 448
pancreas, 66, 69, 252, 280
  cancer of, 74, 80, 81, 109–110, 166, 268, 329
pancreatitis, 69, 80, 81
Pap smear, 172
paralysis, *204–205,* 261
parasites, 66–67, 76, 188, 279, 280
parathyroid glands, 32
Parkinson's disease, *206–*

Parkinson's disease *(cont.)* 207, 209, 233, 313, 411
Parnate, 375
pelvic inflammatory disease (PID), 76, 78, 82, 86, 87, 187, 416–417
  menstrual periods and, 99, 100
pelvis:
  infections of, *88*, 325
  tumors in, 323, 325
penicillin, 47, 194
penile implants, 93, 95, 316
penis, 310–311, 314
  cancer of, *93*, 94
  discharge from, 442
  infections of, 94, 95, *102*, 103
  pain in, 92
peptic ulcer, 150, 162, 252, 410, 418
Pepto-Bismol, 163, 166
pericarditis, *56*, 62, 64
pericardium, 137
  infections of, *126*, 129
peridontitis, 148
perspiration, excessive, *349–353*, 374, 376, 389, 439
pets, 286
Peyronie's disease, 94, 95, *102*, 103
pharynx, cancer of, 415
phenobarbital, 181, 208, 305
phenolphthalein, 400
phenylpropanolamine (PPA), 216, 248, 366, 389

pheochromocytomas, 373, *376*, 378
phlebitis, *38*, *39*, 40, 58, 131
  in legs, 134, *135*, 138, 139
Pickwickian syndrome, *383*, 386
PID, *see* pelvic inflammatory disease
piles, *see* hemorrhoids
pink eye (conjunctivitis), *17*, 18
pituitary gland, 177, 310, 318, 320, 321, 322–323, 357, 377
  overfunctioning of, *21*, 23
  tumors of, *113*, 114, 174–175, 177, 322–323, 337, 338
pleurisy, 54, *57*, 61, 62, 64, 74, 81, 285, 287, 304, 305
pneumonia, *57*, 64, 70, 74, 81, 141, 225, 229, 284, *285*, 287, 289, 304, 305, 426, 440
pneumothorax, *59–61*, 64
poison ivy, *326–327*
poison oak, *326–327*
polio, 260, 263
polyarteritis, 186
polycythemia, *329*, 331, 341, 343
polymyalgia rheumatica, 186
polyps, *86*, 87, 165
  in bladder, 157
  in bowel, 330, *345*
  in cervix, 169

in colon, 271, 274
in nose, 145, 146, *213*, 214
in uterus, 169, 170, 173
in vagina, 172
on vocal cords, 298
see also tumors
postnasal drip, 251, 253
potassium, 251, 393
pregnancy, *95–96*, 97, 108, *127–128*, 129, 169, 174, 176, 249, 251, 253, 304, 317, 319, 333, 449
ectopic, 76, 82, 169, 173
pigmentation and, 345–346, 347
smoking and, 452
toxemia of, *376*, 378
premature ejaculation, *316–317*, 319
priapism, *94*, 95
Prinivil, 282, 313
Procardia, 137
propylthiouracil, 266
prostate gland, 384, 411, 412
cancer of, 32–33, 61, 309, 351, 352, 412, 422–423, *434*
surgery on, 321
prostatitis, *86*, 87, 92–93, 94, 102, 103, 104, 110, 132, 158, 217, 218, 219, 220, 376, 389, 391, 451
pseudopsiesis, 127
psittacosis, 184, *286*, 288
psoriasis, 47, 50, 328, 355, 358, *434*

psychogenic fatigue, 393
ptosis, 237
pulmonary edema, 285, *292*
pulse, 356, 360–369
rapid, 389
medication and, 362, 364, 368, 369
smoking and, 366, 368, 369, 452–453
see also heartbeat, irregular
pus, 400, 401
pyridium, 400

Quibron, 366
quinidine, 142, 243, 277, 422
quinine, 142, 243, 422

radiation therapy, 333, 334, 335, 345, 347
rash, 326, 328, 329, 330, 331, 439, 440
Raynaud's disease, 43–44, 414
rectum, 78, 270
cancer of, 431
embolism in, 111
itching of, 330, 331
lumps in, 132–133
pain in, 85–87
tumors in, 132–133
referred pain, *19*, 24, 31–32, 35–36
Reglan, 305
Reiter's syndrome, 49, 51, *93*, 95
renal failure, 326

reproductive organs, female, 78
  infections of, *101*, 103
reserpine, 137
respiratory tract, 281–306
  infections of, *153*, 287
retinal detachment, *233–234*, 236
Reye's syndrome, 180
rheumatic fever, 25, *48*, 49, 51
rheumatic valve disease, 291
rib cage, *54*, 61, 64
rifampin, 266
ringworm, 334
Ritalin, 385
Rocky Mountain spotted fever, *183*, 186
Rogaine, 333, 338
rubbing alcohol, 293

salicylates, 251
salivary glands, 109, 112
salmonella, 278
salt, 370, 371, 407, 423
schizophrenia, 434
sciatica, *31*, 219
scleroderma, *259*, 263
scopolamine, 305
scrotum:
  cysts in, 131
  varicose veins in, 131, 132
  see also testicles
Seconal, 181
Sectral, 362
sedatives, 181, 271, 312–313
seizures, *202*, 204, 205

brain, 191–195
  medication and, 194, 195
senile dementia, 221–230
sense of smell, loss of, 212–214
sense of taste, loss of, 212–214
sexual intercourse, painful, *100–103*, 317
sexually transmitted diseases, *418*, 438
  see also specific diseases
sexual problems, 307–325
shingles (herpes zoster), 17, 18, 62, 64, *70–71*, 76, 81, 83, 84, 96, 327–328
shortness of breath, 60, 67, *288–294*, 348, 355, 417, 433, 440
shoulder pain, 35–37
sickle cell anemia (SCA), 420–422
sigmoidoscopy, 163–164
silicosis, 437
sinuses, 13–14, 18
  carotid, 198, 203, 305
  infections of, 16, *17–18*, 20
skin, 326–359, 426
  color changes in, *343–348*, 356
  dry, 356, 394
  pale, 348–349
skin tags, rectal, 132, 133
skull fracture, *146*, 147, 149, 150
sleep, 379–396
  alcohol and, 295, 297, 387, 391

sleep apnea, *295–297*, 298, 383–384, 386

sleeping pills, 295, 313, 346, 381, 382, 386, 389, 390, 391, 392

smell, lost sense of, 212–214

smoking, 22, 24, 38, 39, 44, 54, 59, 74, 77, 187, 235, 243, 245, 256, 259, 291–292, 294, 313, 319, 387, 411–412, 415, 429, 445, *450–454*

  coughing and, 153–154, 284, 286, 300–301, 394

  heart rate and, 366, 368, 369

  nausea and, 251, 252, 253, 267

  numbness and, 211, 212

  pregnancy and, 452

  throat and, 298, 300–301, 302

snoring, *294–298*, 384

somnolence, 379–386

sonogram, 172

sores, genital, 441

sore throat, 19, *24–27*, 48, 116, 393, 439

spinal cord, 9, 31, 273, 274

  injuries to, *211*, 212, 217, 310

spine, 30–31, 35, 54, 83, 84

  discs of, 31–32, 35, 36, 82, 84, 219, 221

spleen, 72, 108, 264

  enlargement of, 127

spontaneous pneumothorax, *292–293*, 294

sprain, muscle, 51

starvation, 136, 139

steroids, 74, 151, 176, 266, 340, 343, 366, 372, 375, 418

stillbirth, 452

stimulants, 223, 313, 368, 391

stomach, 73, 74, 77–78, 124, 129, 150, 162, 163, 270, 445

  cancer of, 61, 77, 81, 150, 151, *415*

  ulcers of, *see* ulcers, stomach

stools, 73, 78, 133, 141, 252, 275, 276, 278, 279

  blood in, *162–167*, 272, 276, 394, 431

  color of, 162–163, 272

strain, muscle, 51, 52

strep infections, *25*, 27, 113, 114, 260

streptomycin, 243

stroke, 21, 23, 192, 194, 195, *204–205*, 207, 210, 211, 212, 217, 219, 220, 221, 227, 229, 231, 233, 234, 236, 238, 259, 260, 261, 263, 304, 306, 313, 368, 371, 384, 406, 414, 449

sty, *16–17*, 18

subacute bacterial endocarditis (SBE),

subacute bacterial
endocarditis *(cont.)*
182, 184, 187, 326,
357, 359
subdural hematoma, 14, 16,
225, 227, 229, 384,
386
sulfa drugs, 266
sunburn, 344–345
sundowning effect, 226
swallowing, 25, 259–263,
394, 415, 445
sweating, 349–353, 374,
376, 389, 439
syphilis, 44, 93, 300, 326,
328, 330, 426, *441–
442*
systemic lupus
erythematosus (SLE),
160, 186, *414*

Tagamet, 313, 320
Talwin, 10
tartar, 148
taste, lost sense of, 212–214
Tay-Sachs disease, 425
teeth, 19, 20, 24
brushing of, 148, 153,
156
temperature, body, 178–180
ovulation and, 323
see also fever
temporal arteritis, 13, 16,
18, 235, 237
temporomandibular joint
syndrome (TMJ), 19
tendinitis, 35, 37, 51
tendons, 35, 36, 437
Tenormin, 362, 383

testicles, 309, 310, 320–321,
322
cancer of, 91, 92, *130–
131*, 132
embolism in, 110–111
infections of, 130, 131,
132
injuries to, 89, 91
lumps in, 130–132
pain in, 89–92
self-examination of, 130–
131
varicose veins in, 323–324
testicular torsion, *90–91*,
92, 130
testosterone, 266, 309–310
tetracycline, 346
thalassemia, 425
Theo-Dur, 366
theophylline, 206, 251
thermometers, 179
thiazide diuretics, 182
thirst, *402–407*, 432
Thorazine, 305, 400
throat:
abscesses in, 260, 263
infections of, 260, 263
sore, 19, 24–27 116
thyroid gland, 113, 116–
118, 260, 262, 321,
344
cancer of, 415
eyes and, 115, 116
inflamed, 28, 30
low functioning of, 21,
23, 136, 169, 171,
172, 173, 229, 230,
242, 245, 256, 258,
264, 270, 272, 274,
323, 330, 331, 333,

346, 348, 356, 358,
362–363, 364–365,
369, 383, 386, 389,
393, 394, 396
  nodules on, 117, 118
  overactivity of, 21, 174,
207, 209, 233, 275,
276, 279, 290, 333,
339, 342, 343, 351,
352, 356, 358, 363,
369, 373, 389, 390,
391, 413
tic douloureux (trigeminal
neuralgia), 14, 16
tight-building syndrome,
436–437
tinea capitis, 334
tingling, 40, 210–212, 417
tinnitus, 243
tobacco, see smoking
toenails, 353–359
toes, 39, 41, 43, 44, 47
Tofranil, 194
tolbutamide, 266
tongue, 21–24, 353
  cancer of, 22, 24, 415
  injury to, 22–23
  sore, 21–24
  swollen, 112–114
  tremor of, 21, 23
tonsillitis, 25, 27, 260, 263
toothbrushing, 148, 153,
156
toxemia of pregnancy, 376,
378
tracheitis, 287
tranquilizers, 48, 203, 256,
258, 271, 346, 382,
386, 400, 456

transient ischemic attack
(TIA), 234, 236
tremors, 205–210
  alcohol and, 206, 208–
209, 210
  medication and, 206, 209
  of tongue, 21, 23
trichinosis, 184, 239, 240,
278, 357, 359
trigeminal neuralgia (tic
douloureux), 14, 16
tuberculosis, 51, 154–155,
185, 194, 283–284,
351, 394
Tuinal, 181
tumors, 33, 86, 87, 109,
111, 252, 263, 285,
354, 373, 445
  acoustic neuroma, 244,
246
  in adrenal glands, 174–
175, 177, 338
  in bladder, 157, 438
  in bowel, 77, 271, 272,
274, 330, 394, 395
  in brain, 13, 175, 177,
192, 194, 195, 204,
205, 213, 214, 221,
228, 229, 231, 233,
236, 239, 240, 252,
256, 258, 297, 304,
306, 313, 384
  in breasts, 157
  carcinoid, 276–277, 340,
342, 343
  in cervix, 169
  in colon, 274
  in esophagus, 260, 263
  in heart, 202
  in kidneys, 157

tumors (cont.)
in liver, 268
in lungs, 238
in lymph glands, 340
in nose, 145, 146
in ovaries, 76, 82, 338
in parathyroid glands, 32
in pelvis, 323, 325
pheochromocytomas, 373, 376, 378
in pituitary gland, 113, 114, 174–175, 177, 322–323, 337, 338
in rectum, 132–133
in urinary tract, 157, 161
in uterus, 79, 82, 99, 100
on vocal cords, 298, 303
see also cancer; fibroids, uterine; polyps
Tylenol, 67, 180

ulcerative colitis, 50, 164, 185, 274, 276
ulcers, stomach, 73, 77–78, 81, 82, 87, 162, 256, 261, 390, 434, 445, 450
peptic, 150, 162, 252, 410, 418
ulcers, vaginal, 168, 172
Uniphyl, 366
uremia, 194, 252
ureter, 103
urethra, infection of, 93, 157–158, 159, 161
urinary incontinence, 214–221
urinary tract, 78

infections of, 160, 218–219, 220, 400, 401, 412
tumors in, 157, 161
urination, 273
frequent, 376–377
pain on, 103–105, 159–160
urine, 88, 141, 252, 397–401
blood in, 88, 142, 157–161, 376, 400, 401, 414
color of, 399–400
odor of, 401
Urised, 400
uterus, 78, 321, 413
abnormal vaginal bleeding and, 168–173
cancer of, 170, 171, 173
fibroids in, 169, 170, 171, 173, 217
malpositioned, 32, 34
polyps in, 169, 170, 173
prolapse of, 216
tumors in, 79, 82, 99, 100
uvula, enlarged, 283, 287

vagina, 317, 319, 321
abnormal bleeding from, 168–173
itching of, 329–330, 331, 432
painful intercourse and, 100–103, 317
polyps in, 172
varicocele, 89, 91, 110–111

varicose veins, *38*, 40, 134, 284, 292, 345, 347, 416
  in rectum *see* hemorrhoids
  in scrotum, *131*, 132
  in testicles, 323–324
  in throat, 447
  in vagina, *168*, 172
vascular disease, *39*, 318
vascular spasm, 45
vasopressin, 403–404
Vasotec, 282, 313
veins:
  injuries to, 140
  obstructed, 110–111, 112
  see also phlebitis; varicose veins
verapamil, 271
viral hepatitis, 125, *267*
virilization, 336–338
vision:
  blurring of, 436
  changes in, 12, 13, 17–18, *19*, 323, 406, 417
  medication and, 236
  see also double vision; eyes; farsightedness; nearsightedness
Visken, 362
vitamins, 250, 334, 341, 345, 346, 355, *356*, 358, 389, 400, 401
vitiligo, 344, 347

vocal cords, 298, 299, 300, 301, 302
voice, losing, 298–303
vomiting, 13, *249*, 250, 251, 252, 262, 445–446
  of blood, *150–152*

warts:
  genital, 132
  nasal, 145
  vaginal, *168*, 172
water pills, *see* diuretics
water retention, 133, *256*
weight gain, *253–259*, 272, 377, 394
weight loss, 13, 252, 267–268, 272–273, 276, 285, 371, 376, 389, 432
  drastic, *174*, 177
wheezing, 342, 433
women, life expectancy of, 411–412

yeast infections, 113, 114, *329*, 405

Zantac, 313
Zestril, 282, 313
zinc supplements, 251

ABOUT THE AUTHOR

Isadore Rosenfeld, M.D., is an attending physician at the New York Hospital and Memorial Sloan-Kettering Cancer Center and is the Rossi Distinguished Clinical Professor of Medicine at Cornell University Medical College. He maintains a private practice in Manhattan. A well-known television personality, Dr. Rosenfeld has for years been a health adviser to millions of Americans. He has also served as a consultant to the National Institutes of Health on such task forces as Arteriosclerosis, Sudden Cardiac Death, and Hypertension and is currently a member of the Practicing Physicians Advisory Council to the United States Secretary of Health. In addition to his other bestselling works expressly written for patients—*The Complete Medical Exam, Second Opinion, Modern Prevention,* and *The Best Treatment*—Dr. Rosenfeld writes a monthly health column for *Vogue* magazine and has co-authored many scientific papers and a textbook on cardiology. He has four grown children, two of whom are also authors and one a physician. He lives with his wife, Camilla, in New York City and Westchester County, New York. His main hobby is his granddaughter Rebecca.